Faith, Medical Alchemy and Natural Philosophy

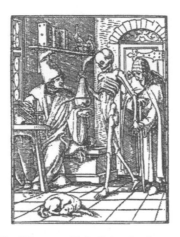

The History of Medicine in Context

Series Editors: Andrew Cunningham and Ole Peter Grell,
Department of History and Philosophy of Science,
University of Cambridge

Titles in this series will include:

Medicine from the Black Death to the French Disease
Roger French et. al.

The Making of the Dentiste, c. 1650-1760
Roger King

*'The Battle for Health': A Political History
of the Socialist Medical Association, 1930-51*
John Stewart

Faith, Medical Alchemy and Natural Philosophy

Johann Moriaen, Reformed Intelligencer, and the Hartlib Circle

J.T. YOUNG

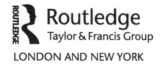

Routledge
Taylor & Francis Group
LONDON AND NEW YORK

First published 1998 by Ashgate Publishing

Reissued 2018 by Routledge
2 Park Square, Milton Park, Abingdon, Oxon, OX14 4RN
711 Third Avenue, New York, NY 10017, USA

Routledge is an imprint of the Taylor & Francis Group, an informa business

Publisher's Note
The publisher has gone to great lengths to ensure the quality of this reprint but points out that some imperfections in the original copies may be apparent.

Disclaimer
The publisher has made every effort to trace copyright holders and welcomes correspondence from those they have been unable to contact.

A Library of Congress record exists under LC control number: 98073999

ISBN 13: 978-1-138-62543-3 (hbk)
ISBN 13: 978-1-138-62546-4 (pbk)
ISBN 13: 978-0-429-45991-7 (ebk)

Contents

List of Abbreviations

ADB: Allgemeine Deutsche Biographie (Leipzig, 1875-1912)

BL: British Library

Blekastad, *Comenius*: Milada Blekastad, *Comenius: Versuch eines Umrisses vom Leben, Werk und Schicksale des Jan Amos Komensky* (Oslo and Prague, 1969)

Bruckner: J. Bruckner, *A Bibliographical Catalogue of seventeenth-century German Books Published in Holland* (The Hague and Paris, 1971)

CSPD: Calendar of State Papers (Domestic Series)

DNB: Dictionary of National Biography (London, 1885-1903)

Doorman: G. Doorman, *Patents for Inventions in the Netherlands during the 16th, 17th and 18th Centuries* (abridged trans. Joh. Meijer, The Hague, 1942)

DSB: Dictionary of Scientific Biography (New York, 1970-80)

Eph 55 (etc.): Hartlib, *Ephemerides* 1655 (etc.)

Figulus Letters: Milada Blekastad (ed.), *Peter Figulus. Letters to Samuel Hartlib 1657-58*, (*Lychnos, Lärdomshistorika Samfundets Årsbok*, 1988)

Grell: Ole Peter Grell, *Dutch Calvinists in Early Stuart London: The Dutch Church in Austin Friars 1603-1642* (Leiden, New York, Copenhagen and Cologne, 1989)

HDC: George Turnbull, *Hartlib, Dury and Comenius: Gleanings from Hartlib's Papers* (Liverpool, 1947)

Hessels: J.H. Hessels (ed.), *Ecclesiæ Londino-Batavæ Archivum* (1887-97)

HP: Hartlib Papers

Kumpera: Jan Kumpera, *Jan Amos Komensky: Poutník na Rozhraní Veku* (Ostrava, 1992)

KK I: Jan Kvacala, *Korrespondence Jana Amosa Komenského* I (Prague, 1897]

KK II: Jan Kvacala, *Korrespondence Jana Amosa Komenského* II (Prague, 1902)

MCG: Monatshefte der Comeniusgesellschaft

MGP I: Jan Kvacala, *Die Pädagogische Reform des Comenius bis zum Ausgange des XVII Jahrhunderts I: Texte: Monumenta Germaniæ Pædagogica* XXVI (Berlin, 1903)

MGP II: Jan Kvacala, *Die Pädagogische Reform des Comenius in Deutschland bis zum Ausgange des XVII Jahrhunderts II: Historischer Überblick, Bibliographie, Namen- und Sachregister: Monumenta Germaniæ Pædagogica* XXXII (Berlin, 1904)

NDB: Neue Deutsche Biographie (Berlin, 1953-94)

NNBW: Nieuw Nederlands Biografisch Woordenboek (Leiden, 1911-37)

Partington: J.R. Partington, *A History of Chemistry* II (*1500-1800*) (London, 1961)

Serrarius: E.G.E. Van Der Wall, *De Mystieke Chiliast Petrus Serrarius (1600-1669) en zijn Wereld* (Leiden, 1987)

SHUR: Mark Greengrass, Michael Leslie and Timothy Raylor (eds.), *Samuel Hartlib and Universal Reformation: Studies in Intellectual Communication* (Cambridge, 1994)

Thorndike: Thorndike, Lynn, *A History of Magic and Experimental Science* V-VIII (*Sixteenth and Seventeenth Centuries*) (New York, 1941-58)

UBA: Universiteitsbibliothek Amsterdam

Unbekannte Briefe: Milada Blekastad (ed.), *Unbekannte Briefe des Comenius und seiner Freunde 1641-1661* (Ratingen and Kastellaun, 1976)

Zibrt: Cenek Zibrt, *Bibliografie Ceské Historie* (Prague, 1912)

Acknowledgments

I would like to thank the following:

Mark Greengrass, who supervised the doctoral research on which this book is based, and gave me much practical help, constructive criticism and moral support.

All my fellow transcribers on the Hartlib Papers Project: Patricia Barry, Margaret Chambers, Judith Crawford, Ekkehard Duisman, William Hitchens, Gwen Smithson and Susan Wallace. Extra thanks to William Hitchens for patiently supplying the shortcomings of my Latin.

Everyone who has corresponded with me about my work or discussed it with me, and/or allowed me access to their own research: especially Susanna Åckerman, Stephen Clucas, Ole Grell, Howard Hotson, Arnulf Link, Martin Mulsow, William Newman and Gerald Toomer.

Thanks especially to Inge Keil, not just for sharing her own expertise and proferring invaluable suggestions, but for consistent encouragement and many personal kindnesses. This book owes more to her than she will probably either realise or admit.

For A.W.Y.

Foreword

The papers of Samuel Hartlib, thought lost for some two and a half centuries, came to light in 1933.[1] Six decades later, their public accessibility was massively increased by the publication on CD-ROM of transcriptions and facsimiles of all the documents in the archive.[2] The research for this book was conducted in tandem with work on this transcription.

Among the various opportunities the papers afford is that of viewing familiar territory from unfamiliar perspectives, gaining access to the viewpoints of little-known and virtually unknown figures. The aim of this study is to contribute to the understanding of the early and middle seventeenth century by presenting in some detail the view from one such hitherto neglected perspective and supplying it with a background.

Hartlib was born in Elblag (Elbing) at the beginning of the century, into a well-connected merchant family of the Reformed religion, to a German father and an English mother. Having studied at Cambridge in 1625-6, he left his home town for good in 1628 and settled in England. He brought with him a positively missionary determination to contribute to a new Reformation, one that would encompass education, learning and religion, changing all three out of recognition. He elaborated a wide assortment of practical schemes for furthering this idealistic vision, foremost among them being the notion of an Office of Address. This was to be a State-funded institution operating as a sort of clearing house of knowledge. It would receive information on all subjects from all quarters, categorise and store it, and pass it on to those best equipped to make use of it for 'the common good'. He was convinced that such fostering of intellectual exchange, or 'intelligencing', was necessary to bring humanity to its preordained inheritance.

Though Hartlib's proposals for the Office of Address, or Council of Learning as it was alternatively known, aroused considerable interest in Parliament, especially under Oliver Cromwell, that interest was never transmuted into the funding that might have realised the vision. The indomitable Hartlib devoted the greater part of his life to fulfilling single-handedly the function he had envisaged for this institution. He made it his business to establish contact with thinkers and practitioners in every field, academic and non-academic, religious and lay; to gather intelligence from them, to log that intelligence, and to pass copies on to others. In the course of three and a half decades, he developed an enormous network of communication and amassed an eclectic store of letters and manuscripts from the most diverse sources and covering an almost limitless range of subjects.

It was in the nature of Hartlib's purpose that his collection should not, in principle, be bounded by religious or political allegiance. In practice, however, his own background in the Reformed faith inevitably affected the contacts he made and the subjects that preoccupied him. The characteristic obsessions of the 'Second Reformation' loom large: millenarianism, encyclopedism, educational theory, 'useful' knowledge.[3] But for all the frequent emphasis laid on practical utility in the papers Hartlib amassed, the underlying and unifying ethos of his collection is spiritualistic: the affirmation of God's providential design in the world, the assertion of man's potential to gain access, through grace, to a more than human understanding of the nature of things, and a palpably horrified rejection of the idea that either mind or matter is on its own sufficient to explain the universe.

Hartlib's principal allies in his great plan for universal reformation were the irenicist John Dury and the Pansophist Jan Amos Comenius. In 1652, these three committed themselves by a 'Christianæ Societatis Pactum' ('pact of Christian union') to cooperate in the prosecution of the scheme.[4] Comenius's task was the reform of education, Dury's the reform and reconciliation of the church, and Hartlib's the reform of knowledge - tasks which interrelated and overlapped one with another. It is not surprising, therefore, that Dury and Comenius should be the individuals best represented, after Hartlib himself, in his surviving papers. After theirs, one of the largest collections of papers by a single hand to be found in the Hartlib archive is comprised by the letters of the German natural philosopher Johann Moriaen (c. 1591-c.1668).[5]

Unlike Dury and Comenius, Moriaen was almost totally unknown between his death and the rediscovery of Hartlib's papers. He published nothing, and he never held any public or academic office. Consequently, he features in no biographical dictionary. He was noticed, if at all, only as a name that occurs occasionally in contemporary correspondence, principally that of Hartlib and another intimate of his circle, the German translator and diplomat Theodore Haak.

Even now, for all the work that has been done on the archive, he remains an extremely obscure figure. The first work to make frequent mention of him is Turnbull's account of the Hartlib Papers, *Hartlib, Dury and Comenius*, though all Turnbull set out to do was to extract statements from his letters which shed light on the activities of better-known figures, principally Comenius. Charles Webster makes occasional references in the same vein in his magisterial study of the Hartlib Papers, *The Great Instauration*.[6] Milada Blekastad has published nine of his letters from the Hartlib archive (also selected for their relevance to Comenius), in generally excellent transcriptions,[7] and some extracts from his work are reproduced by E.G.E. Van Der Wall in her study of the Hebraist J.S. Rittangel.[8] Inge Keil has used part of his correspondence as a primary source for her study of the Augsburg optician Johann Wiesel, whose agent Moriaen was for a time,[9] and William Newman has drawn on his letters in his study of the American alchemist George Starkey.[10] The fullest account of him anywhere to date is the synopsis of his life in E.G.E. Van Der Wall's biography of the chiliast Petrus Serrarius (Pierre Serrurier).[11] Except by these scholars, his correspondence remains an almost wholly untapped source.[12]

Moriaen was born into a Reformed Dutch family living in exile in Nürnberg, and he spent much of the first half of his long life in the service of those Reformed communities that suffered most from the Counter-Reformation and the Thirty Years War (1618-48). From 1619 to 1627, he was a preacher 'under the Cross' with the clandestine Reformed church in Catholic-controlled Cologne. Subsequently he became a principal organiser of relief work for exiles from the Palatinate. Later in life, however, he distanced himself consciously from any denominational allegiance, and portrayed himself less as the servant of any church than as that of God and his fellow man in general. He settled in the Dutch Netherlands in 1638, where he made a living as a merchant and entrepreneur in a variety of fields, while involving himself in further charity work and the dispensing of medicine. It was at this time that he became closely involved with Hartlib's intelligence network, and his vision of public service acquired a new breadth. Instead of merely alleviating the sufferings of particular persecuted or impoverished communities, he began to believe that he could contribute, in his role as intelligencer, to an advancement of learning and discovery of nature that would not only benefit but totally transform the entire world.

Moriaen was no great original thinker or scientist. He made no claims for himself as an innovator, either in practical or theoretical terms. Like Hartlib, he saw his own function as that of a channel of information and ideas. Besides a considerable stock of raw information, what his letters supply is an insight into the workings and ideals of Hartlib's intelligence network, and a means of access to a particular world-view, a particular intellectual context. For the purposes of appreciating such a context, a substantial body of writing by a figure such as Moriaen is valuable precisely because he was *not* exceptional, not 'ahead of his time'. Though he was certainly not unoriginal, he can be taken as far more representative of his period and milieu than any more innovative or influential thinker.

Though Moriaen did practise medicine, probably in an amateur capacity, it was only one interest among many, and his letters provide no new information about the technical and practical aspects of the discipline. In a less literal sense, however, the whole Hartlibian enterprise can be regarded as a medical one. To use an anachronistic analogy, the likes of Moriaen and Hartlib regarded themselves as antibodies in the diseased bodies of Church, School and State. An appreciation of this overarching analogical ideal is essential to any understanding of the context of early modern medicine, particularly alchemical medicine.[13]

This study charts what can be established of Moriaen's personal history, and uses his correspondence as a point of reference for a more general discussion of the ideologies promoted by Hartlib's circle. It focuses on two concepts that were of crucial importance to the movement as a whole and were Moriaen's own principal obsessions. They are two alternative but (it will be argued) closely related attempts to transcend any merely materialist or rationalist view of the world and to gain access to the spiritual dimension: the concepts of Pansophy and alchemy. Through Pansophy, they sought to make learning whole, to heal the fractures in contemporary education and scholarship. Learning, they feared, was crumbling into specialised disciplines which, by losing contact with one another, lost all relevance and vitality. Pansophy would restore their organic unity. Through alchemy, they sought even more ambitiously to cure Creation itself of the diseases that had entered it with the Fall of Man, and to transmute the corrupt human soul.

Note on the Text
All quotations from non-English sources are given in English translations (my own unless otherwise stated). The original text is given in the footnotes. Foreign language interpolations into English passages are given English translations placed immediately after the relevant portion, italicised in square brackets.

In manuscript transcriptions, editorial expansion of any abbreviation is indicated by the use of italics (eg. 'which', 'Hartlib'). Doubtful readings are placed in square brackets with an italicised question mark. The letter 'thorn' (used by this period only in abbreviations of 'the', 'that', etc.) is transcribed *th*. Citations from manuscripts have occasionally been supplied with additional punctuation, placed in square brackets, to aid comprehension or to clarify possible ambiguities. Abridgment of any quotation is indicated thus: [...]. Interlineations are placed within pointed brackets.

Proper nouns are generally given in vernacular, rather than Anglicised or Latinised forms, except where this would entail using another alphabet than the Roman, and except in the cases of countries, geographical areas and cities so well-known in their English form as virtually to constitute part of the language: thus 'Cologne' and 'Danzig' rather than 'Köln' and 'Gdansk', but 'Nürnberg' and 'Leszno' rather than 'Nuremberg' and 'Lissaw'. In the case of personal names, standardisation is rendered virtually impossible by the fact that contemporaries applied none, even to their own names. I have generally tried to use the form favoured by the individual in question where this can be ascertained, and when in doubt have favoured vernacular forms.

Notes

1   Discovered by George Turnbull: for the history of the papers, see 'Introduction' to *SHUR*, 1-26.

2   *The Hartlib Papers on CD-ROM* (UMI, Ann Arbor, 1995).

3   All these subjects will be dealt with in rather more detail in the course of the following study. On the notion of a 'Second Reformation', see *Die Reformierte Konfessionalisierung in Deutschland - Das Problem der 'Zweiten Reformation'*, ed. Heinz Schilling (Gütersloh, 1986), esp. Heinz Schilling, 'Die "Zweite Reformation" als Categorie der Geschichtswissenschaft', 387-437.

4   *HDC*, 363 and 458-60.

5   The only other figures to compare with him in terms of quantity of material preserved are the Parliamentarian Cheney Culpeper, concerning whom see Chapter Seven, and the agriculturalist and mystic John Beale.

6   Charles Webster, *The Great Instauration: Science, Medicine and Reform 1626-1660* (London, 1975).

7   Milada Blekastad (ed.), *Unbekannte Briefe des Comenius und seiner Freunde 1641-1661* (Ratingen and Kastellaun, 1976), 125-50.

8   E.G.E. Van Der Wall, 'Johann Stephan Rittangel's Stay in the Dutch Republic', *Jewish-Christian Relations in the Seventeenth Century*, eds. J. Van Den Berg and E.G.E. Van Der Wall (Dordrecht, Boston and London, 1988), 119-34.

9   Inge Keil, 'Technology Transfer and Scientific Specialization: Johann Wiesel, optician of Augsburg, and the Hartlib circle', *SHUR*, 268-78.

10   William Newman, *Gehennical Fire: The Lives of George Starkey, an Alchemist of Harvard in the Scientific Revolution* (Harvard, 1994).

11   E.G.E. Van Der Wall, *De Mystieke Chiliast Petrus Serrarius (1600-1669) en zijn Wereld* (Leiden, 1987) (*Serrarius*), 99-101, 302-33 and *passim*. This is a work that has been of enormous value to me in the preparation of this study.

12 One short copy extract appears in James Knowlson's 'Jean Le Maire, the Almérie, and the "musique almérique"', *Acta Musicologica* 40 (1968) 86-9, but the article is not concerned with Moriaen himself.

13 See O.P. Grell and Andrew Cunningham (eds.), *Religio Medici. Medicine and Religion in Seventeenth-Century England* (Aldershot, 1996).

PART ONE

Johann Moriaen :

A Biographical Sketch

CHAPTER ONE

Servant of the Church

'Morian [...] is admirably skilful but can bring nothing to perfection but is very inconstant and falls from one thing to another' - Kenelm Digby, cited in *Ephemerides*, 1654, HP 29/4/11A.

Origins and Upbringing

The minister, physician, natural philosopher and would-be alchemical adept Johann Moriaen was born in Nürnberg in the latter half of 1591 or shortly thereafter.[1] His father Frans was almost certainly a Dutch Calvinist exile of comfortable means, and Johann grew up in the tight-knit society-within-a-society of the refugees, who were aliens both by nationality and religion.

In the late sixteenth century, the Free Imperial City of Nürnberg was a commercial centre strategically located at a nexus of major European trade routes. Long before the Reformation, it already had a substantial Dutch population purely on the strength of its economic connections with the Netherlands. This in itself recommended it as a possible destination to the Dutch refugees driven out of their homeland after the Netherlands, at this time hereditary lands of the Habsburgs, fell to Felipe II of Spain in 1556 and the new ruler set about extirpating Protestantism from his dominions. The Nürnberg authorities viewed this influx with mixed feelings. On the one hand, the vast majority of such exiles were Calvinists, and the *Stadtrat* or City Council, though humanistically inclined and averse to rigid dogmatism, did not wish to see the faith of the solidly Lutheran populace tainted with the new heresy, or the city a prey to partisan strife. Nor did it wish to provide the city's great Catholic neighbour Bavaria with an excuse for territorial aggression by overtly fostering a religion that had no legal existence within the Holy Roman Empire under the terms of the 1555 Treaty of Augsburg. On the other hand, the city's market-based economy, which had suffered from the political upheavals of mid-century, stood to benefit from an infusion of skilled artisans and craftsmen. It was precisely from this walk of life that the overwhelming majority of the Dutch refugees hailed - exile being for them, as it was not for unskilled labourers and peasants, a financially viable option. Like a number of other commercial centres in the late sixteenth and early seventeenth centuries,[2] Nürnberg discovered that a measure of religious toleration was good for business.

In 1569, as the notoriously bloody measures of Felipe's new lieutenant the Duke of Alva (appointed Governor 1567) led to a redoubling of the exodus from the Netherlands, the Nürnberg City Council moved from toleration to positive encouragement of the immigrants, or at least of certain selected ones, having spotted an opportunity to capitalise on the textile trade that was being driven out of the Netherlands along with Protestantism. It paid the travelling expenses of and found or even built accommodation for a hand-picked group of skilled workers in this field - dyers, weavers, stitchers and embroiderers - who with their families numbered about forty. Far greater numbers of exiles who arrived of their own accord were also admitted. Many such immigrants acquired Nürnberg citizenship, a stipulation for this being that they should undertake not to set up any separate church or 'sect' within the Lutheran city, or make any attempt to convert or quarrel with any of the native populace. In other words, the city authorities wanted their technical expertise and commercial experience badly enough to be prepared to put up with their obnoxious opinions, provided they in turn were prepared to keep those opinions to themselves. Thus there was from the mid-sixteenth century a substantial and almost exclusively immigrant Calvinist population in Nürnberg, principally Dutch but including French Huguenots and English Puritans, unable (in principle at least) to make any public profession of their faith or conduct any communal worship, but accepting this as the price of shelter in a city where it was at least tacitly accepted that they practised it in private. Though there were periodical investigations of secret religious services being conducted within the Calvinist community, leading to the issuing of threats and admonishments, the authorities were decidedly luke-warm about taking real reprisals against such activity. It was not, however, until 1650, in the wake of the Peace of Westphalia, that a Reformed Church was officially recognised in Nürnberg.[3]

Among these immigrants was a braid-maker by the name of Hans Morianus, who acquired Nürnberg citizenship on 12 April 1581.[4] Two years later, this Morianus featured in a group of nine immigrant citizens and denizens who were summoned before the city court for having had their children baptised in Reformed churches of the Upper Palatinate instead of Lutheran ones in Nürnberg.[5] That they had done so testifies to the tenacity of their faith, since such a journey entailed three days' travelling (with, obviously, a young infant in tow). The City Council admonished its stiff-necked asylum-seekers to stop visiting churches outside the city boundaries, but appears as usual not to have imposed any actual penalties - or to have had much effect on their subsequent conduct.[6]

The surname Morian[us] is a highly unusual one, and it is beyond the bounds of plausible coincidence that this Hans Morianus should not have been related to Moriaen's father Frans and his wife Maria, née von Manten (which is probably a Germanisation of Van Manten).[7] While there is no documentary evidence that the family was Dutch, the Netherlands are far and away the likeliest place of origin for Calvinist immigrants to Nürnberg at this period. The assumption is effectively clinched by the fact that Moriaen consistently spelled his name in the Dutch manner, in preference to the much more Germanic 'Morian' favoured by almost everyone else at the time or since,[8] and that he was fluent in Dutch well before he settled in Amsterdam in 1638.[9] He was not baptised in Nürnberg, which suggests that the family persisted in the practice of sneaking out of Nürnberg to the Upper Palatinate to celebrate communion, weddings and baptisms according to the rites of their own faith.

The few other facts about Moriaen's family discernible from his letters can be quickly summarised. He had at least two sisters. One married the merchant Abraham de Bra, another member of the Nürnberg Dutch community.[10] He left the city in 1633, probably for Amsterdam, and subsequently became a leading figure in the Dutch West India Company.[11]

Another sister married into the Abeele family - a transparently Dutch name.[12] Her husband may well have been related either to the Jan Abeels of Flanders who was an elder of the important Dutch Reformed Church of Austin Friars in London, from 1604 to 1611 or earlier, or the English-born John vanden Abeele who was elder from 1630-36, both of them merchants.[13] Moriaen also had at least one brother, whose daughter in 1649 or 50 married into the family of the renowned Frankfurt printer and engraver Matthias Merian.[14] Other members of his family lived in Cracow, whence Catholic persecution drove them into exile in Danzig.[15]

The first surviving documentary evidence of Moriaen is his matriculation at Heidelberg University in 1611.[16] Later, Moriaen fondly recalled his student days at Heidelberg and his friendship there with Georg Vechner (later a collaborator and editor of Comenius), for whose accommodation he apparently paid.[17] His family evidently had the funds and the will to ensure he was well provided for. Since Moriaen subsequently became a Reformed minister, it is altogether likely that he studied theology, but the records yield no more than the date of matriculation, with no indication of how long he remained in Heidelberg or what degree, if any, he obtained.

Heidelberg, capital of the Palatinate, was a stronghold of Calvinism at this period. The Reformed faith had been imposed on the province in 1562 (and again, after a Lutheran interlude, in 1583), thus gaining for the cause the oldest university in Germany, and one of the most reputable. Though it initially remained academically conservative by comparison with the newly-founded Reformed academies such as Herborn (established 1584), the ethos was changing at the very moment of Moriaen's arrival. In particular, the logical and pedagogical ideas of Bartholomäus Keckermann (1571-1609) were (somewhat belatedly) meeting with an enthusiastic reception. Keckermann had set out to define what he called 'methodical Peripateticism', a synthesis of the traditional Aristotelian logical methodology with the newer and ostensibly anti-Aristotelian ideas of Pierre de la Ramée (Ramus) which had become a standby of Reformed education. Ramism, as Howard Hotson puts it, 'was an instrument adopted in order to achieve a Second Reformation', and Keckermann's achievement was a fusion of 'Ramist clarity with Peripatetic substance'.[18] Keckermann was a founder of the encyclopedic tradition that led through Alsted to Comenius and his notion of Pansophy, of which Moriaen was later to become a prominent champion and supporter. Though there is not a single mention in his surviving correspondence of either Ramus or Keckermann - or, for that matter, Aristotle - his university education took place at the same time Comenius was studying under Alsted in Herborn, just the time when the notions of universal method and encyclopedic knowledge were achieving their greatest vogue, especially in Reformed establishments.[19] It is even possible Moriaen first met Comenius during the latter's brief spell at Heidelberg in 1613, but it is by no means certain Moriaen was still there by then.

Under the Cross

There is no record of Moriaen at all for the next eight years, but at some point during this period he became a minister in Frankfurt am Main. The situation

5

there must have been familiar enough. Like Nürnberg, Frankfurt was an Imperial city under Lutheran control, cautiously and uneasily tolerating a substantial Calvinist minority of largely Dutch origin which was accorded no officially recognised church. Services and sacraments could be delivered only secretly, in private houses, just as they were in Nürnberg. As a boy, Moriaen would have attended such clandestine religious gatherings in his home city; as a young man, he conducted them in Frankfurt.

A new experience for him at this time, which may well have had an impact on his later thought and attitudes, will have been the Jewish ghetto. There was a sizeable Jewish community in Frankfurt, tolerated like the Reformed Christians because it was economically useful, but very much on sufferance and with far more severe circumscriptions. The Jews were subject to a strict curfew, being confined to their ghetto after dark and on Sundays, and at no time permitted to leave it without sporting the stigma of a prominent yellow circle sewn onto their clothing, or to assemble outside it in groups of more than two.[20] No comment whatsoever by Moriaen survives concerning his time in this city, but it is a reasonable conjecture that his experiences or observations in Frankfurt had a bearing on the keen interest he later displayed in Judaism, and the considerable sympathy he showed, by the standards of the day, for its practitioners.

In 1619, at the outbreak of the Thirty Years War, he was summoned by his Church to the still less congenial surroundings of Cologne, one of the most staunchly and intransigently Roman Catholic enclaves of the entire Empire. The records of the German Reformed Church there (henceforth *Protokolle*) note that on 27 February 1619,

> Since the Brothers have decided to summon a third minister, and one by the name of Johannes Moriaen has been suggested to us, who is prepared to be seen next week in Frankfurt, Brothers Wilhelm Engels and Johann Fassing are to arrange for the said Moriaen's preaching to be heard by the leading members of the church, that we may judge whether he might fruitfully serve this congregation.[21]

Apparently his preaching met/with the approval of the church authorities, since two months later he was sent a written summons.[22] His decision to follow it was a brave one. For a Reformed minister to move from Frankfurt to Cologne in 1619 was to exchange, quite deliberately, the frying pan for the fire. The Nürnberg and Frankfurt authorities were prepared to turn a blind eye to Calvinism so long as its adherents maintained a reasonable level of discretion. Cologne wanted no truck with any form of Protestantism at all.

At the time of the first wave of Protestant emigration from the Netherlands in the mid-sixteenth century, Cologne had offered numerous attractions to the exiles: many Dutch traders had business connections there, it was reasonably close to the Netherlands, and it was known for tolerance and hospitality. The Jesuit-led Counter-Reformation soon changed this. The Lutheran and the three rather larger Reformed Churches (German, Dutch and Walloon) found themselves under constant surveillance and at risk of unwelcome attention from the authorities or more orthodox citizens. As Rudolf Löhr, the first modern editor of the *Protokolle*, sums the record up:

From the first onslaught of 1566/1568 until 1627, besides the ambushes of their services reported or merely implied [in the records], the Evangelicals had to endure an unbroken chain of trials, fines, imprisonments and banishments, house searches and house closures.[23]

The full congregation never met at any one time, and from October 1619 on no more than two of the three German ministers ever attended consistorial meetings together.[24] When a service was to be held, the ministers decided which of their flock to call to it, by turns and according to the standard of their behaviour, and secret messages were conveyed to those summoned, informing them of the time and place. Whenever Catholic processions, such as the Corpus Christi day parade, were due to take place, the ministers went discreetly from house to house among their congregation exhorting them to keep well clear of the 'heathen carnival' ('abgöttliche Götzendracht'). When the Reformed Churches, by contrast, decided on a day of prayer and fasting - a standard Protestant strategy for appeasing the wrath of God which was employed about once every three or four months - the same procedure was repeated, firstly to let people know it was happening and secondly to encourage them to observe it.

The elders of the church occupied their position only for a year at a time, after which new elders were elected. This tended to be a cyclical process, former elders being regularly proposed for re-election after four or five years. The ministers never appeared publicly in clerical dress. The locations of the services and even the days on which they were held were frequently changed. The watchword was discretion, and the foremost concern of all members of the church was to avoid drawing attention to themselves.

Despite such conditions, the role of Reformed minister in Cologne may well, in early 1619, have presented brighter prospects to a devout believer in the imminent and ultimate triumph of the Protestant cause than can easily be appreciated with the handicap of hindsight. Bohemia was making its stand against domination by the Catholic Habsburgs and it was fondly supposed by many Protestants that its elected champion, Friedrich V of the Palatinate, would be supported by the might of England under his father-in-law James I. The abundant prophecies of the impending downfall of Antichrist seemed to be borne out by this massive challenge to Catholic domination within the Holy Roman Empire. Moriaen had certainly read the *Fama* and *Confessio* of the Rosicrucians,[25] the one announcing an imminent rebirth of the Evangelical church, the other predicting with positively sadistic glee the downfall of Rome. He also saw the manuscript of the first two parts of *Lux in tenebris*, the visions of Christina Poniatowska and Christoph Kotter, translated into Latin by Comenius, foretelling the restoration of Elector Friedrich and the triumph of Protestantism. That is not of course to say that he uncritically believed them, and his own much later recollection was that he approached *Lux in Tenebris* at least with considerable scepticism.[26] But he can hardly have been unaffected by the emotional and intellectual climate that produced such works, distinctly and deliberately reminiscent of the vengeful optimism and dogged faith of the early Christian Church - another oppressed dissident minority - as expressed in Revelation.

Whether Moriaen shared it or not, the illusion did not last long. The summer of 1620 saw Friedrich's lands in the Palatinate overrun by forces

7

allied to the Emperor, and in November his army in Bohemia was routed by Bavarian-led troops at the Battle of the White Mountain outside Prague. Friedrich and his family fled to the Netherlands, and in 1623 his Electorate was transferred to the Catholic Maximilian of Bavaria. It had rapidly become apparent that the English crown had no intention of engaging for one side or the other, and the position of Protestants in such Catholic strongholds as Cologne, where the Counter-Reformation had in any case already been in full swing for some decades, became more difficult and dangerous than ever. Far from spearheading a Third Reformation, Moriaen and his colleagues can at best have found themselves struggling to sustain the faith of a beleaguered congregation forced to worship in secret and displaying considerable courage in doing so at all. The one thing to be said for Cologne, from a Protestant point of view, was that unlike so much of Germany it avoided becoming a battleground, but in that respect it was a haven securely in hostile hands. It was not until 1802 that public Evangelical worship became possible in the city.[27] That Moriaen stuck to this singularly thankless and dangerous post for a full eight years bespeaks considerable courage and tenacity of purpose on his part.

The contemporary *Protokolle* give some impression of what Moriaen's life must have been like for these eight years. Laconic but vivid, they are records of great value not only for their many historical and biographical details but also for sheer human interest: and they incidentally refute the stereotypical image of Calvinists as humourless. Moriaen's name appears dozens of times over the period of his ministry. In the early years especially, the keepers of the *Protokolle* clearly set out to convey as great a sense of normality as possible, assiduously noting the routine tasks assigned to the church's servants, tasks which would have been the stock-in-trade of a Reformed minister in any location, Geneva as much as Cologne. Moriaen oversaw accounts and dealt with church correspondence; he received and passed on pleas for charitable assistance, both from distressed individuals and other Reformed communities; he catechised aspiring members of the congregation and assessed their suitability in terms of their behaviour and their familiarity with the principles of religion. He frequently attended the consistorial meetings of the three Reformed Churches which took place every few months, and at which common policies were agreed on, the division of labour between the three sister churches allotted and disagreements discussed. Above all, he carried out that most central of a Reformed minister's duties, the supervision of the morals of his flock.

Soon after joining the church, Moriaen was confronted with the rather surprising case of one Jeremias Mist, who wished to marry his late stepfather's widow. Moriaen was appointed to write to the Heidelberg theologian Scultetus for advice. The reply was, as the *Protokolle* drily note, that the proposal was found unacceptable 'in consideration of the fact that the said widow is his mother, or at least is believed to be so'.[28]

Most of the misdemeanours he was called on to admonish were more commonplace:

> It has come to our notice that Johann Mosten, shortly after partaking of holy communion, overburdened himself with drink and thereupon, at

8

home, treated his wife in an unseemly fashion, offending the community
of Christ. To be chastised for this by Brothers Jordan and Moriaen.[29]

One of the worst recidivists in this respect was a certain Matthias Kuiper.
On 1 August 1624, Moriaen was appointed to help arrange a reconciliation
between Kuiper and his wife, whose marital disputes had likewise been
offending the community of Christ.[30] The following December, Kuiper
complained that he was still not being called to the church services, only to be
told the church was unconvinced by his explanation 'that he had only made
advances to his former serving maid in order to test her piety.'[31] Some
months later, being assured that he and his wife were now reconciled,
Moriaen was again sent to tell Kuiper that he could return to the fold if he
promised to remain sober.[32] But by 30 October the wheel had once more
turned full circle:

> Although Matthias Kuiper, on a high oath and with weighty words, on
> the one hand promised to mend his ways and on the other denied his
> faults, matters have turned out otherwise, in that he remains continually
> given to drinking, gambling and frivolity.[33]

Moriaen was again given the seemingly hopeless task of persuading the errant
Kuiper back onto the paths of righteousness.

In the early years of his ministry, indeed, the concern expressed in the
records about 'un-Christian' behaviour on the part of the congregation, such
as drinking, swearing, gambling, quarrelling, fornicating and dancing, rather
outweighs that about Catholic persecution. Dancing particularly concerned
the German church, which appears to have been the most sternly puritanical
of the three. A constant complaint in the records after consistorial meetings
was that the Dutch and Walloon churches considered excommunication an
excessive punishment for persistent dancing, and could not be persuaded to
join the German in a united and uncompromising stance against such
behaviour.

Another recurrent problem was the habit of the congregation of attending
Catholic ceremonies and festivals, or, worse, sending their children to
Catholic schools or tutors. Since there was no official or legal alternative, this
is hardly surprising. Association with Catholics, however, was a matter of
concern not only for its corrupting influence on the individual concerned, but
for the danger it posed to the Reformed community as a whole, especially to
those actually in Church service. When, for instance, the daughter of the
woman appointed to summon catechists took up with a Papist, the Church
was reluctantly obliged to dispense with the mother's services.[34] A careless
or malicious word might let slip the identity of a minister or the location of a
service, as when

> It is reported that Christian Stoffgen, in the presence of a Popish woman,
> unseemingly gave out that he had been dealt with in unfriendly fashion by
> Herr Lauterbach, adding, 'that is how our Elders behave.' Brothers Johann
> and Schütgens to speak with him and chastise him according to their
> findings.[35]

9

The result might be banishment from Cologne of one of the Church's servants, as happened to Johann Kray in 1623,[36] or the arrest of the owner of a house in which services were held. This befell Peter Gülich on 5 March 1627. Faced with the threat of a heavy fine or imprisonment unless he would reveal the names of at least some of the congregation, Gülich was on the point of capitulating, and the Church found itself obliged to spend 300 Imperials from its funds to buy his release.[37] Children of course were particularly susceptible to Papist wiles, and were not admitted to services on the grounds that they were too young for their discretion to be relied on.[38]

In the course of his ministry, Moriaen formed a number of lasting friendships: many of the names that feature regularly in the *Protokolle* recur too in his later correspondence with Hartlib. Among the more respected members of what was in general a well-to-do congregation were the Pergens family. Long before Moriaen's arrival, one Jacob Pergens was Elder for a year (1604),[39] and Leonard Pergens was upbraided for the tiresome sin of dancing.[40] These are almost certainly older relations of the Jacob Pergens, Herr von Vosbergen, who later settled in Amsterdam and became a director of the West India Company, and is frequently mentioned in Moriaen's correspondence with the vague designation 'Vetter' (ie. any male relation beyond the immediate family). His trading contacts would make him a useful channel for conveying parcels of books, minerals, medicines, etc. between England and the Netherlands. Another prominent family was the von Zeuels: Peter and Jacob appear as servants of the church during Moriaen's ministry, and before his arrival, Adam von Zeuel was an elder.[41] Moriaen would later marry this Adam von Zeuel's daughter Odilia. There is frequent mention of the Lauterbach family, who also appear later as relatives of Moriaen.[42] In the tight-knit Reformed community, intermarriage between the larger families was virtually inevitable, so it is hardly surprising that all these names occur in his later correspondence as relations, probably through his marriage to Odilia von Zeuel.

It was also in Cologne that Moriaen became associated with the large Kuffler family. Abraham Kuffler was Elder in 1622 and 1627,[43] and numerous other members of the family are mentioned as attending catechism, delivering their *Glaubensbekenntnis* (confession of [Calvinist] faith) and so forth. At the same time, another Abraham Kuffler of Cologne and his brother Johann Sibertus were in England. These two would later achieve considerable celebrity as inventors, and from the late 1640s onward the fate of Johann Sibertus in particular became inextricably linked with that of Moriaen.

Moriaen's own interest in technological development, particularly in the field of optics, was also established by this time. He is almost certainly the person referred to in a letter of December 1626 from Prince August of Anhalt to the natural philosopher and bibliophile Carl Widemann, mentioning a highly accomplished optician of Cologne with an assistant named Morian.[44] Among his accomplishments was the making of microscopes, albeit relatively basic ones.[45] There is no clue as to the identity of his employer, but he later told the story of a group of Cologne glassmakers who were forced to flee the city because their lenses proved so fragile that they tended to burst spontaneously.[46] The profession of glassmaker may have served as a cover for Moriaen's involvement with the clandestine Reformed Church.[47] There is no doubt, however, that his interest in the subject was genuine and profound, and it remained with him for the rest of his life. His later activity as agent for the German telescope and microscope maker Johann Wiesel will be considered shortly. Moriaen expected more from his lenses, however, than mere magnification: he came to believe that by means of them sunlight itself could be concentrated into a material form and the 'universal spirit' or 'world soul' extracted from it.[48]

His future wife aside, the closest and most enduring relationships Moriaen established were with preachers of the other Reformed Churches. Justinus Van Assche[49] served the Dutch Church in Frankfurt and Cologne simultaneously from October 1622 (some three years after Moriaen's arrival in Cologne) till June 1627 (almost exactly the same time Moriaen left). Hartlib's great friend Dury was with the Walloon Church in Cologne from 1624 to 1626,[50] and was replaced by Pierre Serrurier, or Petrus Serrarius as he is better known, who stayed until 1628.[51] All three were noted for their irenical leanings, and were accused of unorthodoxy by their more doctrinaire co-religionists.

Early in 1624, Van Assche wrote to his friends and future brothers-in-law Jacob and Isaac Beeckman expressing concern about the heterodox opinions of a friend in Cologne. Van Assche's letter is lost, and is known only through Jacob Beeckman's reply, in which the staunchly Reformed Beeckman urged him to keep his distance from such dubious ideas.[52] Neither the friend's name nor the unorthodoxy in question is specified. Since the exchange pre-dates the arrival of either Dury or Serrarius in Cologne, Van Der Wall conjectures that it may refer to Moriaen.[53] This is certainly feasible, though as she stresses herself there is no conclusive proof. As things turned out, however, Moriaen was the only one of the four friends not to become embroiled in public doctrinal disputes.

Van Assche was summoned in 1626 to a new post in Veere, but refused to sign the rigid *Glaubensbekenntnis*, an affirmation of sound doctrinal Calvinism drawn up at the Synod of Dordrecht (Dort). It is a sign of how much laxer his church was than Moriaen's that he had presumably not been required to do so before. This led not only to the appointment's not being ratified but to Van Assche's excommunication - an excommunication which, it appears from Moriaen's correspondence, was still in force thirteen years later.[54] Serrarius, who would later become one of the most spectacularly non-conformist figures of his day, was also removed from his post for unorthodoxy. The precise grounds are unclear, but Van Der Wall, who is the chief authority on this intriguing character, suggests that Serrarius may have rejected the idea of Christ's having assumed human nature.[55]

As for Dury, he spent his life engendering public controversies precisely by dint of his tireless efforts to bring all controversy to an end. Since the studies of Turnbull and Webster established (quite rightly) the centrality of Dury's role in Hartlib's vision of a Great Instauration, it has been all too easy to overlook the fact that this was very much Hartlib's personal opinion, and that to many of his contemporaries Dury's close involvement with his projects seriously compromised their credibility. When the mystic and alchemist Johannes Tanckmar was accused by the Church authorities in Lübeck of promoting unorthodoxy, his friendship with Dury was cited in evidence against him.[56] In November 1639, Van Assche objected, through Moriaen, to a proposed publication of his correspondence with Dury about scriptural analysis, 'for Justinus himself has been removed from the ministry for this reason [public association with ideas deemed unorthodox] and is still excluded from communion'.[57] Though one reason cited is that Van Assche's known unorthodoxy might be seen to taint Dury's endeavours, the letter makes it plain that Van Assche was at least equally worried about the converse: that making his association with Dury public would bring him into greater disrepute. Bringing the work out anonymously would solve nothing, he protested, for Dury's style was so distinctive it would immediately be recognised. If his ideas were to be made public - to which he had no objection - it should be in a separate edition from Dury's.

It is highly probable, though there is no firm evidence, that Moriaen's friendship with another of Hartlib's closest associates, Theodore Haak, also dates from this period.[58] Haak was a translator from the Palatinate, who later settled in England and became a diplomat in the service of Cromwell and a Fellow of the Royal Society. He played a leading role in the organisation of charitable collections for the Palatine refugees, in the promotion of the work of Comenius, and in furthering experimental philosophy through the scientific club known as the '1645 group', including John Wilkins and John Wallis, and of which Haak was certainly a member and may have been the instigator.[59] After studying at Cambridge, Haak spent a year or two in Cologne from the summer of 1626, where he 'joined a group of fellow Protestants and took a regular part in the secret religious meetings which they were holding in a private house.'[60] That is to say, he practised his religion: there was no other sort of Protestant meeting in Cologne. Though there is no mention of Haak in the *Protokolle*, it would be surprising if he and Moriaen did not come into contact in such an environment. Indeed, Haak was in all likelihood part of the audience for Moriaen's sermons.

As time went on, the veneer of ordinariness affected by the Church records became perceptibly thinner. At the beginning of Moriaen's period of service, the days of fasting and atonement were regularly instituted with the formulaic remark that penitence was particularly necessary 'in these fast-changing and dangerous times' ('in diesen geschwinden gefährlichen Zeiten'). By the end of 1625, this had turned to 'on account of great immediate peril and fearsome wrath of God'.[61] The steady trickle of ministers and others in the church's employ requesting demission because they were becoming too well known swells with the passing of time, as does the number detected by the authorities and imprisoned or banished from the city. The elder Jacob Phinor, when he died in 1624, was not replaced due to a lack of suitable candidates - a lack which was expected to become more serious with the passing of time.[62] A recurrent cause of concern was the question of how to reconcile a clean conscience with interrogation under oath if the worst came to the worst. This was discussed on 4 May 1623, but no one could come up with a better idea than that already in practice, that anyone put in such a position should consider him or herself automatically released from the Church and hence able to say honestly that he or she had nothing to do with it.[63] This perhaps proved inadequate to cope with the formula 'are you now or have you ever been', for the same question was raised again, in the 'times now more difficult and dangerous than ever' ('jetzt überaus schwehrlicher und gefährlicher Zeit'), on 26 August 1626, and brothers 'Henricus and Morian' were appointed to search the church records diligently for a previous ruling on the matter that might supply a better solution.[64] (The result of their deliberations is not recorded.) The resolute tone of the earlier entries, and their frequent sardonic humour, gradually give way to a gathering sense of impotent frustration, exemplified by the decision on 1 April 1627:

> In consideration of the great danger and distress increasing here more and more as time goes on, the assembled Brothers are to consider keenly, invoking divine aid, the safest and surest means by which we may conduct our holy worship as diligently as possible, and yet still avoid danger.[65]

By this juncture, Moriaen, who had already stuck to his post a good deal longer than the majority of ministers found possible, had applied to join the swelling exodus. He was released from his duties 'on account of great and most urgent peril' ('aus erheblicher und hochdringender Not') on 29 February 1627 - but with the proviso that he should continue to display his goodwill to the church as opportunity arose.[66] Quite what was meant by this is not altogether clear, but it was evidently more than a rhetorical turn of phrase and involved some sort of practical commitment, since on 1 April he pressed again for his official demission, the other brothers agreeing to refer the matter to their superiors. It was not until 26 May that he was finally, and reluctantly, released:

> Concerning the matter of Brother J, the assembled Brothers have agreed unanimously, in view of his most urgent peril, that although we are most loth to forego his services, we will nonetheless grant his request.[67]

Soon after renouncing his ministry at Cologne, Moriaen returned to his birthplace, Nürnberg, and became involved in setting up and administering charitable collections for the Reformed ministers and teachers, and their families, who had been driven out of the Upper Palatinate by the Bavarian invasion. Nürnberg became the foremost resort of such refugees and the administrative centre for the distribution of funds raised by the international relief effort.[68] Moriaen was, by his own later account, a major player in this for over five years, evidently meaning mid or late 1627 to early 1633.[69]

This charitable collection for exiled Protestant preachers and teachers, who in many cases were literally facing starvation, had been first launched in 1626 as a private enterprise by Johannes Cüner, a former Reformed preacher of Amberg who had himself taken refuge in Nürnberg. Amberg was a town of the Upper Palatinate which had been among those to which Reformed Nürnbergers such as Hans Morianus resorted for baptisms and communion. From the start, however, it was an international operation, applying for and receiving subsidies from sister churches in Switzerland, France, the Netherlands, and England. Various members of the Nürnberg Dutch community soon became involved in the project. Among the merchants who acted as clearing agents in this business, by accepting in their own names the foreign currency donations received and passing on the equivalent amount in Nürnberg guilders to the overseers of the collection, was Moriaen's brother-in-law Abraham de Bra, alongside Jeremias Calandrin and Johann Kendrich, two other names that occur, albeit only in passing, in Moriaen's later correspondence.

On 30 March 1627, the deposed Elector Palatine, Friedrich V, issued a 'royal' decree from his exile in The Hague, 'officially' sanctioning the programme. De Bra, Calandrin and Kendrich all appear shortly after this, no longer as middle-men, but as organisers and overseers of the collection, and were joined in this capacity, according to Neidiger, by the Dutch Nürnberger 'Johann Moriau'. This is an evident (and easily-made) mistranscription of 'Morian'.[70]

As far as the City Council was concerned, of course, the enterprise had no official character whatsoever, and the official approbation of Friedrich, if they knew about it at all, could only serve to make the whole business highly suspect. In 1628, the Council organised an investigation of it. This declared the collection not only illegal but apt to awaken suspicion that Nürnberg was secretly promoting Calvinism, a charge likely to lead to dire reprisals from the Emperor, or to provide Maximilian of Bavaria with an excuse for occupying the city. Charity toward exiles was all well and good (and was, indeed, being organised by the Council itself on a smaller scale), but only under the Council's own aegis. The Council duly admonished the organisers and threatened them with banishment. As had earlier been the case with baptisms and weddings outside Nürnberg or secret Calvinist services within it, however, this seems to have been more a matter of form than a genuine attempt to put a stop to the collection. The 'Dutch' administrators, presumably including Moriaen, discreetly handed their responsibilities over, in name at least, to four ministers and officials from the Palatinate, but by 1631 had as quietly taken them up again. The Council's main concern, it would seem, was to be able to demonstrate if necessary that it was not secretly in league with Friedrich V or actively condoning heresy. It was more important to have these statutes noted in the records than actually to implement them. All it really wanted from the Calvinists was discretion. The one person involved who actually was officially banished from the city, Dr Johann Jakob Heber, himself a Palatine exile and principal overseer of the distribution of funds, did not in fact leave.[71] The collection continued to function until after the end of the war, finally being wound up in 1650. In 1637, indeed, it was given de facto recognition when the Council referred an application from a Palatine serving maid for treatment in a Nürnberg charity hospital to 'the Palatine exiles, they being the patient's countryfolk' ('den pfälzischen Exulanten, als dieser Patientin Landsleuten') and 'the collection and its organisers' ('der Collecta und dero Verwaltern').[72] After what Moriaen had been accustomed to in Cologne, this hardly counted as persecution.

Of all the contributions that reached Nürnberg from the various foreign churches they had appealed to, the most substantial was that from the two Royal Collections in England administered by the Dutch Reformed church at Austin Friars. Hartlib and (especially) Haak were involved in organising these.[73] Despite the obstruction of William Laud, Bishop of London, who was not best pleased to see his sovereign sanctioning what he saw as support for the cause of international Calvinism, the two collections raised close to £10,000 for the relief effort (there was a third Royal Collection in 1635 but Laud, by then Archbishop of Canterbury, kept a much tighter rein on this).[74] It is impossible to say, however, whether Moriaen was already in personal contact with Hartlib by this juncture.

Mystics and Utopists

The cultural and confessional atmosphere of Nürnberg had changed somewhat since Moriaen's childhood. It was still a Free Imperial City and still officially Lutheran, but was becoming known, as were Hamburg, Frankfurt, Lübeck, Rostock and Bremen, as a centre for religious independents. This was perhaps the result of the willingness these free Lutheran cities had earlier shown to admit refugees of various Evangelical hues.

Luther's most revolutionary achievement had been, perhaps, the bringing of the Bible to the people, that they might no longer be duped by the casuistical interpretations set on it by Rome. A perennial source of embarrassment to learned Lutherans in positions of authority, both ecclesiastical and secular, was that instead of uniting joyously in the pure and simple faith that had thus been revealed to them, considerable numbers of the people proceeded to put their own novel interpretations on the sacred texts, and to argue that the Lutheran theologians who sought to suppress their views were indulging in quite as much casuistry and restraint of conscience as the Romanists they had taken over from. In fact, the Lutheran cities were on the whole a great deal milder in their treatment of non-conformists than either Catholic or Calvinist territories, which is the main reason they attracted so many of them.

These Evangelical independents, representing a very broad spectrum of views, and united more by their shared rejection of both Lutheran and Calvinist confessionalisation than by any doctrinal unanimity, are generally lumped together by modern historians under the *faute de mieux* labels 'spiritualist', 'separatist' or (in German) 'Schwärmer'. This last, much like the English 'enthusiast', was a catch-all derogatory term applied promiscuously at the time to the uncategorisably unorthodox. Other contemporary expressions applied in similarly arbitrary fashion were 'Schwenckfeldian', 'Böhmenist' and 'Weigelian', after the mystic writers Caspar Schwenckfeld, Jacob Böhme and Valentin Weigel. Though all these writers had their genuine adherents among the independents, these terms were on the whole used loosely and arbitrarily, often without any clear idea of the doctrines they ostensibly designated.

There are, for obvious reasons, considerable difficulties in establishing the nature and membership of such independent circles, if indeed they can be deemed to have had a sufficiently formalised existence for words such as 'circle' and 'membership' to be applicable to them at all. It is clear, however, that in the Nürnberg of the late 1620s and early 1630s, there were considerable numbers among the populace prepared openly to refuse attendance at Lutheran services. These non-conformists came for the most part from the milieu of the traders and artisans.[75] Many of them must have been children or grandchildren of the Reformed immigrants among whom Moriaen's parents had featured towards the end of the previous century. They had grown a little more confident than their forebears had been of their right to assert an independent religious identity, but also less committed than those forebears to the orthodoxies of Calvinism.

The use of the term 'Schwärmer' for dangerously independent religious thinkers seems to have originated with Luther himself, reflecting his own alarm at some of the forces he had helped unleash. The danger they posed to the establishment was in most cases more perceived than real. A few, such as Ludwig Gifftheil and his disciple Johann Friedrich Münster, preached armed insurrection in the name of the Messiah, but they found few followers.[76] The majority were more concerned with an internalised, pietistic spiritualism, and were quite content to leave the established church to its own devices so long as it extended the same courtesy to them. By definition individualistic, most rejected the very notion of sects and schools. In the case of Nürnberg, there can be no knowing what passed in the private gatherings which undoubtedly took place, but of which no detailed record has survived. However, there is no evidence to suggest that these were more than occasions to discuss and celebrate a doctrinally independent faith, or that the participants either did or desired to challenge the officially established religion of the city.

This was the milieu to which Moriaen returned in (probably) 1627. While such associations provide no conclusive proof of Moriaen's own opinions and still less of his activities, a consistent picture emerges of a man much involved with the doings and writings of these so-called 'enthusiasts' or 'Schwärmer', whose beliefs varied widely on points of detail, but who were generally agreed on the importance of a personal understanding of and relationship with God and the expression and propagation of that faith through practical works of charity and the dissemination of inspirational literature.

It is from Nürnberg that his first surviving letter is addressed: it is to Dury, and dated 22 January 1633.[77] It is a short note in Latin, mainly concerned with an exchange of literature: Moriaen had been enquiring on Dury's behalf after a number of works by the 'spiritualists' Sebastian Franck, Christian Endfelder and Daniel Friedrich, and specified Caspar Warnle as a contact through whom he had tried to obtain them. This Warnle (Werlin, Wörnlein) came from one of the more prominently unconfessionalised Nürnberg families. In January 1648, a church commission considered what to do with a number of 'Weigelians' including Warnle's widow, and recommended banishment, though it is not clear to what extent this advice was acted on.[78]

Later the same year, Moriaen wrote again to Dury that his sister's daughter had married Peter Neefen, adding that Neefen was no stranger to Dury.[79] Neefen, together with Warnle and a few others, belonged to the inner circle of friends of Nikolaus Pfaff, who has been described as the spiritual leader of the Nürnberg non-conformists.[80] Neefen was also particularly close to the radical mystic J.F. Münster, who even hoped that in the event of his wife's death, Neefen would undertake the care and upbringing of his children.[81]

Moriaen's interest in rare and unorthodox mystic literature surfaces again in a letter to Van Assche of 1634, in which he expressed hopes of obtaining a copy of Paul Felgenhauer's *Monarchen-Spiegel* (1633-35). In this work, Felgenhauer accused the rulers of the world of neglecting the higher authorities of Christ and God, and of staining their hands with the blood of innocents. He contrasted the 'empire of the Devil, the Beast and the tyrants of this world' with the reign of Christ in the world to come (the Millennium) and finally with the reign of God in a new incarnation of this world at the end of time.[82] Since the attack on temporal authorities included explicit denunciation of the Emperor Ferdinand, the work later brought down the accusation of lèse-majesté against Felgenhauer.[83] Whether Moriaen was trying to acquire it from or for Van Assche is not clear, but it is evident both men were avid readers and collectors of such books.[84]

However loosely the name of Jacob Böhme may have been invoked by the denouncers of non-conformity, there is no doubt that this mystic visionary genuinely was a source of inspiration for many of the period's less orthodox thinkers, as for some of the radical religious movements that sprang up during the political upheavals in England in the 1640s.[85] Böhme (1575-1624), a cobbler by trade and largely self-educated, preached an intensely personal understanding of God and an almost boundless tolerance to the rest of humanity. His writing is distinguished by an incantatory, biblically inspired and resolutely anti-intellectual lyricism, and by a passionate and transparently sincere desire to communicate a vision individualistic to the point of incommunicability. The themes that recur above all in his work are dissolution of the individual in spiritual communion with the divine, and an empathy not only with all other human beings but the whole of Creation, all of which he maintained was animated by the same divine spirit. It is in connection with Böhme's works, and with the underground literary contacts of Caspar Warnle, that in 1634 Moriaen makes his first appearance in Hartlib's day-book, the *Ephemerides*. Moriaen had recommended Warnle as 'one that could give a Catalogue of all rare books'. The entry goes on to note that the Hamburg patrician Joachim Morsius was a man through whom all the works of Böhme could be obtained, by means of Moriaen.[86]

Of all the many admirers and disseminators of Böhme active in Germany at the period, this Joachim Morsius was among the most enthusiastic (in every sense of the word). How close Moriaen's relationship with him was at this date it is impossible to say. There is no mention of him in any surviving writings by Moriaen. However, there is one surviving mention of Moriaen by Morsius, and since it occurs in a document of some significance and celebrity, a fairly full account of Morsius is necessary to place it in context.[87]

Morsius (1593-1643) was a scholar of some renown, who devoted a great deal of time and energy to attempting to locate and join the Rosicrucians, after the appearance of their two manifestos in 1614 and 1615.[88] In 1616, when he was briefly University librarian at Rostock, an open letter was published urging the entire theological faculty to join the Fraternity. Morsius's authorship is not proven, but he is certainly a candidate.[89] Another open letter, addressed to the Rosicrucians themselves and applying for admission, from one 'Anastasius Philaretus Cosmopolita' of 'Philadelphia' and including quite a detailed description of the author, is almost certainly by Morsius.[90]

Though he never did receive a reply from the Rosicrucians, Morsius's belief in them and taste for literature that blended mysticism and utopiansm never abated. In later years, he found himself in repeated trouble with the authorities of Lübeck and Hamburg for his persistent dissemination of 'enthusiastic' literature such as Böhme's *Weg zu Christo*, Felgenhauer's *Geheimnis vom Tempel des Herrn* and (in particular) Christoph Andreas Raselius's *Trew-Hertzige Buß Posaune* (s.l., 1632), a vehement and decidedly subversive anti-war tract, which accused the German rulers of all denominations, whether Catholic or Protestant (but especially the latter), of squandering the lives and welfare of their subjects on costly and pointless

17

conflicts stirred up only by their own greed, arrogance and prejudices. Besides distributing such literature, Morsius further offended through his association with various suspect figures including Moriaen's friends Dury and Johann Tanckmar.

As well as attracting unfavourable attention from the ecclesiastical authorities, Morsius also found himself in regular trouble with the secular, at the instigation of his own family. This was due to his refusal to adhere to the terms of the pension inherited from his brother Hans at the latter's death in 1629, which were that he should live an 'orderly' life, adopt a 'godfearing' profession,[91] and take back the wife he had left at some time before 1617, claiming she had insulted him.[92]

Morsius of course completely ignored all these stipulations and persisted in demanding his money. After protracted legal wrangling, he was finally committed to the Hamburg lunatic asylum in 1636, where he remained for four years. Whether he really was, in the modern sense of the term, clinically insane, it is now obviously impossible to determine. But it should be said that the Hamburg authorities were in general distinguished, by the standards of the day, by their tolerance and leniency towards the unorthodox, preferring to admonish or at worst banish troublemakers rather than incarcerate them. The 'letter of protest' ('Protestschrift') Morsius published in his own defence in 1634 is a work of quite exceptional incoherence which to say the least provides scant evidence of mental stability.[93]

He was released from the asylum in 1640 after intervention on his behalf by King Christian of Denmark. Three years later, he wrote, apparently out of the blue, to his erstwhile teacher at Rostock University, Joachim Jungius.[94] Jungius, by this time Rector of the Hamburg Gymnasium and a generally respected though sometimes controversial figure in the scientific and educational establishment, had in 1622 founded a short-lived and decidedly secretive scientific research association in Rostock going by the exotic name of 'Societas Ereunetica vel Zetetica'.[95] This group, like just about any private organisation in Germany at this period, had attracted suspicions of Rosicrucianism, and it was even suggested that Jungius was himself the author of the Rosicrucian manifestos.[96] This was enough to make Morsius assume Jungius took the liveliest interest in such matters, and the letter is given over almost entirely to discussion of the Rosicrucians and other secret societies, and to the literature relating to them that Morsius had in his possession. He was particularly keen to know whether Jungius's friend Tassius had obtained

> the third part of the *Dextera Amoris porrecta [Right Hand of Love Offered]* and of the *Imagen Societatis Evangelicæ [Model of an Evangelical Society]*, that is, the *Golden Themis* of the laws of that society, and the Antilian laws, or other details of this society or its members. [97]

This is typical of Morsius's jumbled thinking. The first two works in question, titles both of which he slightly misquotes, are the *Societatis Christianæ Imago* and *Christiani Amoris Dextera Porrecta* (both Tübingen, 1620) of Johann Valentin Andreæ, a Lutheran preacher and acknowledged influence on Comenius, author of the Utopian novel *Christianopolis* (1619) and a fervent promoter of model Christian societies.[98] These two companion

18

pieces constitute a description of (or a proposal for) a loose association of pious spirits dedicating themselves to Christian learning, mutual moral and practical support and charitable works.[99] The two works were subsequently to take on a life of their own when Hartlib, unbeknownst to Andreæ, had them translated into English by John Hall, and used them to promote his own very different visions of Christian assemblies or 'correspondencies'.[100] The *Themis Aurea* which Morsius took for their 'third part' is a totally unrelated work by the mystic Michael Maier, a nobleman of the Palatinate who was certainly involved in some sort of Rosicrucian society in 1611, though whether this was the same group that produced the famous manifestos is another matter.[101] The 'leges Antilianas'[102] are the statutes of yet another society, 'Antilia', which was operative in Nürnberg in the 1620s. Hartlib was associated with this, and Andreæ was aware of it, though he distinguished clearly and carefully between it and his own projected 'Societas Christiana'. The 'leges Antilianas' have never been identified.[103]

For Morsius, however, all these disparate productions related to the same thing and were in turn traceable back to, or at the very least reminiscent of, the original Rosicrucian summons. He told Jungius, 'I have other [such works], and some by the Rosicrucians, which, if I understand by your response that future letters from me will not be unwelcome, shall be added to the foregoing.'[104] Morsius then proceeded, for no apparent reason, to inform Jungius that fourteen years before writing, in 1629, he had visited Andreæ and obtained twelve copies of the *Imago* and *Dextera*, which he had distributed to assorted leading lights in Germany and Scandinavia. Tenth on the list, amid this illustrious company, is 'Ioannes Morian Patric*ius* Noribergensis, pijssim*us* chemic*us*' ('Johann Moriaen, patrician of Nürnberg, most pious chemist').[105]

Here, Morsius's letter provides the source for an error that has passed into a variety of footnotes, the idea that Moriaen was a Nürnberg patrician rather than a first generation immigrant from a family of Dutch artisans or merchants. Though hardly a point of crucial historical importance, it is nicely illustrative of the reliability, or rather the lack of it, of Morsius's evidence. The letter has, naturally enough, attracted a good deal of attention from historians of Rosicrucianism, for its relevance to the distribution of Rosicrucian literature and the continuing debate about Andreæ's alleged authorship of the original Rosicrucian manifestos.[106] These subjects are not at issue here, but it does seem worth pointing out that Morsius's letter cannot be seen as concrete evidence of anything at all beyond the confusion of the man who wrote it.

A striking feature of Morsius's list of addressees is that, with the exception of the name at its head, Herzog (Duke) August the Younger of Wolfenbüttel, not a single figure on it features in any of the several detailed accounts by Andreæ himself of the history of his project for a Christian Society (in which he specifically named numerous individuals he had tried to interest).[107] Andreæ conducted a lengthy correspondence with Herzog August, which in the early 1640s deals extensively with his plans for this society, plans he was hoping might at this date be revived under August's patronage. In 1642, he sent August a presentation copy of the two tracts, bound together, with the Duke's intials embossed on the leather binding.[108] In his letter of thanks, and in a letter to his own agent Georg Philip

Hainhofer, the Duke mentioned having obtained copies of these works through Hainhofer when they first came out in 1620.[109] There is also a personal memo in August's hand to this effect appended to a letter from Andreæ dealing with the tracts.[110] The Duke had indeed commissioned Morsius to obtain various books and manuscripts for him in 1629-1630 - precisely the years in which Morsius claimed to have distributed the works.[111] This raises the question of why, when the works were the subject of so much of his correspondence and he was specifically trying to recall how he had come by them before, he never once mentioned having received copies from Morsius. In Andreæ's side of the correspondence, which is preserved in its entirety and which returns repeatedly to the history of these manifestos and of the society they set out to publicise, there is not one reference to Morsius. If there were a single piece of independent evidence to corroborate any of the claims Morsius made in this letter, it might be taken a little more seriously, but until any such evidence surfaces, it must be reckoned possible that the whole business took place only in Morsius's fevered imagination.

The letter is, however, very suggestive of the impression Moriaen made on Morsius in the 1620s. Moriaen was already a 'most pious chemist', and he evidently struck Morsius as a man interested in mystic literature and the promotion of non-denominational allegiances. Again, Morsius's impressions are in themselves a long way from constituting objective evidence, but in this instance there is corroboration for them. The same impression is given by Moriaen's own account of his earlier association in Nürnberg with the Reformed preacher Georg Sommer,[112] and their discussions about the reform of learning. Sommer thought Moriaen's plans for theology in particular would never be realised in practice, much as he approved of them in theory.[113] Unfortunately, Moriaen was typically reticent as to what these plans might have been, but Sommer's reaction suggests they struck him as too radical ever to find favour with any established church.

Moreover, it is apparent from Moriaen's letters that he was indeed involved with an 'independent' or 'impartial' society ('unpartheÿliche geselschafft') in Nürnberg.[114] It may have been this that Sommer had in mind when he fondly recalled the 'treasured conversations you [Moriaen] held with me in Nürnberg'.[115] Moriaen's sole surviving reference to this society is very vague and fleeting, but does locate the group in Nürnberg and reveal that one of Jacob Andreæ's sons was a member.[116] Jacob Andreæ was Johann Valentin's grandfather, one of the most famous Lutheran preachers of the sixteenth century, so the son in question was probably one of Johann Valentin's numerous uncles.[117]

This association must have been either in Moriaen's teens, before he went to Heidelberg, or, much more probably, after his return to Nürnberg in about 1627. In the latter case, this may well have been the Nürnberg group 'Antilia' with which Hartlib, at this time preparing to leave Elblag for a new life in England, was also associated, if only by correspondence.[118] Whether or not Antilia was the society he joined, Moriaen was certainly aware of it, as appears from his oddly isolated reference over a decade later to an 'Antilianorum socium' ('member of the Antilians') whose exposé of false alchemists Hartlib had sent him.[119] Moriaen's name, however, is mentioned nowhere else in connection with Antilia or any other such society.

20

The history of Antilia, of Rosicrucianism, and the seventeenth-century German vogue for semi-secret societies of various sorts (a trend so marked that the German language has characteristically come up with a single compound noun for it, *Sozietätsbewegung*), is a fascinating and enormously complicated subject which it would explode the limits of this study to deal with in full. It is evident that Moriaen was at least peripherally associated with the *Sozietätsbewegung*, but the evidence is so sparse, so vague, and in the case of Morsius's letter so utterly unreliable, that no exact account of the nature or extent of his involvement can be given. What is abundantly clear, however, is his urgent desire for a new Reformation, a Reformation that would encompass church, school and state, and that at this stage in his life he saw mystic literature and the organisation of Christian societies as part at least of the means to further it. Later he would look to Comenius's scheme of Pansophy and later still to the practice of natural philosophy, in particular to alchemy, to accomplish this goal, but his guiding vision was always the same: the coming dawn of a new era of enlightenment, unity and Christian brotherhood.

Wanderjahre

Moriaen left Nürnberg in March or April 1633, and by late April was in Frankfurt. Here he put his name to two irenical documents that were circulating at the time.[120] Both originate from Hanau and are addressed to the divines of Great Britain by various churchmen with whom Dury had been engaged in negotiations for some two years, principally Johann Daniel Wildius, the Hanau Inspector, and Haak's uncle Paul Tossanus (Toussaint). One is a distinctly unspecific proposal for reconciliation, barely touching on the points of contention and suggesting somewhat vaguely that communication between the British and German churches would be a good thing. The other proposes the compilation of a complete body of practical divinity acceptable to all parties.[121] In both cases, Moriaen's name is a later addition to an original document, indicating only that he approved of the proposals: there is no suggestion that he had anything to do with composing the letters.

He then set off on a tour of the Netherlands. His own account of this, in a further Latin letter to Dury of 19 November 1633, is exceptionally cryptic, reading in its entirety: 'Belgium peragravi' ('I have been through the Netherlands').[122] The exact purpose of the visit remains unclear, though given the central role of De Geer in the Palatine collection, it is more than likely that maintaining contact with him or his agents was at least one of the goals. On a more personal level, Moriaen also took the opportunity to establish contact with other scholars resident there or visiting. He had evidently been a keen and able student of natural philosophy, and especially of optics, in the course of his career to this date, since he showed enough familiarity with recent developments in this field to make an impression on two leading experts in it, Isaac Beeckman and René Descartes.

Beeckman met him in Dordrecht on 24 August 1633, and made a note of his account of a *perpetuum mobile* which Johann Sibertus Kuffler had tried to sell to Duke Wolfgang-Wilhelm of Neuburg.[123] Kuffler and his younger brother Abraham were members of the extensive Kuffler family Moriaen had known so well as a preacher with the Cologne church. They had been based in England from around 1620, and married two daughters of the (then) celebrated emigré Dutch inventor Cornelijs Drebbel; the *perpetuum mobile* in question was in fact (like a number of 'their' inventions) the work of their father-in-law, or perhaps a modification of it. According to Beeckman's account of Moriaen's report, the Duke was so impressed with Kuffler's model that he had been willing to offer ten thousand Imperials for a full-scale realisation but was dissuaded by his advisors. In the event, however, Kuffler did set up such a machine for him that year,[124] and Moriaen himself in 1640 mentioned the Drebbel/Kuffler *perpetuum mobile* in Pfalz-Neuburg.[125]

In recording Moriaen's account, Beeckman rather implied - as a great many people who mentioned him implied - that he thought him somewhat gullible. Moriaen did not understand how the mechanism worked but thought it had something to do with mercury: Beeckman, however, suspected that Moriaen had fallen for a ruse, the mention of mercury being a red herring used by Kuffler to mislead potential imitators.[126]

Beeckman took a more respectful interest in Moriaen's views on lens-grinding,[127] as did René Descartes, who thought it worth telling his friend Constantin Huygens that

> Some time ago, an honest man of Nürnberg by the name of Mr Moriaen, who was passing this way, told me he had often ground spherical lenses which had proved very good; he also admitted that in doing so he made use of two movements, now applying one part of his model to the glass and now another, which is all very well for spherical lenses, since all parts of a sphere have an equal curvature, but as you know better than I it is not the same for hyperbolic lenses, in which the edges are markedly different from the centre. [128]

This is surely the same encounter Moriaen himself recalled in tellingly different terms when warning the mathematician John Pell, through Hartlib, not to become involved in Descartes' schemes:

> I would assure him [Pell] that he will only waste much time and effort on it in vain. What he [Descartes] is looking for is still uncertain and, besides, only a point of detail. It is demonstrable on paper, but the workman cannot put it into practice, as the event will show them. I have done somewhat in these matters, and I understand the techniques so far as they are known and practised at this time. Five years ago, M. Descartes pressed me very eagerly to lend him a hand with the realisation of his project, but I could see no possibility of it, as they too have found so far in their work.[129]

That each man comes out of his own report sounding rather cleverer than the other is not in itself very surprising: more telling is the difference in the rationales behind this. Whereas Descartes' version has Moriaen 'admitting' that he lacked the skill to grind hyperbolic lenses, Moriaen's has Descartes obstinately persisting with a hypothesis that had not stood up to practical experiment. This was to become something of a refrain in Moriaen's reflections on natural philosophy, placing him firmly in the Hartlibian camp of experimental research. Deeply mistrustful both of 'book learning' as opposed to experiment and of theory divorced from practice, these thinkers interpreted Nature by the twin lights recommended by Bacon, the Book of God's Works and the Book of God's Word. For them, Descartes' resolutely deductive thought, though admirable for breaking with scholasticism, threatened to replace it with as great a vanity, that of shutting oneself up in the labyrinth of fallible human reason.[130]

From the Netherlands, Moriaen returned to Cologne. Here on 6 October 1633, under the auspices of the secret church he had so long served, he was married to Odilia von Zeuel, the sister of his former colleague Peter.[131] Of Odilia, virtually nothing else is known at all. Her presence is barely felt in the correspondence except as someone receiving or sending greetings, or whose ill health interfered with Moriaen's work and curtailed the time he had available for writing (which does at least imply he made some effort to tend her). The tone of his references to her is generally affectionate and solicitous, but no impression is given of her character or the closeness of the marriage.

Mystifyingly, a letter from Moriaen to Dury apparently dated 19 November, though the date has been altered and is ambiguous, refers to the marriage as imminent. Perhaps Moriaen was having one of his frequent bouts of absent-mindedness and meant to write September.[132] In the same letter, he informed Dury that he had 'frustrated, or, rather, freed' himself of his Nürnberg citizenship.[133] Though the letter bears no address, it must have been sent from Cologne.

Given that he had so urgently needed to flee the city six years previously, it is a little surprising that he should then have settled in Cologne for a further two and a half years. However, his involvement with the Reformed Church was henceforth purely as a lay member: there is no further mention of his service in the *Protokolle*. Moriaen's letters from this period supply the earliest surviving evidence of an interest that was to be his consuming passion in later years: Paracelsian chemistry. By the end of 1635 at least, he was producing chemical medicines for sale through Abraham de Bra. Advice and materials were supplied him by Van Assche, who had returned to his original profession as a physician after being dismissed from the church, and was now practising in Amsterdam. It was not, however, a straightforward teacher-pupil relationship, more an exchange between equals: though eager to receive his friend's recommendations, Moriaen was confident enough of his own abilities to query or challenge them in some instances. There is reference too to the authority of Johann Hartmann (1568-1631), who at Marburg in 1609 became the first professor of chemistry (specifically iatrochemistry) in Europe. Whether Moriaen was actually earning his living as a medical practitioner is not clear, but it is obvious that the prospect of financial recompense provided at least some incentive. Physic provides the classic example of a field in which the profit motive and charitable service of one's neighbour could be reconciled. He was working on the 'Elixir proprietatis Paracelsi', and also on medical preparations of juniper berries and bezoar stone, both staples of the Paracelsian tradition, and told Van Assche:

> I have been busy making Bezoar for some time, and a few days ago sent about 1/4lb. to Mr de Bra, that not only our friends but others too might

be [served?] by it [...] were any profit to come from my work, it would
encourage me the more to [delve into?] the secrets of Nature.[134]

This was an interest that remained with him throughout his life, and
several of Hartlib's correspondents referred to him specifically as a medical
practitioner, though there is no evidence that he possessed any medical
qualification, and the title 'Dr' was never applied to him.[135] The available
evidence provides no means of gauging his success as a physician, either
from his own point of view or that of his patients. However, a rather
crestfallen report that the glasses in which he was rectifying some medicine
had burst apart and that he could not understand what he had done wrong
suggests that initially at least it was less than overwhelming.[136]

Odilia Moriaen's two brothers, Adam and Peter, were living with or near
the couple in Cologne. Though there is no mention whatsoever of the von
Zeuels in any account of the scientific literature of the period, it is obvious that
Peter at least was a committed Paracelsian, and in Moriaen's eyes a proficient
one. In 1651, Moriaen cited him as a vital source of information on
alchemical matters with whom he had hoped to collaborate on the 'great work'
(transmutation), a plan frustrated by Peter's death.[137] A visit from him in
1642 was sufficient excuse for a two month lapse in the correspondence, 'we
found so much to do both in our joint affairs and my private ones that I was
able to think of nothing else'.[138] The letter does not specify what these affairs
were that were of such consuming interest, but it is altogether likely that
alchemy featured among them. It is quite conceivable, indeed, that Peter von
Zeuel's alchemical and iatrochemical expertise constituted part of his sister's
attraction.

Adam von Zeuel, despite his new brother-in-law's medical prowess, died
not long before 24 November 1635,[139] and it may be that the Moriaens
benefited financially from this event. This would account for Moriaen's
deciding about a year later to move to Amsterdam and becoming a seemingly
successful financial speculator. It would also explain his later rather odd
remark that he had at some point acquired some farmlands 'with my wife',[140]
which I can only construe as meaning that the lands came along with the wife
through an inheritance or a dowry. Again in 1640 he mentioned his hopes of
improving 'our lands' ('vnseren landguttern') by applying some of the
methods of Hartlib's protegé, the agriculturalist Gabriel Plattes.[141] This
striking and very unusual inclusion of Odilia in a first person plural,
effectively acknowledging her as co-proprietor, strongly suggests the lands
belonged originally to her family. In this case, they would presumably have
been in the region of Cologne, and have suffered badly from the Thirty Years
War: Moriaen mentioned that, like most such lands in these war-torn times,
they yielded very little.[142]

Moriaen had decided to move by January 1637, when he wrote to Van
Assche that they planned to arrive in early or mid-May.[143] He added,
however, that Odilia was pregnant,[144] and that Peter von Zeuel, who had
earlier been suffering from an abdominal disorder[145] and was evidently still in
poor health, could not be abandoned until a wife had been found to take care
of him.[146] These considerations detained the Moriaens in Cologne for over a
year. Their daughter Maria Elisabeth (named after Johann's and Odilia's
mothers in that order) was baptised into the German Reformed Church there

on 13 June 1637.[147] The best part of another year elapsed before a wife was found to tend Peter von Zeuel, who married Gertraud Breyers on 12 March 1638.[148]

It was probably soon after this that the move was finally made. At the date of his first surviving letter to Hartlib, dated Amsterdam, 13 December 1638, Moriaen owed his friend replies to three letters. The excuse he gave for his failure to reply was lack of time due to his wife's and his own recent illnesses and the upheaval of their departure from Cologne. One at least of Hartlib's letters must, then, have been received before that departure, and the earliest of them is mentioned as being dated 13 July 1638. Some three months later, Moriaen wrote that he could not comment on a treatise on magnets until it was sent on to him from Cologne, where he had left it behind: again this powerfully suggests that the move was a relatively recent event, and that Hartlib had been sending him materials to Cologne.[149] Settled at last, Moriaen now embarked on a new career as a businessman and on what was initially at least a rather more stable phase of his life than the fifteen or so years spent in the service of the Reformed Church and its exiled ministers.

Notes

1   The only indication of his date of birth is his mention in a letter to Benjamin Worsley of 2 July 1651 that he was nearly sixty at the time of writing: 'id unum tantum addam me prope sexagenuarium esse' (HP 9/16/10A).

2   The most notable examples are Hamburg and - after it had shaken off Spanish dominion at the turn of the century - the Dutch Netherlands. See Joachim Whaley, *Religious Toleration and Social Change in Hamburg 1529-1819* (Cambridge, London, New York, New Rochelle and Sidney, 1985).

3   See Hans Neidiger, 'Die Entstehung der evangelisch-reformierten Gemeinde in Nürnberg als rechtsgeschichtliches Problem', *Mitteilungen des Vereins für Geschichte der Stadt Nürnberg* XLIII (1952), 225-340. My account of Nürnberg at the time of Moriaen's birth is heavily indebted to Neidiger's fascinating study, which far transcends the bounds of its somewhat dry-sounding self-appointed brief.

4   Kurt Pilz, 'Nürnberg und die Niederlande', *Mitteilungen des Vereins für Geschichte der Stadt Nürnberg* 43 (1952), 1-153, 156.

5   Neidiger, 'Die Entstehung der evangelisch-reformierten Gemeinde in Nürnberg', 258.

6   Ibid., 258-9.

7   The names of Moriaen's parents are to be found in the record of his marriage to Odilia von Zeuel, *Protokolle der hochdeutsch-reformierten Gemeinde zu Köln 1599-1754* II (Cologne, 1990), 476, no. 947.13.

8   There are only two signatures to non-Latin holograph letters spelled 'Morian'. Latin letters have to be considered separately, since it was normal to use the Latin form of a name when writing in that language (Hartlib for instance becoming Hartlibius, and Dury Duræus), but even when writing in Latin Moriaen occasionally used the Dutch form. A significant exception to the general preference for the spelling 'Morian' is provided by Dury, who was brought up in the Netherlands: he used both forms, but marginally preferred the Dutch.

9   Four holograph letters in Dutch (to Justinus Van Assche) date from before his move (UBA N65a-d).

10 Moriaen to Hartlib, 5 April 1640, HP 37/62A, referring to de Bra as 'schwager' (brother-in-law). Though the term could be used more loosely in the seventeenth century than it is now, there also survives a letter to Hartlib of 22 April 1661 from one Isaac de Bra - doubtless Abraham's son - enclosing a (now lost) recommendation 'from my uncle Johann Moriaen' ('meÿnes herrn Ohman Ioh: Moriaen') (HP 27/41/1A).

11 Neidiger, 'Die Entstehung der evangelisch-reformierten Gemeinde in Köln', 270.

12 The evidence for this is, again, the existence of a nephew, Jean Abeel, who, writing from Amsterdam on 10 April 1659, sent Hartlib £3 'van mynnen waerden Oom Iohan Morian' ('from my worthy uncle Johann Moriaen') (HP 27/44/2A).

13 See Ole Peter Grell, *Dutch Calvinists in Early Stuart London: The Dutch Church in Austin Friars 1603-1642* (Leiden, New York, Copenhagen and Cologne, 1989), 257, and J.H. Hessels (ed.), *Ecclesiæ Londino-Batavæ Archivum* (London, 1887-97) III, *passim*. Neither of these can have been the husband, for their marriages are recorded (ibid., 270), but a family connection is altogether likely. There was also another Jan Abeel at Austin Friars at least between 1648 and 1656 (Hessels III, nos. 3013 and 3043).

14 Moriaen to Hartlib, 22 July 1650, HP 37/156A.

15 Moriaen to Hartlib, 23 January 1640, HP 37/53A.

16 G. Toepke, *Die Matrikel der Universität Heidelberg von 1386 bis 1662* (Heidelberg, 1886), II, 254, entry 84.

17 Moriaen to Hartlib, 23 June 1639, HP 37/27B. Georg Vechner matriculated at Heidelberg two months after Moriaen, on 8 July 1611 (*Matrikel der Universität Heidelberg*, II, 254, entry 118).

18 Howard Hotson, *Johann Heinrich Alsted: Encyclopedism, Millennarianism and the Second Reformation in Germany* (PhD thesis, Oxford, 1991), 41 and 82. For a fuller account of Keckermann and his impact, see the second chapter of this thesis, pp.52-90. On Ramus and his impact, see Walter J. Ong, *Ramus, Method and the Decay of Dialogue: From the Art of Discourse to the Art of Reason* (Cambridge, Mass., 1958).

19 Ibid., 82-5. See Chapter Four, sections 1 and 2 for a fuller discussion.

20 See Gerald Lyman Soliday, *A Community in Conflict: Frankfurt Society in the Seventeenth and Early Eighteenth Centuries* (Hanover, New Hampshire, 1974).

21 'Weil die Brüder sich entschlossen den dritten Diener zu berufen, und uns einer mit Namen Johannes Morian vorgeschlagen wird, welcher sich auf die zukünftige Woch wird finden lassen zu (Frankfurt); als sollen die Brüder Wilhelm Engels und Johan Fassing Anordnung tun, daß gemelter Morian in seiner Predigt von den vornehmsten Gliedern der Kirche angehöret werde, damit man abnehmen möge, ob er dieser Gemeinde würde früchtbarlich dienen können.' - *Protokolle* I, 235, no. 750. The *Protokolle* are a fascinating document, but unfortunately are published in a massively modernised and standardised form with what appear to be somewhat *ad hoc* editorial policies: it is never made clear what the bracketing of (Frankfurt) indicates, though I would guess it is editorial expansion, perhaps of 'Ffort', a common abbreviation of the name.

22 *Protokolle* I, 235, no. 752, 25 April 1619.

23 'Vom ersten Schlag, 1566/1568, über berichtete oder nur angedeutete Überfälle auf Predigten [...] ist es bis 1627 eine fortwährende Kette von Verhören, Geldstrafen, Haft und Stadtverweisungen, von Hausdurchsuchungen und Hausverschließungen, worunter die Evangelischen zu leiden haben.' - Rudolf Löhr, 'Zur Geschichte der vier heimlichen Kölner Gemeinden', *Protokolle* IV, 11-33, esp. 16-17 (prepared for

publication by Dieter Kastner: Löhr died before completing his work). See also A. Rosenkranz, *Das Evangelische Rheinland: ein rheinisches Gemeinde- und Pfarrerbuch* I (Düsseldorf, 1956), esp. p.376. Rosenkranz gives the name of the 'third minister' in Cologne from 1619-27 as Johann Moreau, which must be a variant form or a mistranscription of 'Morian'.

24   *Protokolle* I, 243, no. 775. On 29 July 1626, the maximum number was further reduced to one (pp.327-8, no. 1040).

25   *Fama Fraternitatis des löblichen Ordens des Rosenkreutzes* (Cassel, 1614) and *Confessio Fraternitatis oder Bekanntnuß der löblichen Bruderschafft deß hochgeehrten Rosen Creutzes* (1615).

26   Moriaen to Hartlib, 19 Feb./1 March 1658, HP 31/18/7B.

27   Löhr, 'Zur Geschichte der Vier Heimlichen Kölner Gemeinden', *Protokolle* IV, 11-33, 19.

28   'in Ansehung gedachte Witwe seine Mutter sei oder zum wenigsten dafür gehalten werde' - *Protokolle* I, 238-40, nos. 762 and 767 (3 and 31 July 1619).

29   'Wir kommen in Erfahrung, daß Johann Mosten bald nach dem Gebrauch des heiligen Abendmahls sich mit dem Trank überladen und darüber zu Hause gegen seine Hausfrau ungebührlich verhalten, dadurch die Gemeinde Christi geärgert. Soll deswegen bestraft werden von Bruder Jordan und Morian' - *Protokolle* I, 259, no. 838 (16 June 1621).

30   *Protokolle* I, 299, no. 966.

31   'daß er seiner gewesenen Magd nachgangen, hab er allein getan, sie zu versuchen, ob sie fromm wäre oder nicht' - *Protokolle* I, 302, no. 977.

32   *Protokolle* I, 309-10, no. 1000 (7 Aug. 1625).

33   'Matthias Kuiper ob [...] er [...] mit hohem Eid und teuren Worten einsteils Besserung angelobet, andern Teils seine Mängel verneinet, so haben danach die Sachen anderes befunden, daß er dem Saufen, Spielen und Leichtfertigkeit unaufhörlich nachhanget' - *Protokolle* I, 312, no. 1006.

34   *Protokolle* I, 327, no. 1037 (8 July 1626).

35   'Christian Stoffgen wird berüchtigt, daß er in Gegenwart einer Päpstischer Frauen sich ungebührlich verlauten lassen, daß er von D. Lauterbach unfreundlich tractiert wurde, und dabei gesagt, 'so tun unsere Eltesten'. Soll darüber von Bruder Johann und Schütgens angesprochen und nach Befindung gestrafet werden' - *Protokolle* I, 305, no. 988 (6 March 1625).

36   *Protokolle* I, 282, no. 919 (5 July 1623).

37   *Protokolle* I, 335, no. 1056.

38   *Protokolle* I, 242, no. 774 (10 Oct. 1619).

39   *Protokolle* I, 118, no. 286.1.

40   *Protokolle* I, 122, no. 303 (14 June 1606).

41   *Protokolle* I, 118, no. 286.1 (he took over from Jacob Pergens at the end of 1605).

42   He is mentioned several times in Moriaen's correspondence and seems to have been something of an inventor. *Eph 1640* refers to a 'Luterbach Mr Morians cozen' who has designed a folding table; Mersenne in Sept. 1640 told Haak that 'Mr Lauterbach vostre amy' had visited him bringing an unspecified invention of Thomas Harrison (*Correspondance de Mersenne* XI, 415; HP 18/2/24A), and Comenius told Hartlib on 13 Dec. 1656 that Lauterbach had presented him with a copy of his 'brachygraphia' (shorthand) (Blekastad, *Unbekannte Briefe*, 31; HP 7/111/27A). Blekastad suggests the Glogau syndic Johann Lauterbach, but with no other evidence than the name.

43   *Protokolle* II, 275, no. 898, and 332, nos. 1048-9.

44   'zue Cölln einer seii sehr perfect Inn solchen [optischen] Sachen, der hab ainen gesellen Morian genandt' - August von Anhalt to Widemann, 13 Dec. 1626, Niedersächsische Landesbibliothek Hannover, MS iv 341, 861, cit. Inge Keil, 'Technology transfer and scientific specialization: Johann Wiesel, optician of Augsburg, and the Hartlib circle', *SHUR*, 268-278, 272, n.18.

45   As appears from his letter to Hevelius, 9 April 1650, Observatoire de Paris *Corr. Hev.* AC I,2, fol. 215v, ref. Inge Keil, 'Technology transfer and scientific specialization: Johann Wiesel, optician of Augsburg, and the Hartlib Circle', *SHUR*, 268-78, 275.

46   Moriaen to [Worsley?], 4 May 1657, HP 42/2/7B.

47   As Inge Keil suggests, 'Technology transfer and scientific specialization', 272.

48   See Chapter Five, section 2, for a detailed discussion of Moriaen's ideas on this notion, and his reports of experiments to demonstrate it.

49   See *NNBW* I, 187-8; *Journal tenu par Isaac Beeckman* (ed. Cornelijs de Waard) I (The Hague, 1939), 219, n.2 and II (1942), 175-6, n.3; E.G.E. Van Der Wall, *Serrarius*, 39-42 and *passim*.

50   See J. Minton Batten's hagiographical *John Dury, Advocate of Christian Reunion* (Chicago, 1944); Karl Brauer, *Die Unionstätigkeit John Duries unter dem Protektorat Cromwells* (Marburg, 1907); G. Westin, *Negotiations about Church Unity 1628-1634* (Upsala, 1932); George Turnbull, *Hartlib, Dury and Comenius: Gleanings from Hartlib's Papers (HDC)* (Liverpool and London, 1947); Anthony Milton, '"The Unchanged Peacemaker"? John Dury and the politics of irenicism in England 1628-43', *Samuel Hartlib and Universal Reformation*, ed. M. Greengrass, M. Leslie and T. Raylor, (Cambridge, 1994) (*SHUR*), 95-117.

51   See Van Der Wall, *Serrarius*, and 'The Amsterdam Millenarian Petrus Serrarius (1600-1669) and the Anglo-Dutch Circle of Philo-Judaists', *Jewish Christian Relations in the Seventeenth Century: Studies and Documents*, ed. J. Van Den Berg and E.G.E. Van Der Wall (Dordrecht, Boston and London, 1988), 73-94.

52   Jacob Beeckman to Van Assche, 31 March 1624, *Journal tenu par Isaac Beeckman*, ed. Cornelijs de Waard (The Hague, 1939-53) IV, 79-80.

53.   Van Der Wall, *Serrarius*, 40-1.

54   Moriaen to Hartlib, 14 November 1639, HP 37/47B.

55   Van Der Wall, *Serrarius*, 45-50.

56   See Caspar Heinrich Starck, *Lübeckische Kirchen-Geschichte* (Hamburg, 1724), 785-811, partially reproduced in Steiner, *Morsius*, 48-57.

57   'denn Er selbsten Iustinus vmb dieser vrsach willen des ministerij entsezet worden vnd annoch von der Communion abgehalten wird' - Moriaen to Hartlib, 14 Nov. 1639, HP 37/47B.

58   See Pamela R. Barnett, *Theodore Haak, FRS (1605-1690): The First German Translator of* Paradise Lost (The Hague, 1962). The book is a fund of information on the Hartlib circle and gives a vivid impression of their milieu.

59   See Webster, *Great Instauration*, 54, for details.

60   Barnett, *Haak*, 13.

61   'wegen großer gegenwärtiger Not und schrecklichen Zorn Gottes' - *Protokolle* I, 312, no. 1006.

62   'weil es uns allbereit an Personen mangelt, und je länger, je mehr ermangeln wird' - *Protokolle* I, 297, no. 960.

63   *Protokolle* I, 280, no. 913.

64   *Protokolle* I, 328-9, no. 1042.

65 'In Betrachtung der großen Gefahr und Not, die an diesem Ort je länger je mehr zunimmt, wollen sich die sämtlichen Brüder mit Anrufung göttlicher Hilf auf die allerheilsamsten und sichersten Mittel eifrig bedenken, wie wir möchten unsern Gottesdienst besten Fleißes verrichten, und gleichwohl Gefahr wohl vermieden bleibe' - *Protokolle* I, 336, no. 1057.

66 'daß gleichwohl er uns seine Gutwilligkeit, solang es Gelegenheit gibt, wolle wiederfahren lassen' - *Protokolle* I, 334, no. 1055.

67 'Über die Gelegenheit Bruder J haben die sämtlichen Brüder aus Betrachtung hochdringender Not einmütiglich dahin geschlossen, daß, ob wir wohl sehr ungern seines Dienstes entbehren wollten, dennoch ihm auf sein Begehren zu willfahren' - *Protokolle* I, 337, no. 1060.

68 Grell, *Dutch Calvinists*, 186-7; Barnett, *Haak*, 21.

69 Moriaen to Hartlib, 3 October 1641, HP 37/88B. Turnbull, confusing English and German usage of the perfect tense, takes this to mean the five years up to and including 1641 (*HDC*, 355), an error followed by Blekastad (*Comenius*, 328).

70 Hans Neidiger, 'Die Entstehung der evangelisch-reformierten Gemeinda in Nürnberg' (see n. 3 above), 270.

71 Ibid., 271-3. My account of the Nürnberg collection is again heavily indebted to Neidiger's excellent article, esp. pp.269-75.

72 Ibid., 273.

73 Cf. Ole Peter Grell, *Dutch Calvinists in Early Stuart London*, ch. 5 ('The Collections for the Palatinate'), 176-223, Barnett, *Haak*, 21-3, and Hessels III, nos. 2141 and 2244. Haak acted as representative in England for the Lower Palatine refugees.

74 Grell, *Dutch Calvinists*, 206-7 and 223.

75 See Richard van Dülmen, 'Schwärmer und Separatisten in Nürnberg (1618-1648)', *Archiv für Kulturgeschichte* 55 (1973), 107-37, esp. 115. Van Dülmen is overly inclined to take passing mentions in letters as evidence of close and formalised contacts, and consequently gives an impression of more organised and active resistance to orthodoxy than his evidence warrants. The essay is nonetheless a valuable account of unofficial religion in Nürnberg at the period and the (not very effective) measures taken to suppress it.

76 See Van Der Wall, *Serrarius*, 112-14.

77 HP 9/15/1A-B.

78 Van Dülmen, 'Schwärmer und Separatisten in Nürnberg', 132-4, esp. n.96 which quotes extensively from the commission's findings.

79 Moriaen to Dury, 19 Sept. 1633, HP 9/15/3A: 'Nuptias neptis meæ ex sorore, cum Petro Neefio tibi non ignoto celebravi'.

80 Van Dülmen, 'Schwärmer und Separatisten in Nürnberg', 115.

81 Van Dülmen, 'Schwärmer und Separatisten in Nürnberg', 116, n.50, and 119. On J.F. Münster, see Van Der Wall, *Serrarius*, 112-114.

82 See Ernst Georg Wolters, 'Paul Felgenhauers Leben und Wirken', *Jahrbuch der Gesellschaft für Niedersächsische Kirchengeschichte* 54 (1956), 63-84, and 55 (1957), 54-94, esp. part 2, 72-3.

83 Ibid., part 2, p.69.

84 UBA N65a (10 March 1634), a letter principally devoted to alchemy, but which concludes 'als ul den monarchen Speigel oock *per dominum* Serrarium (quem ex me ut salutes rogo) niet tewege brengen can so moet ick dien in de toecomende missie bestellen' ('if you cannot obtain the *Monarchenspiegel* through Mr Serrarius (to

whom please send my regards), I can order it at the next [Frankfurt] Fair'). Van der Wall (100) takes this to mean that Moriaen was trying to obtain the work through Van Assche, but the implication could equally be that Moriaen would try to get it for Van Assche if Serrarius could not.

85   See Margaret Lewis Bailey, *Milton and Jakob Boehme: A Study of German Mysticism in Seventeenth-Century England* (New York, 1964), and Christopher Hill, *The World Turned Upside Down: Radical Ideas during the English Revolution* (London, 1972).

86   *Ephemerides 1634 (Eph 34)*, HP 29/2/12A-B.

87   The principle source on Morsius is Heinrich Schneider, *Joachim Morsius und sein Kreis: zur Geistesgeschichte des Siebzehnten Jahrhunderts* (Lübeck, 1929), which repeats or supersedes everything about him in Rudolf Kayser, 'Joachim Morsius', *MCG* VI (1897), 307-19, and Will-Erich Peuckert, *Die Rosenkreuzer. Zur Geschichte einer Reformation* (Jena, 1928).

88   *Fama Fraternitatis Deß Löblichen Ordens des Rosenkreutzes* and *Confessio Fraternitatis*. Textually, much the best modern edition is provided by Richard van Dülmen in *Quellen und Forschungen zur Württembergischen Kirchengeschichte* Bd. 6 (Stuttgart, 1973), which unlike all its predecessors makes no attempt to modernise or 'correct' the original text. The introduction and notes, however, are perfunctory and often inaccurate. The colossal impact of the Rosicrucian manifestos, and the complex question of their origins and authorship, have been discussed and debated respectively at daunting length ever since the works were first published, and there is still no scholarly consensus in sight. Many later myths have their origin in Gottfried Arnold's wonderfully vivid but not overly reliable *Unpartheyische Kirchen- und Ketzer-Historien* (Schaffhausen, 1740-42) vol. II, book 7, ch. 18, and vol. III, book 4, ch. 25. Will-Erich Peuckert's *Die Rosenkreuzer. Zur Geschichte einer Reformation* (Jena, 1928) is a book rich in useful references and imaginative speculation but very short on reliability: Peuckert has a particularly annoying habit of not distinguishing quotation from narrative, so that what appears to be (modernised) citation of a source sometimes turns out to be his own invention or commentary, and vice versa. Frances Yates, in *The Rosicrucian Enlightenment* (London, 1975), also tends to let her imagination run away with her, and her thesis that the Rosicrucians were formed as part of the support mechanism for Friedrich V of the Palatinate has subsequently been disproved, but the book contains much of interest, and depicts with singular vividness the extraordinary contemporary reaction to the *Fama* and *Confessio*. Probably the soberest account is J.W. Montgomery's chapter on 'Andreæ and the Occult Tradition' in *Cross and Crucible: Johann Valentin Andreæ (1586-1654), Phoenix of the Theologians* (The Hague, 1973) I, 158-255. See also Paul Arnold, *Histoire des Rose-Croix et les origines de la franc' maçonnerie* (Paris, 1955); *Die Erbe des Christian Rosenkreuz: Vorträge gehalten anläßlich des Amsterdamer Symposiums 18-20 November 1986* (no editor named) (Amsterdam, 1986), especially Adam McLean, 'The Impact of the Rosicrucian Manifestos in Britain' (170-179); and Susanna Åkerman, *Queen Christina of Sweden and her Circle: The Transformation of a seventeenth-century philosophical libertine* (Leiden, 1991), especially Chapter Seven, 'Neo-Stoic Pan-Protestants and the Monarchy'. I have not been able to consult Roland Edighoffer, *Rose Croix et société idéale selon Jean Valentin Andreæ* (Paris, 1995), or Susanna Åkerman's forthcoming *Rose Cross over the Baltic*, except for a draft version of Chapter One, for access to which I am much indebted to Dr Åkerman.

89   G.F. Guhrauer, *Joachim Jungius und sein Zeitalter* (Stuttgart and Tübingen, 1850), 67; Schneider, *Morsius*, 30-1.

90   Schneider, *Morsius*, 31-2, including a summary of the letter.

91 The rest of the family were jewellers; Morsius was an itinerant scholar who seems never to have held down any position for long.

92 The lady in question, of whom no more is known than that her maiden name was Telsen, would perhaps have placed a slightly different emphasis on the quaint assertion of Morsius's biographer that 'it seems a likely conjecture that the woman was unable to come to terms with his restless, fantastical nature, which, in its continual yearning quest for the new, never attained to a firm, masculine clarity' ('Die Vermutung liegt nahe, daß die Frau sich nicht in sein unruhiges, phantastisches Wesen zu finden wußte, das immer nach Neuem sehnsüchtig ausschauend nie zu einer festen männlichen Klarheit gelangte') - Schneider, *Morsius*, 64.

93 Morsius, *COPIA Einer kurtzen eylfertigen/ doch Rechtmässiger Ablehnung vnd Protestation [...] in justissimâ causâ Morsiana* ('Philadelphia', 1634).

94 Morsius to Jungius, 26 Aug. 1643, Stadts- und Universitätsbibliothek Hamburg, 98.19-22; transcript in Schneider, *Morsius*, 57-62, following R. Avé-Lallemant, *Des Dr. Joachim Jungius Briefwechsel*, (Lübeck, 1863). An earlier transcript by Guhrauer (*Jungius*, 232-5) contains a great many errors; Avé-Lallemant's is much superior. Quotations here are from the original manuscript.

95 Guhrauer, *Jungius*, 69-71.

96 See Guhrauer, *Jungius*, 56-67, and Peuckert, *Die Rosenkreuzer*, 88-9 and 228-30 on the suggestion of Jungius's involvement with Rosicrucianism. Not even Peuckert, who can generally be relied on to find evidence of Rosicrucian mysticism almost anywhere, takes the idea very seriously.

97 'tertiam partem Dextræ amoris porrectæ & Imaginis Societatis Evangelicæ, Themidem videlicet auream de legibus illius societatis, vnd leges Antilianas [...] oder andre particularia de istâ societate ac socijs' - SUBH 98.19v.

98 The best and fullest account of Andreæ, which contains an extensive bibliography, is J.W. Montgomery's *Cross and Crucible: Johann Valentin Andreæ (1586-1654), Phoenix of the Theologians* (The Hague, 1973); see also Andreæ's *Selbstbiographie*, translated from the Latin manuscript *Vita ab ipso conscripta* by David Christoph Seybold (Winterthur, 1799). On his relations with Comenius, see Comenius, *Opera Didactica Omnia* (Amsterdam, 1657; facsimile reproduction Prague, 1957) I, 283-4, and Ludwig Keller's fanciful extrapolations from this, 'Johann Valentin Andreæ und Comenius', *MCG* I (1893), 229-41.

99 Turnbull discovered copies of the two tracts in question, which were long supposed lost, among the Hartlib papers (HP 25/2/1A-B and 6A-20B, and 55/19/1A-15A), and published them with a valuable introduction in *Zeitschrift für deutsche Philologie* (*ZfdPh*) 73 (1954), 407-32. He followed this with a reprint of Hall's English translation in *ZfdPh* 74 (1955), 151-85. A printed version of the originals was later discovered in the HAB, Wolfenbüttel, by Roland Edighoffer: see his 'Deux écrits de Johann Valentin Andreæ retrouvés ou le nouveau *Neveu de Rameau*', *Etudes Germaniques* (Oct.-Dec. 1975), 466-70.

100 Turnbull, 'John Hall's letters to Samuel Hartlib', *Review of English Studies* New Series IV (1953), 221-33. They were published as *A Modell of a Christian Society* and *The Right Hand of Christian Love Offered*, with a dedication to Hartlib, in 1647.

101 See McLean, 'The Impact of the Rosicrucian Manifestos in Britain' (see n. 88 above).

102 Not, as Guhrauer reads, 'Andilianos', a mistake taken over, with a surprised '(sic!)', by Turnbull ('Johann Valentin Andreæs *Societas Christiana*', *ZfdPh* 73, 410).

103 Cf. Turnbull, 'Johann Valentin Andreæs *Societas Christiana*', 409-10.

104 'habeo alia, & de Rhodostauroticis singularia, si intellexero ex responsorijs vestris, literas meas vobis non ingratas futuras, quæ superioribus addenda erunt' - SUBH 98.21v.

105 SUBH 98.20v. The twelve alleged recipients are enumerated in detail. They are: Herzog August the Younger of Braunschweig-Wolfenbüttel; Prince Moritz of Hessen, the great patron of alchemists; Duke Frederick of Schleswig-Holstein; Prince Ludwig of Anhalt, founder of the literary 'Fruchtbringende Gesellschaft'; Holger Rosenkrantz, the King of Denmark's former privy counsellor; Johann Adler Salvius, a Swedish diplomat; Henricus a Qualen, a Danish noble; Laurens Grammendorf, a leading German lawyer and theologian; Wendelin Sybelist, a spagyrist who had been personal doctor to the Russian Czar; Moriaen; Johann Jakob Pömer, a Nürnberg patrician associated with Antilia, and Georg Brasch, a Lutheran pastor who - ironically enough - represented Lüneburg at the conventicle arranged in 1633 by the churches of Hamburg, Lübeck and Lüneburg to discuss ways of dealing with such enthusiasts as Felgenhauer, Raselius, Tanckmar and Morsius (see Caspar Heinrich Starck, *Lübeckische Kirchen-Geschichte*, 797-8 and 977-80).

106 His authorship is strongly contested by J. Kvacala, *J.V. Andreäs Antheil an Geheimen Gesellschaften* (Jurjew, 1899), which like so much of Kvacala's work stands up as well now as it did a hundred years ago; R. Kienast, *Johann Valentin Andreæ und die vier echten Rosenkreutzer-Schriften* (Leipzig, 1926); J.W. Montgomery, *Cross and Crucible: Johann Valentin Andreæ, Phoenix of the Theologians* (The Hague, 1963). For important supplementary evidence, see Wolf-Dieter Otte, 'Ein Einwand gegen Johann Valentin Andreäs Verfasserschaft der Confessio Fraternitatis R.C.' *Wolfenbüttler Beiträge* 3 (1978), 97-113. For summaries of the evidence presented on either side and full bibliographies of the issue, see Montgomery, op. cit., who comes out against Andreæ's authorship, Frances Yates, *The Rosicrucian Enlightenment* (London, 1972), who suspends judgment, and Susanna Åckerman, *Rose Cross Over the Baltic* (forthcoming), who favours the attribution.

107 In his autobiography, his letters to Herzog August in the Herzog August Bibliothek, Wolfenbüttel, his funeral oration on his friend Wilhelm von der Wense who first proposed the scheme (in *Amicorum singularium clarissimorum Funera*, Lüneburg, 1642), and a letter to Comenius of 16 Sept. 1629 (Comenius, *Opera Didactica Omnia*, Amsterdam, 1657, I, 284). A letter from Andreæ to August of 27 June 1642, HAB 65.1 Extrav. fol. 21r-23v, includes a list (admittedly obviously incomplete) of the 'Pauci, ad quos **Christianj amoris dextera porrecta** pervenit' ('the few whom the *Right Hand of Christian Love* reached': Andreæ's emphasis is very apparent in the original). Though often interpreted as a membership list of the *Societas Christiana*, this is surely only a punning account of which individuals Andreæ was aware had received copies of the work. It is reproduced in *MGP I*, 184, but Kvacala mysteriously transcribes 'Daniel Hizler' as 'Daniel Hikler' and 'Baltas. B. Roggendorffij' as 'Baltas. B. Seckendorffius', errors uncharacteristically taken over by Montgomery (*Cross and Crucible* I, 176). A few members of the society who do not appear on this list are mentioned in the funeral oration on Wense and the autobiography. See Montgomery, (*Cross and Crucible* I, 176) for details.

108 The copy is still held in the Herzog August Bibliothek and is the only known copy of the original edition.

109 August to Andreæ, 26 July 1642, HAB 236.1 Extrav. fol. 30r; August to Hainhofer, 19/29 July 1642, HAB 236.1 Extrav. fol. 12r

110 Andreæ's letter is dated 27 June 1642: HAB 65.1 Extrav. fol. 23v; transcript in *MGP I*, 184.

111 August to Hainhofer, 9 Jan. and 22 May 1630, HAB 149.6 Extrav. fol. 214r and 214v-215r.

112 Sommer was (according to this same letter) a minister in the Upper Palatinate at some date before 1639, by which time he was in church service in Danzig. Dury had contacted him in 1633 via Haak's uncle Paul Tossanus seeking support for his ecumenical projects (HP 5/53/9A-B).

113 Moriaen to Hartlib, 23 June 1639, HP 37/28B.

114 Moriaen to Hartlib, 13 Dec. 1638, HP 37/1B.

115 'lieben discursen so der herr mit mir zue Nurmberg gepflogen' - Sommer to Moriaen, as quoted by the latter in a letter to Hartlib, 23 June 1639, HP 37/28A.

116 HP 37/1B.

117 One of Jacob Andreæ's sons was called Jacob after him, but Moriaen was almost certainly referring to the much more famous preacher.

118 Turnbull, 'John Hall's letters to Hartlib'.

119 Moriaen to Hartlib, 24 March 1639, HP 37/14A.

120 Copies at HP 59/10/53A-60B, 24 Feb. 1633, and 59/10/113A-116B, n.d. Both were signed by Moriaen on 23 April. See *HDC*, 146, n.1, and 153.

121 Published with an English translation in Dury's *The Earnest Breathings of Forreign Protestants* (London, 1658).

122 HP 9/15/3A.

123 De Waard, *Journal tenu par Isaac Beeckman* III (The Hague, 1945), 302.

124 See *NNBW*, II, 736 (which misprints the date as 1663).

125 Moriaen to Hartlib, 23 Jan. 1640, HP 37/54A.

126 He may well have been right, but a contemporary account of Drebbel's device also implies some sort of chemical process at work: Drebbel 'extracted a fierie spirit, out of the minerall matter, joininge the same with his proper aire, which encluded in the Axeltree, being hollow, carrieth the wheeles, making a continual rotation or revolution' (Thomas Tymme, *Dialogue Philosophicall* (London, 1612): summary and extracts in Harris, *The Two Netherlanders*, 152-5). Harris believes the device to have been powered by variations in temperature and air pressure, though how this could have yielded the regularity claimed for the device it is difficult to see.

127 *Journal tenu par Isaac Beeckman* III, 300 (24 Aug. 1633) and 381 (1 July 1634).

128 'Il y a quelque temps qu'un honnête homme de Nüremberg, nommé M. Morian, passant par ici [Utrecht], me dit qu'il avait souvent taillé sur le tour des verres sphériques qui s'étaient trouvés fort bons; mais il m'avoua aussi qu'il s'y servait de deux mouvements, appliquant tantôt une partie de son modele contre le milieu du verre, tantôt une autre; ce qui est bon pour les verres sphériques, à cause que toutes les parties d'un globe sont également courbées, mais, comme vous savez mieux que moi, ce n'est pas la même de l'hyperbole, dont les côtés sont fort différents du milieu' - 8 Dec. 1635, *Correspondence of Descartes and Constantin Huygens*, ed. Leon Roth (Oxford, 1926), 9.

129 'Ich will ihn [Pell] woll versichern das viel zeit vnd muhe nur vergeblich zuebringen [...] wird[.] was Er suchet ist noch vngewiß vnd darzue nur ein particular stuckh. [...] Auß diesem fundament der parabolæ ist es meines erachtens nicht zue practiziern. auff dem pappier kan mans woll demonstrirn aber der artifex kans nicht præstirn, wie sie mit der that woll finden werden. [...] Ich hab in diesen sachen auch etwas gethan vnd verstehe die handarbeit so weit sie dieser zeit vblich vnd bekand ist H des Cartes hatt mich berait vor 5 Iahren sehr eyferig ersucht das Ich ihme die handt bieten vnd sein furhaben ins werckh richten wolte, Ich sehe aber darzue keine müglichkeit, wie sie auch bißher im werckh selber erfahren haben' - Moriaen to Hartlib, 14 November

1639, HP 37/47A. This report of a meeting 'five years ago' ties in plausibly enough with Descartes' 'some time' before December 1635.

130   The response to Descartes in the Hartlib circle was by no means uniformly negative, and his mathematical gifts in particular were generally recognised and admired. But the approach I have outlined was the prevalent one, the more so as time went on. Comenius in particular, after some initial interest, became increasingly hostile to Descartes, whose approach he thought likely to lead to atheism. He wrote a refutation of Descartes and Copernicus which was destroyed in the siege of Leszno (*Comenius*, 549) and a satirical pamphlet *Cartesius cum sua naturali philosophia a mechanicis eversus* (*Descartes and his natural philosophy overthrown by craftsmen*) (1659: *Comenius*, 593, and see also pp.640-641).

131   *Protokolle* II, 476, no. 947.13.

132   HP 9/15/3A-B. The date is given, bewilderingly, as 'Ao 1633 Ad 16 19 9b; both '1633' and '16' have been altered, and '19' could debatably be read as '29'. Dury has noted on the back 'Sc*ripsit* 19. 9bris (written 19 November)'.

133   HP 9/15/3A: 'Noribergâ solvi civitatis Iure me frustravi aut liberavi potius'.

134   'so hebbe ene tyt lang met t'Bezoardicum maeken besig geweest, en hebbe voor enige daegen aen Monsieur de Bra ontrent _lb daerof gesonden, om niet alleen de vrienden maer oock andere daermede te [*illeg.*] [...] dat oock een wat profyt van mynen arbeyt quaem dat soude mij incourageren om de Naturæ wonders t'[*illeg.*]' - Moriaen to Van Assche, 6 September 1636, UBA N65c.

135   For instance Appelius to Hartlib, 12 June 1644, mentioning 'H Morian, vnd andere Medici' ('Herr Moriaen and other physicians') (HP 55/1/8A), Rand to Hartlib, 10 Jan. 1653, HP 62/17/4A, and Hübner[?] to ?, 30 July 1655, HP 63/14/31B.

136   Moriaen to Van Assche, 17 January 1637, UBA N65d.

137   Moriaen to Worsley, 9 June 1651, HP 9/16/7A. A fuller account of Moriaen's alchemical project and von Zeuel's putative involvement is given below, p. 227.

138   'haben wir so woll in vnseren gemeinen als meinen priuatsachen so viel zue thun gefund*en* das Ich auff nichts anderß gedenkh*en* können' - Moriaen to Hartlib, 2 August 1640, HP 37/66A.

139   Moriaen's letter of that date to Van Assche, UBA N65b.

140   'ich mit meiner haußfr. dz mehrertheil an landgutern bekom*m*en habe' - Moriaen to ?, 21 July 1639, HP 37/35A.

141   Moriaen to Hartlib, 2 August 1640, HP 37/66B.

142   Moriaen to ?, 21 July 1639, HP 37/35A.

143   Moriaen to Van Assche, 17 Jan. 1637, UBA N65d: 'maeken wy rekenninge tegen t'beginsel of $\frac{1}{2}$ Mey te geliggen God geue tot syns naems eer genadige uytcoomste'.

144   Ibid. 'het heeft God belieft myn beminde huysvrouw met de hote van lyfsvrücht te segenen'.

145   Moriaen to Van Assche, 24 Nov. 1635, UBA N65b, with the news that 'het onsen God ook belieft heeft onsen Broeder Adam van Zeuel uyt dese werelt te nehmen ende onsen noch resterenden Broeder Pet. v Z. met de beginseln van malo Eupochondriaco te gesoeken daeraen hy nu over 3 weken te bedde ligt'.

146   Moriaen to Van Assche, 17 Jan. 1637, UBA N65d: 'so lang Monsr: van Zeu: niet getrouwt is so haeken hem niet te verlaeten'.

147   *Protokolle* II, 511, no. 989.9. There were no less than five witnesses: Abraham de Bra's wife (so Moriaen's sister if this is not a different Abraham de Bra), standing in for Elisabeth de Famars, Maria Mitz, Magdalena Bergens (ie. Pergens), Maria Hildebier (standing in for the Lauterbachs), and Odilia's brother Peter.

148   *Protokolle* II, 480, no. 952.2.
149   Moriaen to Hartlib, 24 March 1639, HP 37/13B. This was probably John Pell's manuscript 'meditationes de causâ diminutionis magneticæ', a copy of which he sent to Mersenne on 24 Jan. 1640, mentioning that he had earlier sent the original to Hartlib (*Correspondance de Mersenne* IX, 59). Moriaen did not say in so many words that he had had the piece from Hartlib, but this is the obvious implication.

CHAPTER TWO

Servant of God

'[Moriaen] is taxed for nothing so much as with *the* general fault of all honest men too much charity or overmuch credulity' - Hartlib to John Winthrop, 16 March 1660, HP 7/7/3A.

In A Free Country

Moriaen had mixed feelings about his new home, the United Provinces. He was certainly not unduly proud of his Dutch parentage. Though there were many individuals of that nationality among his closest friends, notably Justinus Van Assche, Louis de Geer and the Collegiant Adam Boreel, his remarks on the nation as a whole suggest he thought them a vain people, jealous of their academic and cultural reputation and stinting of their money, adept at capitalising financially and intellectually on other people's talents and ideas, but loth to give credit where it was due. He advised against bringing Comenius to the Netherlands on the grounds that he would meet with envy if not outright slander from the country's own scholars:

> These lands are greedy for fame and love the renown of their learned people and useful inventions. Though there are many among them who love and seek only the art [of advancing knowledge], yet are there not a few who consider it demeaning that a foreigner should know more than they and invent something new.[1]

G.J. Vossius in particular, he went on (Professor of History at the Athenæum Illustre), had dismissed Comenius as unlearned: a half-learned Dutchman could do more, and Vossius himself twice as much if he cared to.[2] He considered that John Pell (an Englishman) was shabbily treated as Mathematics Professor at the Athenæum, and warned that Christian Rave (a German) would meet with the same fate if he accepted an invitation to Amsterdam: 'once they have people [here] they pay them no attention; were they prepared to work for nothing, or indeed to pay for the privilege, they would be men fit for this city'.[3]

On the other hand, he warmly approved the liberty of conscience and lack of censorship which so distinguished the Dutch Netherlands, and especially the capital, rejoicing that 'we are in a free country here' ('man ist hier in einem freÿen land').[4] This was the country in which both the deposed Calvinist Elector Palatine and the deposed Catholic Queen of England took refuge, where Collegiants and Anabaptists were tolerated and where the largest Jewish community in Europe was free to practise its faith in public. Deploring the censorship imposed on Joachim Jungius by the Hamburg school authorities and on Comenius by his own church, Moriaen repeatedly contrasted the situation in the Dutch Netherlands: 'here one is free to believe and to write whatever one can or will'.[5]

He settled in Amsterdam as a man of some means, and a number of incidental comments suggest that his principal investment was in the fishing industry. He remarked so phlegmatically on the seizure of three ships in which he had an interest - one at least of which was a fishing vessel - by Dunkirk privateers in 1640 and 1642 that it seems fairly safe to assume he had considerable other assets besides.[6] Though he in fact referred to the ships as 'his', it is extremely unlikely that he owned them outright: normal practice was for a syndicate to raise funds for trading expeditions, especially in the high-risk fishing industry, and to divide the profit (or loss) accordingly.[7] Two weeks after the second incident he asked for Hartlib's help in the recovery of yet another ship, also taken by privateers and sold by them in England, in which he stood to inherit a one-sixteenth share (whether from the Moriaens or the von Zeuels is not clear).[8]

A further indication that things were going well for him financially during the early years in Amsterdam is his remark in March 1639 that he was now in a position to devote himself exclusively to raising funds for Comenius and his collaborators).[9] He was no more specific than this, but the obvious implication is that he was no longer burdened with earning a living. Possibly he had inherited some money; possibly he had been successful (or lucky) in his business ventures. It was certainly possible for investors to rise from fairly modest means to quite spectacular wealth in the market economy of the mid-seventeenth century Netherlands. On 15 August 1643 he bought 2600 guilders (about £260) worth of shares in the Dutch West India Company. He finally cashed them in, having fallen on hard times, in 1658.[10] This is no vast sum, but probably represents only a portion of his total investments.

Maria Elisabeth Moriaen, the daughter born in 1637, died of an unspecified illness at the age of just over two. She was, according to Moriaen's stoical report of the event, the couple's only child.[11] Not one extant letter makes any reference to subsequent offspring, and the concern Moriaen expressed after narrowly surviving a serious illness in 1657 as to what would become of his wife should he die strongly suggests he left no heirs.[12] One of the very few extant letters addressed to him, from 1651, concludes with greetings to his wife and friends but makes no mention of any other family.[13]

Besides his business activities, Moriaen had three main occupations during his early years in Amsterdam. First and foremost, he became Hartlib's principal agent in the Netherlands for the drive to raise financial support for and interest in the Moravian thinker Comenius and his educational reform programme. This will be discussed in detail in Chapter Four. His other principal concerns were the printing industry and the conversion of the Jews.

Writers from all over Europe looked to Amsterdam to publish works that would be banned in their native countries. Moriaen promptly associated himself with the leading printers in Amsterdam, Willem Jansz Blaeu, Johann Jansson and Lodewijk Elsevier. As has been mentioned, he was also friendly with the Frankfurt printer Matthias Merian the Elder, and he was quick to make the acquaintance of another German, Hans Fabel, when the latter set up a press in Amsterdam in 1646. Moriaen was particularly impressed with Fabel, who specialised in works of a mystical and alchemical nature, such as Franckenberg, Tschesch, Böhme, Raselius and above all Felgenhauer[14] - all very reminiscent of the type of literature Moriaen had been discussing with Dury and Van Assche, and obtaining from Morsius, during his stay in Nürnberg. In 1648, Fabel also printed a work by Hartlib's brother, *Georgii Hartlibii Exulis Diarium Christianum*,[15] though this (rather surprisingly) is unmentioned anywhere in Moriaen's surviving correspondence. Through these various contacts, and no doubt also through old acquaintances in Frankfurt who could keep him advised of what was on show at the city's annual book fair, he became one of Hartlib's principal informants on what was being published in Germany and the Netherlands, and a major supplier of continental literature. The names of Böhme and Felgenhauer recur once again in the commissions sent him by Hartlib and Haak, as does that of the similarly unorthodox spagyrist and prophet Sophronius Kozack.[16]

He also commissioned a number of publications on Hartlib's and Dury's behalf and oversaw their printing. Costs were lower in Amsterdam than in England, and there was less likelihood of interference from the censors, though the problem still remained of having the works brought into England after they had been printed. Most of the works commissioned were intended to publicise Comenius's pansophic work or Dury's irenic projects. Hardly any of the pieces mentioned have been preserved, which suggests they were brief pamphlets issued in cheap editions for widespread and possibly free distribution by the intelligencers in England.

It was Moriaen who commissioned the 1639 Elzevier edition of Comenius's *Prodromus Pansophiæ*, and he consulted with Hartlib about any alterations to be made in the new 1640 edition of the *Janua Linguarum*.[17] There is repeated mention of a planned Amsterdam edition of the English mathematician William Oughtred's *Clavis Mathematica*, though this seems never to have appeared, probably because of Oughtred's failure to send over his revisions and additions.[18]

In many instances, it is impossible to tell whether proposed printings in fact took place. This is the case with Hübner's *Idea Politica*, which Moriaen was keen to print but the author apparently deemed unworthy of publication,[19] and with Dury's *Analysis Demonstrativa*.[20] Other works that certainly did go to press under Moriaen's auspices include a *Paranesin* ('Exhortation') by Dury, which Moriaen also spoke of having translated (probably into German or Dutch, possibly Latin). This may well be the same work as *An Exhortation for the Worke of Education Intended by Mr Comenius*, published through Moriaen along with *The Duties of Such as Wish for the Advancement of True Religion*, an *Answer to the Lutherans*, and an unspecified 'dissertatio didactica', all by Dury.[21] Of all these works, the only one now known to survive in printed form is the *Duties*, a later edition of which is noted in Wing's *Short Title Catalogue*.[22] A number of other works were also entrusted to Moriaen, but their titles are not recorded. Indeed, Moriaen considered Hartlib's passion for publishing somewhat excessive: 'I cannot see, indeed, what purpose is served by so many pieces directed to the same purpose'.[23] However, he did as he was asked, and 1640 in particular saw a steady flow of tracts from the Amsterdam presses sent across by Moriaen into London.

One large batch of works, evidently by Dury and including the above-mentioned *Duties* and *Exhortation*, was impounded by the English authorities acting under instructions from the Church. Dury at this time, as Anthony Milton puts it, had 'both sides [Anglican and Puritan] scrutinizing him for lack of zeal', and was extremely uneasy about receiving politically sensitive material, such as an anti-Laudian petition of March 1640, by post from Hartlib.[24] Suspicion had been aroused in the case of the pamphlets by another piece of carelessness on Moriaen's part: the works had been bound under the wrong titles.[25] Moriaen's letters suggest that this was indeed a genuine error rather than a deliberate piece of camouflage. It is of course possible that the letters were themselves adapted to take account of the possibility they too might be intercepted, but the remarks about the unchristian and untimely zeal of the impounders hardly sound calculated to reassure official eavesdroppers.[26] In any case, it is understandable that the authorities should have wondered what was being brought into the country under an apparent disguise. Moriaen's indignant declaration that a title is neither here nor there, and that this was a typical piece of petty-minded interference on the part of the tiresome bishops, is less than reasonable:

> so the child has been wrongly christened, is that so terrible? No one is done any harm by it. I can scarcely imagine that the bishops will meet with the applause of any sensible politician for their untimely zeal (so far as the contents are concerned).[27]

In due course, the works were indeed found to be innocuous and were released, but not until Hartlib had been put to a deal of trouble to negotiate this outcome. Dury, who was in Hamburg at the time, sent a rather ingratiating letter about the affair to Philip Warwick, the Bishop of London's secretary, thanking him for ordering their release. The whole point of this, as he told Hartlib, was 'to Cleere my self of all suspicions which might fall upon me'.[28] In the letter to Warwick, Dury castigated Moriaen (without naming him) for his inefficiency, and rather implausibly denied that Dury himself knew anything at all about the printing and shipping of his works:

> although the harmelesse matter contained in them so farre as my conceptions were unaltered, needeth no Apologie; yet the fashion of their habit, the place whence they came, the company which came with them, et the forme of theire conveiance being somewhat suspicious in these doubtfull times, et I being ignorant et innocent of all this, who neverthelesse hadd might a been[29] a sufferer thereby in the judgment of superiours: therefore your courtesie deserveth thancks et due acknowledgment from having freed me from the appearance of guilt which the irregular proceeding of imprudent, though well meaning persons, was like to bring upon me.[30]

This did not prevent Dury from employing Moriaen two years later to print his now lost *Answer to the Lutherans*, and in the case of this work there can be no doubt whatsoever that publication occurred at his own request, since he repeatedly mentioned the fact himself and complained about the delays in bringing the work out - delays for which Moriaen apparently blamed the dilatoriness of the printer (which printer this was is nowhere specified).[31] When it finally appeared in October 1642, it turned out that Moriaen had botched the job again. Dury was thoroughly disappointed and annoyed:

> Mr Moriaen hath caused the Epistolicall Dissertation to bee printed, but

so incorrectly *that* it is a shame to see it: & without any preface; so *that* I
shall be taken for the putter of it forth, by euery one *that* seeth it; I would
rather it hadde not at all beene putte to the presse, then so abused.[32]

Having blamed the delays on the printer, Moriaen now rather lamely blamed
the errors on a scribe, who had presumably been employed to produce a more
legible version of the manuscript for the benefit of the printer and typesetters
(who would probably not have understood English). Moriaen had checked
the edition not against the original but the transcription.[33] After 1642, Hartlib
and Dury looked elsewhere to have their productions brought to light by
agents whose skill and efficiency were better answerable to their zeal.

Moriaen and the Jews

Moriaen also cultivated contacts with Amsterdam's substantial Jewish
community. The exceptional tolerance with which Jews were treated in the
Dutch Netherlands, being allowed to maintain synagogues openly and to
associate freely with any Christians who cared to let them do so, made the
capital a focal point for Christian-Jewish contacts. Moriaen took full
advantage of this fact, as did his friends Van Assche and Serrarius, who had
both moved to Amsterdam ahead of him. As Dury later remarked with regard
to the activities of the Hebraist Christian Rave in promoting such dialogue,

> I conceiue *that* Amsterdam where there is a Synagogue of Iewes, & a
> Constant waye of Correspondencie towards the orientall parts of the world;
> & where there are some alreddie in a public waye intending the promotion
> of those studies; will bee a place more fit for his abode then any in
> england, except somethinge extraordinarie were done by those of London
> for the aduancement of vniuersall Learning.[34]

How far Moriaen's scholarly interest in Judaism extended is not at all
clear. He mentioned having lent the Hebraist J.H. Bisterfeld his concordance
of Hebrew, and spoke of plans for Bisterfeld to teach him his 'method of
investigating the true meaning of Hebrew roots' ('methodum inquirendi veram
radicum Hebr*aicarum* significationem'),[35] which argues at least an interest in
studying the language, but gives no firm evidence as to how far he had
progressed. There is also an intriguing reference to someone Moriaen called
'my Hebrew' ('Mein Hebræus'), possibly a convert, with whom he had been
discussing religion, and who had drawn his attention to a passage in a Jewish
text about the sufferings of the Messiah for the sins of the whole human race
('de passionibus Messiæ pro peccatis totius generis humanj').[36] This delight
in finding supposed prefigurations of Christianity in the parent religion is very
much like Serrarius's response to the highly unorthodox opinion of Rabbi
Nathan Shapira that the Messiah had been revealed in Jesus among others:

> When I heard these things, my bowels were inwardly stirred within me and
> it seemed to me that I did not hear a Jew, but a Christian, and a Christian
> of no mean understanding, who did relish the things of the Spirit and was
> admitted to the inward mysteries of our religion.[37]

Serrarius was one of the foremost promoters, on the Christian side, of communication between the two camps. He came to believe that the Jewish expectation of a coming Messiah and the Christian expectation of Christ's return were simply two sides of the same coin, and that though the Jews had failed to recognise their Saviour on his first visit, they would not make the same mistake again. This synthesis of Christian Millenarianism and Jewish Messianism was an area where a number of less orthodox figures from either faith found common doctrinal ground. Serrarius eventually became so involved with Messianism that he went half-way to accepting the self-proclaimed Jewish Messiah Sabatai Sevi, who launched his mission in 1665, though Serrarius saw him only as a precursor of the true Second Coming, a sort of latterday John the Baptist. Even Sevi's subsequent public conversion to Islam was seen by Serrarius as a part of the providential scheme and failed to shake his faith.[38]

While there is nothing in Moriaen's letters to suggest that his sympathy for Judaism went nearly so far as this, he was certainly interested in the Jews and concerned like Serrarius 'to gain them through kindness',[39] by presenting them with the human face of Christianity. He was particularly keen to see a Hebrew version of Comenius's *Janua Linguarum* brought out, for as will be discussed he saw Comenius's educational and philosophic method as a far more effective means toward the reconciliation of different faiths than doctrinal dispute. He and Van Assche were even involved in a charitable collection for the Amsterdam Jews in 1643 - a most remarkable activity for a respectable Amsterdam merchant to be engaged in at this period. Popkin describes the fund raising efforts in 1657 by Dury, Serrarius and other Millenarians for the visiting Rabbi Nathan Shapira of Jerusalem on behalf of Palestinian Jews as 'the first known case of a Christian venture of this kind for Jews',[40] but this collection for the Amsterdam Jews preceded it by fourteen years. Whether Moriaen and Van Assche had a hand in organising it or merely contributed is uncertain: the only record of the business is a mention in a letter from Moriaen to his friend, stating that some of the Jews had become suspicious about the way the money was being distributed.[41] Moriaen asked Van Assche to send a detailed account of how much he had given and exactly to whom, so that any doubts could be cleared up, at least so far as his part in the matter went.

For many Christians, a major impetus to such endeavours was the belief that the conversion of the Jews was prophesied in the Bible. The key text here was Romans 11, especially verses 23, 26 and 27:

> And they [the Jews] also, if they abide not still in unbelief, shall be graffed in: for God is able to graff them in again. [...]
> And so all Israel shall be saved: as it is written, There shall come out of Sion the Deliverer, and shall turn away ungodliness from Jacob [ie. Israel]:
> For this is my covenant unto them, when I shall take away their sins.

Paul's somewhat ambivalent thinking on this point, moving as it does from the conditional possibility of Jewish redemption to confident prediction of it, in fact allows of a number of interpretations. To a doctrinally uncommitted reader, it looks very much like an unresolved struggle on the author's part to reconcile his sense of his own Jewish origins with his commitment to the new faith. The chapter begins: 'Hath God cast away his people? God forbid. For I also am an Israelite'. Paul sought to resolve this conflict by deciding that the rest of his nation was destined to follow him in his conversion. For his Christian readers in the seventeenth century, however, the passage of course represented not Paul's private difficulties but a divine prophecy. To the Millenarians looking to the fulfilment of all Biblical prophecy in the near future, conversion of the Jews thus became a major desideratum. So did the completion of the Jewish diaspora, for it was believed that the scattering of the Jews to all corners of the earth was also destined to precede the Millennium. This was another point on which Millenarians and Messianists found common ground, and is why both the circle around Menasseh ben Israel and that around Hartlib were so excited by the reports that began to come out in 1650 that the native Americans were of Hebrew descent.[42] (No comment by Moriaen on this notion survives.) Menasseh made this a keynote of his bid to have the Jews readmitted to England. The diaspora was already much further advanced than anyone had realised: England and Spain were practically the only places left without a Jewish population (or at least without an officially recognised one). The Christian Millenarians added to this a providential role for England not only in the completion of the diaspora but also in the conversion of the Jews.

One of the reasons the Jews rejected Christianity, it was argued, was that even where they were not actively persecuted or oppressed by its adherents, they saw it practised in such corrupt and absurd forms that there was little incentive for them to study it more closely or seriously. Once the Jews saw the true faith being practised in truly godly fashion, as it was in England, they would be far more likely to take it seriously.[43] In the Reformed Dutch Netherlands, for instance, while there had not been quite such a spate of conversions as might have been hoped for, there were a number of Jews - such as Menasseh, Jehudah Leon and Moriaen's anonymous 'Hebrew' - who were at least willing to consider the arguments and look at the evidence.

The promotion of Jewish-Christian dialogue, particularly at an intellectual and academic level, was a favourite project of Hartlib and especially of Dury. They petitioned Parliament in 1649 for £1000 to set up, as part of a new University of London,[44] a College of Jewish Studies (to be attended exclusively by Christian scholars), with a view to increasing Christian knowledge and awareness of Jewish language, culture, customs and beliefs, the better to be able to enter into a dialogue with the Jews and to explain to them that Christianity, far from being a rejection of their faith, was its culmination.[45] They were in regular contact with Menasseh (who despite his failure to see the light was proposed as one of the professors) about plans for this college and for the readmission of the Jews to England, and Moriaen was frequently used as an intermediary in these exchanges.[46] It was through Moriaen that one hundred copies of Menasseh's *Spes Israelis* were sent to England in 1650, though in his only surviving mention of this he lamented that they had failed to arrive. Moriaen could no longer remember by which shipper he had sent them, but Menasseh had offered to send another hundred to replace them.[47] What became of the lost copies, however, is not revealed. Clearly Moriaen was in close contact with this leading figure in the promotion of Judaeo-Christian dialogue. Regrettably, and rather surprisingly, this is the only mention of him in Moriaen's surviving correspondence, beyond two very fleeting references earlier in 1650 to letters forwarded by Moriaen from Dury to Menasseh, and to Christian Rave's purchase of Menasseh's Hebrew press.[48] Presumably he sent most of his news of Menasseh to Dury and trusted him to pass any relevant information on to Hartlib. On 29 April 1654, Dury wrote to Hartlib from Amsterdam that Menasseh 'intends to come ouer to sollicit a freedome for his nation to liue in England [...] if he come hee will make his addresse to you by Mr Moriaens direction'.[49]

Moriaen also became involved with all the Christian figures who loomed largest in the plans for the College of Jewish Studies. Johann Stephan Rittangel (1606-52) had lived a long time among Jewish communities in Eastern Europe and, it was said, at some time shared their faith. Dury even stated that 'in *Asia* and some part of *Europe* [he] hath been above twenty years conversant with them, and a doctor in their Synagogues'.[50] Moriaen too, some time before meeting him, heard from Bisterfeld of a learned 'Rabbi Rittungal',[51] which looks very much like a slightly skewed form of his name. The German biographer J.C. Adelung, in his notice on Rittangel, claims the story that he was born or converted to Judaism is unfounded, that he himself always denied it and that 'not even his enemies ever accused him of such a thing'.[52] But Dury, Bisterfeld and Moriaen were by no means his enemies, and were under this impression well before 1652, when (according to Adelung) the 'accusation' was first made (by the Königsberg Consistory). The possibility remains, of course, that Bisterfeld, Dury and Moriaen were mistaken; on the other hand, if the story was true, it would not be surprising that in 1652 Rittangel found it expedient to deny the fact.

He was Professor of Oriental Languages at Königsberg in the 1640s, and in 1641 set off on a visit to Amsterdam to supervise the publication of his manuscripts. However, the ship he was travelling on was attacked by privateers, and his manuscripts and many personal effects lost. Furthermore, in the wake of the attack, the ship put in at England, presumably having been left in no condition to continue its journey, and Rittangel found himself unexpectedly in London. Here he was eagerly taken up by Hartlib and Dury. This was precisely the moment when they thought their grand design for religious reconciliation and educational and scientific reform was on the point of bearing fruit in England. Comenius had at last been persuaded to join them in London, and the newly-convened Parliament was looking favourably on their plans.[53] The sudden and unlooked-for appearance of a brilliant Hebraist seemed nothing short of providential. They set about promoting him as a reconciler of Jews and Christians and an indispensible source of information on the former.[54]

Rittangel, however, appears to have been less impressed by his new friends and benefactors then they, at least initially, were by him. He left England in November 1641 and proceeded with his original plan to go to Amsterdam, where Moriaen took him under his wing. In the letters relating to Rittangel, the high ideals of Jewish-Christian reconciliation and the propagation of knowledge are repeatedly interrupted by references to the incongruously mundane detail of Rittangel's bed, which had for some reason been left behind in London and which Hartlib was supposed to forward. Rittangel became thoroughly despondent about his missing bed, and according to Moriaen came to the conclusion 'that by not forwarding his effects you [Hartlib] are trying to hold him up, here as there'.[55] A likely explanation of this remark is that the ever-optimistic Hartlib had been holding out to Rittangel glowing prospects of Parliamentary sponsorship for his work, and that the failure of any such sponsorship to materialise led the Hebraist to think Hartlib was merely dallying with him. Certainly Moriaen was still hoping there might be some support forthcoming for Rittangel from the English Parliament, in return perhaps for the dedication of his work, some months after his departure from England.[56]

Rittangel was a particular authority on the Caraite, or Caraean, Jews, among whom he had apparently lived. The Caraites were a sect who rejected the Talmud (ie. the post-Biblical Jewish oral tradition), a stance in which some Protestant commentators saw a parallel with their own rejection of the Scripturally unsanctioned 'innovations' of Rome. By the same token, Caraites were often seen as prime targets for conversion to 'true' Christianity: as Hartlib wrote to Worthington, they were 'such as begin to look towards their engraffing again'.[57] Hartlib's papers include a sympathetic account of them by Rittangel, in which he stressed their favourable disposition to Christian teaching and their respect for New Testament figures, and claimed (somewhat implausibly, since the sect did not come into being until the eighth century AD), that according to their own literature, their schism with the Pharisees first arose because the Caraites tried to protect Christ from them.[58]

Rittangel's principal occupation in Amsterdam was the preparation of an edition of the Cabbalistic *Sefer Yezirah*, or 'Book of Creation',[59] which explained a method of mystic contemplation based on the ten *sefirot*, or primordial numbers, and the twenty-two Hebrew letters. A Hebrew manuscript of this was obtained, probably through Moriaen, from the merchant and Hebrew scholar Gerebrand Anslo, who had studied under Menasseh ben Israel. First, Rittangel had to transcribe the entire work so that he could return the precious original to its owner, and then he set about translating it into Latin and annotating it. Moriaen followed his work on the project closely and reported to Hartlib on his progress. Interestingly enough, he saw the work not only as a means of increasing Christian awareness of Jewish traditions and beliefs, but as containing important religious truths in its own right:

> I am firmly assured that such Rabbinical secrets, particularly those concerning the doctrine of the Trinity, have never before been brought to light, and I likewise have no doubt that it will be possible to use his work as usefully against the anti-Trinitarians as against the Jews.[60]

It was evidently his view that, since the Christian faith was implicit in the Jewish, or at least in the pre-Christian form of the Jewish, a true exposition of Jewish texts could only serve to demonstrate the truths of the daughter faith. The *Yezirah* was in fact written at some time between the second and sixth centuries AD, but was believed to be contemporaneous with the patriarch Abraham, if not actually to have been set down by him. It was Moriaen who arranged for publication of Rittangel's translation, through his old friend Johann Jansson, in 1642.[61] Rittangel also considered undertaking a translation of another Cabbalistic work, the *Ticcunei Zoar*, though he seems never to have got round to this.[62]

During the eight months or so Rittangel spent in Amsterdam, Moriaen found him lodgings, raised money for him (he specifically mentioned supplying fifty Imperials, though whether from another collection or out of his own pocket is not clear), and did his best to keep his spirits up. This last undertaking seems to have been a lost cause. To be fair, Rittangel had had more than his share of bad luck, and moreover was missing his wife and young child, left behind in Königsberg. But Moriaen soon came to find him insufferably melancholic and thoroughly tiresome, as he repeatedly complained both to Hartlib and Van Assche.[63] It has to be said that Rittangel's report on the Caraites, mentioned above, does not say much for his sense of proportion or his humility. He claimed that the Caraites had advised the King of Poland that if he wished to know more about them, he could do no better than to read Rittangel's work, and that Rittangel himself, after acting as interpreter, so impressed the King and his confessors that

> I was often obliged to dine with them, and to hear it said, in the presence
> of persons of high rank, 'This is the only man for Oriental languages, his
> like is not to be found in all Europe![64]

After Rittangel's return to Königsberg in mid-1642, his association with the circle fizzled out in mutual disappointment. Looking back on the business some five years later, Moriaen observed of Rittangel, 'he is so bizarre that there is little or nothing to be done with him'.[65] Nonetheless, he continued to do his best for the man and to promote his studies, distributing copies of the *Yezirah* through Van Assche and Dury (and no doubt other contacts besides),[66] but without undue success: in 1657, he had to send fifty unsold copies back to the author (and, furthermore, payment for another fifty he had never seen, 'in order to have peace from him').[67] As he put it in a typical little burst of homely philosophy, 'merely for the sake of the sweet honey, one must sometimes patiently endure the stinging of the bees'.[68]

Moriaen had higher hopes of the young Hebraist Georg Gentius (1618-87), another protegé of the same Anslo who lent Rittangel his copy of the *Yezirah*. Anslo, however, imposed on his patronage the condition that he be made sole dedicatee of any of Gentius's work, thus cutting him off from any other possible source of income.[69] Both Gentius and Moriaen considered this an entirely unreasonable attitude, saying more about Anslo's regard for himself than about his concern for the common good. Through Hartlib, Moriaen tried to arrange a secret patronage deal with James Ussher, Bishop of Armagh and Primate of all Ireland. Ussher, however, turned out not to be interested. Gentius, who was planning a visit to the Middle East in the service of the Turkish Ambassador to the Netherlands, was also seen as a possible means of contact with the Caraites, despite Rittangel's characteristic warning that no one else would be able to win their trust in the way that he had.[70] There was even talk of Rittangel's joining him to provide an introduction, but again nothing came of this. On his return from Constantinople after a visit of no less than eight years, Gentius pursued a career as diplomat and interpreter in the service of Johann Georg of Saxony, with no further involvement in such schemes.

By at least 1647, Moriaen had become acquainted with another Hebraist, the Dutch patrician Adam Boreel, who he suggested might be better suited than Rittangel to provide the bridge of learning and correspondency that would span the gulf of mutual ignorance separating the two religions.[71] The only problem was that he was expensive.

In fact, Boreel was already known to the circle. A letter from Dury to Hartlib of 31 August 1646 contains extensive details about him, which have been summarised by Popkin in his study of Christian-Jewish contacts in Amsterdam.[72] Boreel, according to Dury, had supported the Amsterdam Rabbi Jacob Jehuda Leon while the latter produced an exact scale model of the Temple of Solomon according to the specifications in Ezra, a model which subsequently brought Leon considerable fame (and profit) and provided a popular attraction as he took to going on tour with it and charging fees for viewings. Its fame was such that Leon became known by the pseudonym 'Templo'. Boreel learned Portuguese in order to be able to communicate with Leon, who did not speak Latin, and elicited his help in producing a punctuated and annotated edition of the *Mishna*, or Jewish Oral Law, which was published not under Boreel's (or Leon's) name, but that of Joseph ben Israel, with a preface by his brother Menasseh, 'because if it should bee put forth under the name, or by the Industrie of any Christian, it would not bee of Credit amongst them [the Jews]'.[73] It was Boreel's intention to produce similar versions of other sacred Jewish texts, and also Latin translations for the benefit of Christian scholars, and Spanish ones for the benefit of European Jews who did not know Latin or Hebrew. Boreel had also, apparently, produced a treatise

> to demonstrat the Divinitie of the Histories of the New testament by all the Arguments by w*h*ich they [the Jews] beleeue the old testament to be deliuered by God unto their nation.[74]

This was precisely the sort of labour Dury and Hartlib hoped their College of Jewish Studies might promote: Dury was most anxious to see state funding provided 'that this man & such as are qualified in this kind might bee sent for & employed in these workes wherunto God hath eminently fitted them'. For

> no doubt the tyme doth draw near of their Calling; & these preparatifs are cleer presages of the purpose of God in this worke for when hee doth beginne to fitte meanes for the discouerie of their errors <&> for the Manifestation of the Truth of Christianitie [...] it is a cleer token *that* hee intends to take the vaile from of their faces.[75]

This letter of Dury's provides an excellent example of the essentially colonialist attitude adopted towards the Jews by those Christians who are frequently termed 'philo-Semites'. This expression is semantic nonsense on at least two counts. Firstly, their attention was directed not at Semites in general but at Jews in particular. The absurd use of the word 'Semite' to mean 'Jew' can only stem from an uneasy sense that the word 'Jew' is a term of abuse, and, paradoxically, can only enhance the potential for the word 'Jew' to be used as such.[76] This objection is avoided by the term 'philo-Judaism', which has less to be said against it. But although it is true that genuine friendships between Jews and Christians did occur, and there were a number of Christian scholars with a real interest in and extensive knowledge of Jewish culture, the motive force on the Christian side behind such interests and such friendships was almost invariably the desire to convert. Unless love (the Greek *phileein*, whence the prefix *philo-*) is understood as the desire to annihilate the individuality of the beloved, it does not provide a very good account of the type of relationship envisaged by the 'philo-Judaists'.

The purpose of Boreel's work on the *Mishna*, as Dury described it, was

> that the Common sort of Iewes might know what the Constitutions of their Religion is, & also that the Learned sort of Christians upon the same discouerie might bee able to know how to deale with them for their Conuiction.[77]

So far as the Christians were concerned, Jewish-Christian relations were a strictly one-way traffic, the Jews constituting the object of attention and the Christians being the people who did all the studying, all the proselytising and all the persuading. The Jews were viewed as raw material that the Christians might mould into their own image.

The proprietorial tone so noticeable in Moriaen's mention of 'my Hebrew' is still more marked in Dury's letter on Boreel. Leon is referred to as 'his Iewe' and 'The Iewe which hee made use of'.[78] My point in stressing this is not to condemn Dury, Moriaen and their ilk for an attitude that to them would have seemed self-evidently right and to call for no justification; it is rather to urge that that attitude be recognised for what it was, intellectual colonialism, and not mistaken for an early form of liberalism or humanism.

Technology Exchanges

In the late 1640s, Moriaen's financial situation was deteriorating. In letters to both Van Assche and Hartlib he bemoaned the declining value of his West India Company shares.[79] By the end of 1647, he was complaining bitterly about the expense of receiving so many letters, and especially about the exorbitant charges levied on those from England: he was spending as much on correspondence, he claimed, as on household necessaries.[80] In February 1648 he was pursuing his various debtors, and particularly asking Hartlib's help in persuading Christian Rave, who was then in England, to settle up with him.

The precise cause of this collapse is not altogether clear. Moriaen himself repeatedly put it down to his excessive Christian charity: 'I have indeed, as my friends maintain, if judged by outward appearances and worldly wisdom, acted according to the proverb and "used myself up in serving others"'.[81] This is not mere specious self-justification. Moriaen genuinely was given to loaning large sums without security, and he did lose by it. Comenius benefited for several years from an interest-free loan of 100 Imperials.[82] Moriaen's friend Budæus died owing him 1000 guilders (about £100).[83] His support for Rittangel, despite his personal antipathy to the man, has already been mentioned. 1644 saw him prepared to loan an unnamed friend 'another 2000 thalers'. He complained that 'this was very difficult for me, but not wishing to abandon him I had resolved to help him', [84] though on this occasion a brother-in-law (probably de Bra) relieved him of this burden. In early 1647 he was supporting a son of his friend Matthias Merian, who was apprenticed to an Amsterdam engraver, and wrote with obvious embarrassment that this was proving something of a financial strain on him.[85] Christian Rave owed him something in the region of 300 guilders.[86] Visited by the somewhat shady English inventor William Wheeler[87] in 1650, Moriaen went so far as to borrow £13 himself in order that he might lend it to Wheeler: a fortnight's loan was agreed on, but six months later he had still not seen his money.[88]

This all adds up to evidence that Moriaen was not merely indulging in pious rhetoric in his frequently repeated assertion that it is more blessed to give than to receive. However, it was also at this period that he became deeply involved in an assortment of expensive alchemical projects, together with the German natural philosophers J.R. Glauber, J.S. Kuffler and Antony Grill, the English Benjamin Worsley and (possibly) the American George Starkey. While these undertakings, which will be considered in detail in Chapter Seven, were probably not the initial cause of his financial decline, they certainly set the seal on it. Things took an abrupt turn for the worse in 1650, when he declared himself virtually ruined:

> faced with such unbearable damage and loss, I must seriously consider and diligently busy myself with the question of how to set my affairs in order before I die, and thus retain and redeem my good name, which next to my good conscience is my greatest treasure on earth.[89]

It may well have been this reversal of fortune that moved Moriaen to set himself up at just this time as an informal agent for technologists and inventors, finding many of his customers through Hartlib. He presumably received a commission for his pains, and this may have helped him keep his head above water.

Moriaen's various contacts with the scientific communities of Germany and the Netherlands, cultivated at least since his days in Cologne, made him a valuable source of news and personal introductions, promoting the very considerable input from mainland Europe to English science and technology. Especially under the Commonwealth and Protectorate, England seemed a promising location for the professional freelance inventor. The new regime was eager to promote technological advance, and showed every sign of being favourably disposed to Hartlib's schemes for State-sponsored promotion of such inventors and projectors.

In the event, the assorted and ultimately fatal teething troubles of the new Republic meant that these worthy intentions were seldom translated into practical measures and hard cash, but Hartlib was not to be daunted. After repeated disappointments during the reign of Oliver Cromwell, he saw new hope in his son and successor Richard. Eleven days after the former's death, he wrote to Boyle that 'I suppose, that his Highness, that now is, will perhaps more favour designs of such a nature, than his deceased father, otherwise of very glorious memory'.[90] Boyle apparently shared the view: Hartlib a little later declared himself 'wondrous glad, that you have written of the present protector's intentions for countenancing and advancing of universal useful learning in due time'.[91] Hartlib's unquenchable optimism, as relayed by friends such as Moriaen, did much to enhance the apparent prospects and to encourage the influx of foreign scientists and inventors.

The first German inventor to use Moriaen as an agent was the optician Johann Wiesel (c.1583-1662).[92] A Protestant from the Palatinate, Wiesel had moved to Augsburg by 1621, where he gained citizenship by marrying the daughter of a local craftsman, and founded what was possibly the first optical workshop in Germany to specialise in the production of telescopes and microscopes. As early as 1625, he was noted for the production of burning-mirrors, lenses and other instruments. He was 'probably the first optician in Europe to make use of a third lens - the field lens - in his microscopes to give a greater field of vision'.[93] After the Swedish occupation of Augsburg in 1632, he produced optical instruments for the Swedish King Gustavus Adolfus; by 1650 his clients included Maximilian of Bavaria and the University of Paris.[94] It may have been through Hartlib's and Moriaen's mutual friend the mathematician John Pell, who in the late 1640s was eagerly investigating developments in optics on the Continent, that Moriaen first learned of Wiesel.[95]

Through friends such as Johann Hevelius and Constantijn Huygens, but above all through Hartlib, Moriaen helped spread Wiesel's fame around northern Europe and across the water to England. It was through him that Wiesel's telescopes and microscopes first reached these shores. His customers included the astronomer Hevelius and the cartographer Joan Blaeu on the mainland, and Robert Boyle, Benjamin Worsley and one Mr Sotherby in England.[96] He also sent news of Wiesel's newly-invented binoculars and ophthalmoscope,[97] the latter being an instrument which represented a major advance in the investigation and treatment of defects of the eye.

Moriaen must have been very useful to both Wiesel and his clients as a middle man and a trustworthy agent by way of whom the valuable and fragile instruments could be conveyed, and payment for them settled. However, as with his printing commissions from Dury, and despite his own previous experience as an optical instrument maker, he evinced a certain tendency to bungle. A telescope for Worsley reached Moriaen with one of its lenses loose, so he glued it into place with lime. This piece of well-meant interference spoiled the telescope, as the lens had to be removable in order to be kept clean. It was supposed to be kept in place by an adjustable screw. Moreover, Wiesel surmised, Moriaen had not fixed the lens into the right place. Whether Worsley managed to mend the instrument himself according to Wiesel's directions or had to send it all the way back to Augsburg to be fixed (as Wiesel offered) is not clear.[98]

The publicity material Wiesel sent through Moriaen strikingly reflects the popular attitude to microscopes and telescopes, which were recognised by relatively few for their enormous potential to expand the scope of scientific enquiry, but much more widely sought after as 'curiosities' or sources of entertainment. Boyle was regarded as exceptional in that he 'cares not for optical niceties but as they are subordinate to Natural Philosophy'.[99] Describing his microscope, for instance, Wiesel remarked not on its potential utility for medicine and science but its sensation value: 'it makes a flea as big as a tortoise; whoever sees such a thing through this little instrument cannot but be truly horrified'.[100] The sort of games that could be played are suggested by Wiesel's directions for viewing a small picture at a distance through his daytime telescope in such a way as to make it appear life-size, 'which it is an extraordinary pleasure to behold'.[101] However, when the client in question (possibly Worsley) tried to set up this party piece, it failed. Wiesel concluded that this was because he had specified the relevant measurements in Augsburg ells, and that English ells were different. Apparently frivolous pastimes such as these played their role alongside weightier pieces of international scientific cooperation in bringing about the standardisation of weights and measures. Wiesel, ever the pragmatist, sent over a piece of string to indicate the precise distance required.

Wiesel's telescopes and microscopes enjoyed a very high reputation in England when they began to arrive at mid-century. In time they were surpassed by native products, but as Inge Keil shows, Wiesel was imitated before he was superseded, and (as Hartlib reported to Hevelius) it was precisely the desire to outdo the German that stimulated the great English opticians such as Richard Reeve to their finest efforts.[102]

Friedrich Clodius, a Paracelsian iatrochemist who had at some point lived as a guest in Moriaen's house,[103] moved to England in 1652 with a letter of recommendation from Moriaen,[104] though he had been known to Hartlib (probably through Moriaen) at least since the previous year.[105] He at first gave the impression of living up to his personal and professional credentials so well that he gained not only the confidence of Hartlib and friends such as Boyle, but also the hand of Hartlib's daughter Mary, probably in late summer 1653. Boyle wrote fulsomely to him in congratulation: though Clodius had earlier declared he would never marry, being wedded to his chemical calling,

> I cannot conclude you less a servant to philosophy, by choosing a mistress in his [Hartlib's] family; and I cannot but look upon it as an act of his grand design to oblige this nation, that he hath found this way to detain you among us.[106]

He installed himself in his father-in-law's house and converted the back kitchen into a laboratory which he used as the headquarters of his 'Chemical Council'. This was an association headed by Clodius and Kenelm Digby, with which Boyle was also involved, devoted to the production of chemical medicines and the quest for the great iatrochemical arcana, elixir, alcahest, lapis and ludus.[107] Though (as will be seen) the addition of Clodius to the family subsequently proved to be a very mixed blessing, he was certainly an important figure in the scientific community of England in the 1650s and 60s.

It was Moriaen too who recommended the multi-talented inventor J.S. Kuffler and the chemists Remeus Franck, Peter Stahl and (probably) Albert Otto Faber, all of whom settled in England between 1654 and 1661.[108] Hartlib obviously passed on Moriaen's recommendation of Stahl to Boyle, whose protegé Stahl became. He shared Boyle's house in Oxford for a time, and later gave private chemistry lessons there.[109]

Remeus Franck or Franken was an apothecary who had lived at some point with Moriaen and moved to England in 1654, where he was given lodgings in Hartlib's household. His *Nottwendige Anmerckung vnd Betrachtung Allen Gelehrten vnd wohlerfahrnen Männern/ welche die CHIRURGIAM Handhaben/ erhalten vnd derselben sich gebrauchen* (Amsterdam, 1653),[110] appeared in William Rand's English translation as 'A short and easie Method of Surgery, for the curing of all fresh Wounds or other Hurts' in Hartlib's *Chymical, Medicinal, and Chyrurgical Addresses* of 1655. It describes five 'chirurgical balsams', which, the English version concludes, 'are to be bought of *Remeus Franck*, who is to be found at Mr *Hartlib's* house, neer Charing-cross, over against Angel Court'.[111] The content of the balsams is, of course, not specified, but the treatments Franck offered probably were a genuine advance on contemporary surgical practice, especially as applied to the poor, if only in that he stressed the importance of hygiene and advised against amputation except as a last resort. In a chilling evocation of the current state of surgery, Franck suggested that 'Governours and Magistrates' should recommend his balsams to their hospitals, not only out of charity but also because

> it would prove likewise very beneficial and profitable unto themselves, when the maimed persons shall depart the sooner from the Hospitals, and the cries of the distressed shall not so long vex their ears, by reason that many violent and offensive practices of Chyrurgery, in such cases usual, shall by this Method be avoided.[112]

It would seem that Franck had previously been employed by Moriaen as a laboratory assistant, and was passed on by him to Clodius - or, possibly, he had worked for Clodius at the time the latter lived with Moriaen, and went on to join him in England. It is in any case quite clear both from Moriaen's letters and Hartlib's that he was acting under orders. Moriaen told Hartlib that he would 'send you Remeus at once, with the chirurgical balsams'[113] (that he referred to the man by his first name is in itself very suggestive of Franck's subordinate position). A few days later, Hartlib told Boyle that Clodius 'hath written for an expert ancient old laborant, which hath lived with Mr. *Morian*, who is like to be here very shortly'.[114] Hardly anything is known of Franck's activities in England beyond this publication and the attempted marketing of the balsams, but it would seem that this did not meet with a resounding success. Six years later, in 1660, Franck had obviously moved on (or died), and Hartlib told Winthrop,

> Of the Medicinall and chyrurgicall Balsams, I could never obtain the communication [of the recipe, presumably]. But some many potts and glasses full were left at my house; but no creature comming to ask for them, they were sent back into the place from whence they came.[115]

At some point between the end of April and 16 October 1654 Moriaen moved to Arnhem,[116] where he took up residence on the estate of Hulkestein as a guest of the Kuffler brothers, who had a dye works there.[117] A possible reason for Moriaen's being invited is that in 1654 J.S. Kuffler planned to return to England as (he thought) a guest of Parliament, to demonstrate various inventions including his torpedo, or 'dreadfull Engine for *the* speedy & effectuall destroying of shipping in a Moment', and to discuss terms should his secrets be deemed worth purchasing. This information is preserved in a petition to Richard Cromwell giving a history of Kuffler's attempts to sell his inventions to England and the various assurances he had received, which he hoped Cromwell would honour.[118]

The *Calendar of State Papers* makes no mention of any such invitation issued at this period, but it hardly seems likely Kuffler made the whole story up later merely to impress Richard Cromwell, who after all was singularly well placed to verify the claims. Was Kuffler perhaps misled, just as Comenius and perhaps Rittangel earlier had been,[119] by over-enthusiastic private assurances from Hartlib or his friends in Parliament that the State was well-disposed to Kuffler's project and keen for him to visit? This must remain a conjecture, as there is no firm evidence that Hartlib was in contact with Kuffler as early as May 1653.[120] According to the petition, Hartlib had 'from time to time Corresponded with yr Pet*itioner* for applying his said Invention [the torpedo] to *the* use of *the* State of England', but there is no indication of when such correspondence began. Hartlib had, however, taken an enthusiastic interest in Kuffler's inventions since at least 1635,[121] and was certainly his main promoter in England from late 1654 onwards.

If the time spans cited in Kuffler's account are at all accurate, he must have set out for England in early or mid-1654. He had received the invitation, he claimed, shortly after May 1653, and had initially intended to set sail at once, but was prevented by a 'sicknesse w*h*ich continued vpon his family for neare 12 months together'. Mid-1654 is just the end of the period during which Moriaen is known to have remained in Amsterdam. It seems likely that Moriaen, as an experienced chemist and long-standing friend of the family, was invited to become a partner in the business and to supervise the dye-works during J.S. Kuffler's absence, either on his own or together with Kuffler's brother Abraham.[122] This would have enabled Moriaen to realise some much-needed cash by selling his house in Amsterdam while still keeping a roof over his head.

Kuffler did not, however, reach England in 1654, for

> being come neare to *the* Lands end [he] by a suddaine Tempest was driven back into *the* Low-Countries, where hee continued vpward of a yeare, hee being informed by some frinds of *the* change of *the* Government in England about *that* time, wh*i*ch made it not soe convenient a season [...] to make his application in.[123]

There is an anomaly here, in that the 'change of government', i.e. the announcement of the Protectorate, occurred in December 1653, and it is hardly conceivable Kuffler did not hear of it until the middle of the following year. A rather likelier if not very edifying reason for this being 'not soe convenient a season' to sell arms in is that the first Anglo-Dutch War had come to an end in April 1654.

Kuffler returned to Arnhem, where a correspondent from Cleves (possibly Hübner) met both him and Moriaen in July 1655.[124] All the surviving extracts from Moriaen's letters of that year represent part of a campaign to arouse interest in England in Kuffler's inventions and to guarantee him a market should he decide to undertake the crossing again. Ideally, he hoped to interest the State itself in the person of Oliver Cromwell, and Moriaen specifically asked Hartlib to approach the Protector with these proposals.[125] Several of the letters exist in two or more versions representing different stages of Hartlib's editing, showing how he adapted a personal letter into a formal petition, mainly by dint of excising personal details (including Kuffler's name) from Moriaen's reports.

The torpedo was not, initially, the main item on offer, or at any rate not the one Moriaen was keenest to promote. The principal subject of Moriaen's publicity was Kuffler's portable ovens, in one of which, it was claimed, 2000 pounds of bread could be baked in a single day.[126] These were designed primarily for armies to take with them on campaigns, and could also be used on board ship. Moriaen also promoted a device of Kuffler's for purifying water by distillation, an operation of obvious use to a maritime nation such as England. Neither Moriaen nor Kuffler had any qualms about explaining that Kuffler had originally designed his ovens towards the end of his earlier stay in England and had intended to offer them to Charles I, but that his project had been cut short by the outbreak of the 'troubles' in 1642. As in almost every mention of them in Hartlib's papers, the 'troubles' are referred to with politic caution almost as if they had been a natural disaster which all concerned had simply weathered as best they could, having played no part at all in either their origin or outcome.

Hartlib applied himself with his customary vigour to making Kuffler's inventions known both to Cromwell and to friends such as Worsley who had influence with the managers of the State economy.[127] There was, however, dispiritingly little response. Moriaen's letters reveal a mounting frustration, and considerable tetchiness with Worsley when he expressed doubts about the viability of the water-purifier.[128] He was even more annoyed when his erstwhile protegé, Hartlib's son-in-law Clodius, turned against his old benefactor by responding to the publicity about the ovens in a decidedly luke-warm, if not positively disparaging fashion, maintaining somewhat unsubtly that he could do a great deal better himself:

> Now, Sir, I am assured that my invention is of a higher order than Herr Kuffler's, and I know very well how to prove my point without spending 1000 guilders. I do not know how it comes about that I have the good fortune to understand pyrotechnics rather well. Without wishing to boast, I do not believe that there is a man in Europe who has a digesting oven that can burn longer and on fewer coals than mine.[129]

But for all his own prowess, Clodius declared himself keen to receive further details of Kuffler's method. He did not consider that he should have to pay for this, as his intention, he claimed, was to improve on the design, for Kuffler's own benefit. If Clodius was such an expert on ovens, retorted Moriaen bluntly, then why did he not present his own products to the public instead of merely passing judgment on other peoples'? Moriaen may well have had a gullible side to his character, but in this instance he did not fail to draw the obvious inference; nor did he balk at telling Clodius precisely what he thought of such behaviour: 'should I take for myself [the fruits of] another man's sweat and labour? Far be it from me'.[130]

This was precisely the attitude that so bedevilled Hartlib's attempts to institute mechanisms for the dissemination of knowledge. For people to be willing to communicate their discoveries, they had to be guaranteed a just recompense for their labour and ingenuity, yet such guarantees became impossible as soon as the knowledge was in the public domain. The security provided by a patent, assuming one could be obtained, was largely theoretical, and Kuffler remarked through Moriaen that he could see little point in taking the necessary trouble, especially not when a product was being pitched at the State as a whole rather than at private individuals.[131] Very few patents were issued under the Protectorate anyway, thanks to a backlash against the notion of monopolies.[132] Moreover, patent law was in many respects antithetical to the Hartlibian ideal of the free dissemination of learning and inventions in the interest of the common good.[133] The problem remained, however, of securing the rewards for ingenuity that both justice and expediency demanded. Moriaen's ideal (if rather naive) solution would seem to have been self-regulation by an honest and God-fearing populace, and to see that ideal being undermined by his own protegé must have been a bitter pill to swallow.

The first mention of Kuffler's torpedo occurs in July 1655, some months after Moriaen had begun promoting the ovens. This was probably (like many of the Kufflers' projects) a development of an invention originally made by Drebbel, whose torpedo designed for Charles I had been used with some success at the siege of La Rochelle in 1626-8.[134] Moriaen had grave qualms about recommending a project explicitly designed to inflict death and destruction, but tried to reassure himself that its deterrent value would make it an instrument of peace rather than war, even managing to find Scriptural authority for the view:

> And I look on the matter in this light, that it will rather serve to prevent bloodletting than to spill blood. For as Scripture itself reminds us, no one goes so thoughtlessly into battle, but that he first considers his own and his enemy's might, and whether he may prevail against it. If not, he sends to him from afar and sues for peace.[135]

In the event, it was the torpedo that aroused most interest from the English authorities, and Moriaen's continuing unease about the invention reveals that he had not succeeded in convincing himself on this point.

Eventually, Kuffler set out again in the first half of 1656,[136] despite not having received the assurances he had hoped for that the journey would be made worth his while, and was joined in the summer by his family (this time definitely including Abraham, who died in London the following year).[137]

On arriving in England, Kuffler was at once, like almost all the technologists recommended by Moriaen who crossed to this country, given hospitality, encouragement and practical assistance by Hartlib and his friends. Hartlib arranged a loan of £100 from his friend the Puritan educationalist Ezerell Tonge, while Hartlib at the same time committed himself in a legal document to

> produce in writing & deliver vnto the said Mr. Tonge, such Testimonialls concerning Dr. Küffeler his abilities [...&] concerning the reality & certaintie of the Experiments [...] as shall vnto wise & indiferent men be of satisfaction.[138]

It was no doubt to fulfill this requirement that about three weeks later Moriaen sent over a fulsome testimonial for Kuffler, which Hartlib had translated into English.[139] The idea was evidently that Hartlib's petitioning on Kuffler's behalf could be expected to yield such results as would make Tonge's £100 a safe investment. Hartlib further promised that he would diligently attend & sollicite his Highnesse [Cromwell], *the* Councill, *the* Secretary of Estate, & such other Persons, & use such other meanes, *that* may most probably bringe the said Experiments to their desired effect, for the benefitt of this Commonwealth.[140]

Tonge for his part was at the time a prime mover in schemes for a new college at Durham, which it was hoped would become a third university, and which was to promote the Hartlibian ethos of 'useful knowledge', with a strong emphasis on such subjects as husbandry, medicine and chemistry, at once spreading learning and true religion to the remoter provinces, and breaking the stranglehold of the traditional academics at Oxford and Cambridge on the nation's intellectual life.[141] When the college obtained its charter, with Oliver Cromwell's blessing, in 1657, the senior appointments consisted almost exclusively of Hartlib's associates and protegés. Tonge featured as a schoolmaster and fellow, and Kuffler as a professor, presumably of medicine and/or chemistry.[142] However, he never occupied his chair, apparently preferring to pursue the promotion of his various inventions. Events proved him wise, since after the Protector's death, Richard Cromwell (for all the hopes invested by Hartlib and Boyle in him as a patron of learning) bowed meekly to pressure from the established universities and declined to grant Durham equal status. After a promising start, the new college faded quickly into oblivion.[143]

Hartlib introduced Kuffler to Cromwell around the beginning of 1657, but beyond Kuffler's being 'received in friendly fashion' ('freundlich empfangen') by the Protector,[144] nothing seems to have come of the meeting. At some point that year he also set up a maltings (for whatever else Kuffler may have been, he was certainly resourceful), but again without any apparent success.[145] Not until 13 May 1658, some two years after his arrival, was he finally given an opportunity to demonstrate his torpedo. Moriaen, Hartlib, Boyle and Brereton all waited in mildly horrified anticipation to see what the outcome would be; Brereton at least was present at the display, which took place at Woolwich. Moriaen, as Hartlib told Boyle, hoped that Kuffler 'may not blow up a good conscience to get riches by such means'.[146] The demonstration, in the event, was a failure, a fact Moriaen attributed to divine disapproval: 'it may be, then, that God is not pleased with this undertaking and therefore prevents its success'.[147] Boyle apparently shared these misgivings, for Moriaen added a few weeks later, 'I am of one mind with Mr Boyle, and should rather recommend and wish well to any undertaking but this'.[148] Kuffler would never have become engaged in such an enterprise, he repeatedly stressed, if not driven by financial extremity. Hartlib, indeed, seems to have been rather keener than most of his correspondents to see this warlike device promoted, so long at least as it was to remain in the hands of the godly nation he had made his home.[149]

A second demonstration, however, which took place at Deptford on 4 August 1658, was by all accounts a spectacular success. According to an anonymous German report in Hartlib's papers, the torpedo immediately blew a breach of over nine yards in the ship it was aimed at, sinking it instantly. The writer described it as a 'splendid arcanum for the destruction of humankind', claiming it could also be used on land to annihilate entire regiments at a stroke, and that 'it seems to have been granted the English by a wondrous providence'.[150] A few days later, Hartlib mentioned to Boyle that 'Dr Kuffler was with me on Monday, telling in what words you had congratulated the success of his terrible destroying invention'.[151] Moriaen's earlier remarks would seem to suggest that these words were not entirely approbatory.

According to Kuffler's later petition to Richard Cromwell, the Protector was so impressed with this devastating device, which as Hartlib put it would 'enable any one Nation that should bee first Master of it, to give the Laws to other Nations at Sea',[152] that he offered the truly magnificent sum of ten thousand pounds for it, £5000 for the proof and a further £5000 for a full revelation.[153] Cromwell having died the following month, however, the matter had been left in abeyance, and the purpose of Kuffler's petition was to claim the £5000 he was owed and renew the offer of full disclosure for a further £5000. This contrasts rather dramatically with the remark made twice by Moriaen that he had been offered £1000 for a demonstration and a further £1000 for a full revelation, Moriaen's opinion being that he should settle for the one thousand and consign the horrible secret to oblivion.[154]

Whatever the true figure Kuffler had been offered, Richard Cromwell proved no more scrupulous about honouring his late father's promises in the case of the torpedo than in that of Durham College. Kuffler never did receive his award, and as Moriaen and Boyle had hoped, the workings of the 'terrible destroying invention' were never revealed. Subsequent approaches to Charles II, though they did lead to an preliminary inspection by Pepys, also remained fruitless.[155] By April 1659, Hartlib was trying to secure Kuffler a post as physician to Boyle's elder brother Lord Broghill, for 'now he dares not go upon the streets to follow his business, for fear of being arrested. But such a protection would save him from all his creditors'.[156] Kuffler was now engaged on yet another new project, involving fertilisers, and Hartlib played adroitly on Boyle's moral unease about the earlier scheme: if Kuffler could find sponsorship for his agricultural plans, 'he would willingly desist from all eager pursuits about his dreadful and destroying machine'.[157]

Thanks probably to this or a similar petition from Hartlib, Kuffler managed to weather the storm. Though Hartlib was still complaining as late as March 1660 that he could not prevail upon the state to take the interest it should in any of Kuffler's proposals,[158] he seems to have found a sufficient private market for his dyes, fertilisers and ovens to get by. He was still making, or at least displaying, his ovens in 1666, at the age of over seventy: John Evelyn on 1 August that year 'went to Dr. Keffler [...] to see his yron ovens, made portable (formerly) for the Pr. of Orange's army'[159]

However various, and in many cases limited, the success of these inventors may have been from a personal point of view, their practical and theoretical expertise represented an important contribution to intellectual life and technological advance in England. Throughout the 1650s, Moriaen, in his discreet fashion, was a principal instigator and conveyor of such contributions. While the distasteful but unavoidable subject of money frequently came to the fore and hindered or compromised the ideal of a 'free and generous communication', communication there certainly was, and he and Hartlib between them were a major channel for it.

The Godly Entrepreneur

The estate of Hulkestein, where Moriaen was now settled, did not belong to the Kufflers. The fragmentary accounts of the estate in the Rijksarchief, Arnhem show that from 1599 to 1666 it belonged to the Van De Sande family, whence it passed to a nephew, Johan Brantsen.[160] There is no mention in the surviving records of either Kuffler or Moriaen, nor of the dye works. Kuffler rented Hulkestein, and in his absence, Moriaen was standing surety for him.[161] How Moviaen was able to stand this surety, if he was as destitute as he claimed, is a moot point. Poverty short of outright starvation is a relative concept, and there is no suggestion he was starving: he even got by until 1658 without selling his West India shares. But he was certainly no longer in the situation to which he had been accustomed, and was in a state of constant anxiety as he waited to hear news of Kuffler's success in England.

The suggestion that Moriaen had gone to Arnhem to superintend, and indeed probably to take a share in, the Kufflers' dye-works is supported by Moriaen's at first referring to it as 'our dye-works' ('unßere färbereÿ'), presumably meaning his and the Kufflers'. By the beginning of 1658, this had run into the doldrums, and Moriaen had consequently had no income whatsoever since the previous September, when the merchant he had been dealing with had declined to renew his contract.[162] He put his failure on the market down to his inability to dye in more than one colour (probably the 'Bow scarlet' the Kufflers had imported into the Netherlands from their father-in-law Drebbel's dye-works at Stratford-le-Bow). However, he was unable to find anyone who could teach him to branch out, until a young Nürnberger happened by on his way from England offering to teach him all the arts of dyeing at a remarkably low rate (less than 12 Imperials). Moriaen was immediately moved to stake all his remaining money and any more he could by any means raise on relaunching the business. This latest piece of improvidence was enough to move Odilia Moriaen to emerge for once from the historical shadows by protesting about it strongly enough for her husband to consider it worth mentioning her qualms to Hartlib. Even after he had lectured her on the manifest operation of the hand of God in the matter, he had to admit that he won her 'consent' only with difficulty.[163]

From this point in the letters onwards, 'our dye-works' becomes 'my dye-works', suggesting that Kuffler had abandoned what appeared to be a sinking ship, perhaps handing over his stake in the business to Moriaen in lieu of his debts to him. He may already have resolved to settle again in England, this time for good. It is impossible, however, to be certain exactly what the financial arrangements were, as no documents have survived and Moriaen's letters are extremely vague about such details.

Virtually nothing else is revealed of the Nürnberg master dyer, who remains nameless and is hardly mentioned again: though Moriaen originally envisaged sharing the profits with him, it seems the young man simply sold his expertise and went on his way. Presumably Hartlib had met him in England and suggested he visit Moriaen, for Moriaen expressed his effusive thanks to God and Hartlib in roughly equal proportions. This is characteristic of their providential view of things: Moriaen could, with the utmost seriousness, see the encounter as a clear indication that God was guiding his affairs and also view Hartlib as God's chosen instrument. In the philosophical terms of the day, Hartlib was a 'secondary cause', and amply deserved recognition as such, but the prime mover in all matters was God. It is a clearer manifestation of the attitude earlier taken to the intelligence his circle received from Hartlib on the eve of the Civil Wars, 'for which we are thankful to God and Your Honour'.[164] Similarly, when Dury reached England in time for Comenius's arrival in 1641, it must have been obvious that the immediate impulse for his coming (as for Comenius's) was an urgent summons from Hartlib, but Moriaen still saw their coming together as 'a singular providence of God and a good omen'.[165]

There followed a string of letters of increasing urgency and proportionately decreasing subtlety bewailing Moriaen's lack of capital resources for the venture and fear that all would fail for want of a long term loan of a mere £200. Hartlib did his best to help his friend. He told Boyle in February 1658 that he had

> shot an arrow of charity at random toward Zurich [which] lighted upon our resident there Mr Pell, who hearing of his [Moriaen's] very low condition, and to have been assisted with 3l sterling by Dr Vnmussig, ordered, that the sum of 10l sterling, should be made over to that worthy man out of the pension, which the state doth pay him quarterly.[166]

Consequently, Hartlib added, he did not wish to press Moriaen for medicine from Glauber, lest Moriaen should suspect an ulterior motive behind Hartlib's petitioning on his behalf, or stint himself for Hartlib's sake:

> if I should beg a few doses of the Glauberian medicine, Mr Morian might happily think, that I desired to be gratified this way, which truly is far from my spirit and intentions. But I am confident, if I should venture such a request upon him, he would certainly pay for the medicine whatever it should cost, out of those supplies, which have been procured, by the blessing of God, upon my hearty recommendations.[167]

Whether or not Boyle responded to the hint implicit in this story is not recorded, but many of Hartlib's friends and acquaintances did. The £3 from Unmüssig was acknowledged in August 1657.[168] Comenius, Rulice and Hartlib himself all contributed.[169] The MP and Neoplatonist thinker John Sadler was moved to send £10, asking in return only that Moriaen use his contacts in the printing industry to obtain Heinrich Bunting's rare *Itinerarium Sacrum* for him.[170] Hartlib hoped to make Moriaen a beneficiary of his projected Council for Learning, hopes for which were constantly being revived (and re-dashed) in the late 1650s. Exactly what sort of a role Hartlib had in mind for him is unclear, but it was probably that of local agent and intelligencer. He appears, however, on none of Hartlib's surviving draft lists of prospective members of the Council.

The Council of Learning turned out to be another of Hartlib's pies in the sky, but the donations he sent or elicited seem to have been sufficient to enable Moriaen to relaunch the business with some success. Moriaen, now well into his sixties, threw himself into this small cottage industry with a religious fervour of striking intensity. Indeed, to an age accustomed to see material and spiritual gain as utterly distinct if not outright antithetical, it can seem comically incongruous. There is a veritable deluge of references to 'God's gracious providence', the 'wondrous care God has for me' and the like:[171] the enterprise begins to sound more like a mystical pilgrimage than a business venture:

> I am led in wondrous fashion and know not whither, but I shall follow my
> guide in blind obedience; let him look to it; whatever it may please him
> to be or to become in me, I shall be content with it.[172]

But this quasi-mystical approach is characteristically combined with a shrewd eye to a business opportunity. At one point, he announced that, despite being quite without funds or security, he had purchased all the necessary equipment and taken on an overseer and an unspecified number of hands on two year contracts. An almost identical diatribe to the one just quoted, stressing once again that he was acting not according to human reason but 'with childish trust and in blind obedience to the hand of God that guides me',[173] is followed immediately by the remark that this was just the moment to catch the springtime orders from the local merchants before they sent their cloth to their usual dyers in the province of Holland. To Moriaen, there was manifestly no discontinuity between the two thoughts. Like his old friends the De Geers, though obviously on a far smaller scale, Moriaen might be viewed as an archetype of the godly entrepreneur.

The highly ambivalent relationship in the Dutch 'Golden Age' of a ruggedly Calvinist ethos with an economy thriving principally - and spectacularly - on trade and speculation is analysed with great wit and originality in Simon Schama's *The Embarrassment of Riches*. That ambivalence is encapsulated in Schama's delightful declension, 'I invest, he speculates, they gamble'[174]. Some dextrous ethical juggling was called for, Schama suggests, when unprecedented economic expansion driven largely by the manipulation and exploitation of markets coincided with a religious ethos that stressed primarily the virtues of penitence and self-denial, while the culture of the 'self-made man' sat ill with Calvinist notions of predestination. Christ's warnings about the camel and the eye of the needle,[175] about the rich man and Lazarus,[176] could not easily be ignored in such a society. Against these, however, could be set the parable of the talents,[177] or the injunction to cast one's bread upon the waters.[178] The sin, then (or so the rationalisation went), was not to make money but to hoard it: the root of all evil is not money itself but the love of it.[179] Furthermore, disposable income provided a means of performing those good works that could not possibly guarantee membership of the elect but might very well be a sign of it. Conspicuous expenditure, wise investment and public philanthropy became, according to Schama, the standard strategies by which the wealthy Dutch, and especially those who were becoming wealthier, sought to square their ethos with their income.

The level of Moriaen's expenditure is not ascertainable, but by 1651, for all his claims of impecunity, he was living on the Princengracht, in one of the grand new buildings that still distinguish Amsterdam three and a half centuries later with their imposing blend of opulence and sobriety, embodiments of the conflicting ideals of the godly entrepreneur.[180] As he later ruefully remarked, 'time was I was myself well provided-for'.[181] He collected Oriental manuscripts and other rarities; he was able in the 1640s to leave home on tours lasting weeks or months; he could offer substantial loans to Comenius, Rave and others, and he could risk very considerable sums on speculative alchemical ventures.[182]

One of many tightropes the godly entrepreneur had to walk was that of accepting what Schama calls the 'providentially distributed opulence' of high return on a risky investment[183] without falling into the sin of improvident gambling. For all the time he had spent in Cologne warning parishioners such as Kuiper against the evil of games of chance, Moriaen seems to have taken a fairly elastic view of the distinction. Fishing and, especially, whaling, which appear to have represented his major investments in his early Amsterdam years at least, were notoriously high-risk ventures, with potential profits running high but a fair risk of total loss, partly on account of the inherent dangerousness of the activity, partly because of the ceaseless depredations of privateers. The same willingness to run risks is abundantly evident in his venture with the dye-works.

Of all the rationales for making money, directing it into good works naturally represented the least morally complicated. A man earning ten thousand Imperials a year could contribute more, quantitatively, to the public weal with ten percent of his income than a man earning one thousand could with fifty percent of his. The widow's mite was not, of course, to be despised, but it was still only a mite.

The attitude of Louis de Geer to the getting and redistributing of worldly wealth provides a striking insight into the mentality of the godly entrepreneur. De Geer declined to take out insurance on any of his ships or family, giving the equivalent sums instead to charity, principally to the refugees from the Palatinate and the Spanish Netherlands. Moriaen remarked that the poor share proportionately in his profit.[184] Blekastad suggests that by this means de Geer had 'bought himself Gods grace in dangerous undertakings'.[185] This, however, is something of an over-simplification. It should not be supposed de Geer was trying to strike a deal with God. He knew very well that any covenants between Creator and creature were for the former alone to draw up. The gesture was more one of proffered sacrifice, for the Lord to take or not as he saw fit. When in due course de Geer was relieved of nine ships to the value of some fifty thousand guilders,[186] his reaction was probably very like that of Moriaen after his crash in the late 1640s: personal distress and concern for his dependents, tempered by acquiescence to God's will and a patient willingness to watch and wait until divine Providence should offer an opportunity to recoup the loss and resume the former works of charity. Job provided a precedent at once cautionary and reassuring.

Once Moriaen had launched his new dye-works, he promptly returned to a favoured charitable practice of his age, the dispensing of medicine. He was delighted to acquire as a nearish neighbour in Arnhem the Paracelsian iatrochemist André Niclaus Bonet, personal physician to the Elector of Brandenburg. Thanks to the ten pounds Hartlib had procured him from Sadler, he wrote in June 1658, he had been able to buy coals and set up a cauldron, so that 'next week I can and must help those people who have waited a long time now for our aid, but whom for want of a cauldron we have not been able to help'.[187] While it is unclear what exactly Moriaen was cooking up in his philanthropic cauldron, the likeliest explanation by far is some sort of chemical medicine, for this stress on 'helping many' seems to rule out the possibility of its being merely a part of the dyeing equipment. In July 1658, Moriaen approached Bonet for advice and assistance, 'for several patients afflicted with the falling sickness [epilepsy] have applied to me'.[188] This is an unequivocal indication that he was operating some sort of medical practice alongside his dye-works.

There is another hiatus in the surviving holograph letters between July 1658 and January 1662, though it is obvious the two men remained in touch,[189] so no personal account of Moriaen's affairs is available, but numerous remarks from other sources suggest that his circumstances were at least comfortable again by early 1659. The clearest indication of this is that he went some way to returning the favours the now increasingly hard-pressed Hartlib had shown him, sending £3.8/- through his nephew Jan Abeel on 18 April 1659,[190] and another £3 in March 1661.[191] Already by February 1659 he was in a position to send the overseer of his works to Amsterdam on business, and the following month was considering having a special 'optical lantern' made for himself.[192] In mid-1659 he revisited Amsterdam at least twice, lodging at Glauber's house,[193] which suggests that the dye-works was running well enough for him to entrust it to the supervision of his employees and/or his wife. The physician, alchemist and diplomat Friedrich Kretschmar, who met him during this stay in the capital, thought him 'stattlich':[194] an ambiguously complimentary term tending to suggest an air of prosperity. In March 1660, Hartlib strongly implied an upturn in his fortunes, and neatly epitomised the image of the godly entrepreneur, when he told John Winthrop that

> Honest Mr Morian is still alive not far from Arnheim, having erected a new dying of colours in grain &c whereby he maintains him*self* and hopes to prosper in time to be able to serve *the* good of many.[195]

A measure of financial security thus recovered, Moriaen must have been free to redouble his interests in optics, alchemy and chemical medicine, the main themes of the fragmentary remains of his letters of 1659. He was particularly concerned to find someone who might provide relief for Hartlib, who by this point was in continual agony from what he described as 'my three most tormenting diseases',[196] to wit haemmorhoids, what he took to be an ulcer either of the bladder or the testicles, and what he took to be a stone either in the liver or the kidneys. In his last years, he was taking increasingly desperate remedies for an increasingly desperate condition, and there can be little doubt that many of his treatments did him more harm than the ailments themselves. Peter Stahl, a chemist and iatrochemist who was shortly to come to England armed with a recommendation from Moriaen,[197] sent over some 'spirit of salt' (hydrochloric acid) for Hartlib's treatment which the patient was distressed to find had a tendency to dissolve the glass bottles it was kept in. What worried Hartlib seems to have been the fact that he had consequently lost a substantial amount of the medicine, not the thought of what it was doing to his innards.[198] Poleman was having made for him a whalebone catheter through which he might painlessly (Poleman claimed) inject into his bladder an acid distilled from four to five week old urine, in order to dissolve the stone.[199] In December 1661, Moriaen's young friend Albert Otto Faber[200] moved to England armed with a variety of treatments for Hartlib. He presented him with an amulet made from a urine-moistened cloth rubbed in 'sympathetic powder', a 'Primum Ens des Saurbrunnens' ('primary essence of the mineral spring') to be taken in beer or Spanish wine on an empty stomach, and 'a pound of the true *ludus Paracelsi,* such as is to be found in Antwerp according to Helmont's directions, and which I was given by Moriaen'.[201]

The last surviving letter of the correspondence - a stray holograph which may well be indeed the last written - makes melancholy reading, and suggests that Moriaen may have contributed - indirectly, inadvertently and probably mercifully - to Hartlib's death. Hartlib had received, obviously through Moriaen's recommendation, a medicine from one 'Herr Kreußner', who is mentioned nowhere else in the papers and of whom I can find no other trace. Nor is there any indication of the medicine's content: Moriaen did not know what it consisted of, only that it had proved efficacious in other cases. All that is clear is that it was causing Hartlib even greater pain than he was accustomed to. Moriaen was embarrassed, distressed, and unable to suggest anything but prayer. Two months later Hartlib was dead.

His death effectively brings to a close Moriaen's recordable history. This same last letter also contains the news that Moriaen was preparing to leave Arnhem and return to the province of Holland, but it has not been possible to ascertain whether the plan was carried out. The very manuscript of this last letter, which is badly damaged, seems to embody Moriaen's disappearance from historical record. The text becomes increasingly fragmented and illegible, finally breaking off altogether as the bottom of the paper is torn off through the middle of the last farewell. The signature is entirely missing.

The proposed move suggests perhaps that the dye-works had been successful enough for Moriaen, who was now about seventy, to retire at last on the profits, but without further evidence no definite conclusions can be drawn. What is certain is that in spite of all his complaints about his ill health and failing strength, he survived for several more years. The history of his whereabouts and activities for this period is a complete blank. There remains only the report sent by a downcast and ailing Theodore Haak to John Winthrop on 22 June 1670, in reply to the latter's 'kinde & large letter to me last year'. This constitutes a catalogue of woe including a lawsuit and a serious illness, but principally the death of 'my dear wife' and

> a sad traine of many other troubles to me; besides *the* losse of many very speciall ffrends in severall parts, & especially of that dear & worthy frend of ours Mr Moriaen, whom I had so great a Desire to have seen once more. He & his wife soon deceased one after another, & I am informed that all his goods & those many excell*ent* curiosities & rarities he was master of were suddenly sold, distracted, scattered.[202]

Winthrop's letter being lost, the obvious inference is that the events related in Haak's may have occured at any point between early 1669 and the date of the letter, 22 June 1670.[203] But this is to assume that Haak was informed of Moriaen's death straightaway and that he recalled perfectly the sequence of events over a particularly unhappy period during much of which he was seriously ill. A circumstantial clue suggests Moriaen's death occurred in

1668. Amongst the 'curiosities and rarities he was master of' was an Arabic manuscript of the Greek mathematician Apollonius Pergæus belonging to Christian Rave, which Rave sent him in 1651 to forward to Claude Hardy in Paris.[204] Hardy never received it, and as late as 1669 Rave was still complaining about the detention of his manuscript by certain unnamed persons.[205] But by then the manuscript was in the hands of Thomas Marshall, later Rector of Lincoln College, Oxford, who had purchased it from the Amsterdam bookseller Ratelband almost certainly in the first half of 1668 and certainly not later than 24 June.[206] Rave was evidently not aware of this and perhaps thought Moriaen still had it. That Moriaen was deeply concerned about Rave's unpaid debts to him a few years before he was sent the paper has already been mentioned, and whether they were ever settled in full remains uncertain. It is conceivable, then, that he detained Rave's manuscript as security against them, though obviously any number of other explanations are feasible. If this was indeed the case, the fact that the manuscript materialised in an Amsterdam bookshop in the first half of 1668 strongly suggests that this is when Moriaen died.

During the nearly eighty years of his life, Moriaen had been closely involved with some of the leading figures in the intellectual life of the day, foremost among them Hartlib, Dury, Comenius and J.R. Glauber. He had also been acquainted with a host of figures now largely forgotten but whose ideas and activities seemed at the time hardly less important, and a knowledge of whom is essential to a full understanding of the thought of the period on its own terms. He was personally and practically involved in promoting new technology and ideas, above all the concepts of Pansophy and alchemy. His fortuitously preserved letters present a unique individual perspective on a whole mental world.

Notes

1   'Diese lande sindt ehrgierig vnd lieben den ruhm von gelehrten leuthen vnd nuzlichen Inventis zue haben, wie nun Ihrer viel sindt die allein die kunst lieben vnd suchen also sindt deren nicht wenig welche es ihnen eine verkleinerung halten das ein frembder etwas mehr als sie wißen vnd was newes erfinden solle' - Moriaen to Hartlib, 17 January 1639, HP 37/4A.

2   Ibid., paraphrased in *HDC*, 343. Rulice had written in similar terms of Vossius's judgment a year earlier (quoted by Turnbull from HP 36/1/3B-4A).

3   'wan man die leuthe hatt so achtet man Ihrer nicht[;] wan sie vmbsonst arbeiten oder geltt zuegeben wolten das weren männer fur diese Statt' - Moriaen to Hartlib, 24 October 1647, HP 37/123A.

4   Moriaen to Hartlib, 31 March 1639, HP 37/16B.

5   'hie hatt man freÿheit zue glauben vnd zue schreiben was man nur will oder kan' - Moriaen to Hartlib, 20 Oct. 1639, HP 37/44B. The controversies concerning Jungius and Comenius are discussed in Chapter Three, section 2.

6   2 Aug. 1640, HP 37/66B: 'So gleich iezund bekom Ich aduis das die Duynkerker mir ein Schiff dz auff den fischfang auß war abgenommen', and 27 March 1642, HP 37/106A, on the seizure of two more.

7   Cf. A. Th. Van Deursen, *Plain Lives in a Golden Age*, 19-22.

8   Moriaen to Hartlib, 15 April 1642, HP 37/107A.

9   'Ich nun fortan all mein werkh von diesen dingen machen kan' - Moriaen to Hartlib,

31 March 1639, HP 37/15A.

10 Gemeendearchief Arnhem, RA 513 Fol. 101, 19 July 1658; it is this document that records the date of purchase.

11 Moriaen to Hartlib, 12 August 1639, HP 37/36B-37A; the death is described as having happened since his last letter to Hartlib, which was dated 21 July. References in *Correspondance de Mersenne* XI, 308, 420, 421, to a 'fils de Mr. Morian' whom the editors identify as Moriaen's son are mistranscriptions: copies of the same letters in the Hartlib archive clearly read 'Merian', and the figure in question is almost certainly Matthias Merian the Younger of the Frankfurt family of printers and engravers.

12 Moriaen to Hartlib, July 1657: 'sie würde sich hier under frembden und ganz allein ohne rath und trost von menschen befinden, niemand würde viel nach ihr umbsehen' (HP 42/2/14A)

13 Christian Rave to Moriaen, 12 Nov. 1651, Bodleian MS. Lat. misc. c.17 Fol. 42: 'Tua Castiss. Uxorem et Amicos omnes meo quæso nomine diligentissime salutabis'. The only contrary evidence is the description of him, in the above-mentioned document concerning the selling back of his West India shares, as 'Iean Moriaen den ouden'. It is possible, however, that the younger 'Iean Moriaen' was not a son but the 'Cous: Ioh: Moriaen' whom 'Iean den ouden' had much earlier recommended to the care of Justinus Van Assche in Amsterdam (UBA N65d, 17 January 1637, cf. n.1). There were certainly other Moriaens in Arnhem, where he was by then living: the court ordered the paying in of debts to one 'Christina Morians', wife of the engineer and surveyor Isaac van Geelkerch, in May 1661, especially those relating to 'Moriaens erfschap' (the Moriaen inheritance) (Gemeendearchief Arnhem, RA 513, fol. 226, 6 May 1661). There was also a 'Haus Moriaen' in the centre of the town, though Johann was not living there. Unfortunately, the records are so fragmentary (and, in the case of the legal documents, in such an appallingly bad scribal hand) that no more can be deduced about this Christina and her inheritance, nor what connection Moriaen had with the house that bore his family's name.

14 See J. Bruckner, *A Bibliographical Catalogue of Seventeenth-Century German Books Published in Holland* (The Hague and Paris, 1971), *passim*.

15 Bruckner, no. 167. Bruckner somewhat mystifyingly gives Samuel Hartlib as the author.

16 On 5 Nov. 1640 Moriaen promised to obtain unspecified works by Böhme for Haak, and by Felgenhauer and Kozack for Hartlib (HP 37/70A). On Felgenhauer, see below, pp. 87-8; on Kozack, Jöcher II, 2154; Van Der Wall, *Serrarius*, 105-7, and Blekastad, *Comenius*, 340, 350, 378-9. Hartlib received four unspecified works of Kozack from Moriaen the following January (Hartlib's accounts, HP 23/12/2B), and there is a partial MS copy of Kozack's *Liber Spagyriæ* at HP 25/20/1A-44B.

17 Moriaen to Hartlib, 3 November 1639, HP 37/46A.

18 As late as July 1650, Moriaen was still complaining that Oughtred was failing to send material for the edition that had first been proposed at least ten years earlier (HP 37/164A). The work finally came out in 1652 in Oxford.

19 Moriaen to Hartlib, 7 March 1639, HP 37/10B. This work, mentioned several times in Moriaen's correspondence, is almost certainly the unattributed Latin 'Idea Politicæ' preserved in a scribal copy at HP 26/24/1A-8B, in the form of a letter to Hartlib dated 1 July 1638.

20 Moriaen to Hartlib, 30 June 1639, HP 37/31A. The *Analysis Demonstrativa*, which survives in manuscript, is discussed in some detail below, pp. 118-20.

21 HP 37/21A, 31A, 36B, 100A.

22   Wing, no. 2907B: the edition listed is dated Edinburgh, 1659. Moriaen's came out in Aug. 1639 (as he told Hartlib on 12 August, HP 37/36B).

23   'Ich kan zwar nicht absehen was so viel verscheidene zue einem zweckh gerichtete schreiben nuzen können' - Moriaen to Hartlib, 12 Aug. 1639, HP 37/36B.

24   Milton, 'The Unchanged Peacemaker?', 109-110, and see Dury to Hartlib, 31 March 1640, HP 2/2/10A. Milton also refers to the business of the impounded pamphlets, but with the minor error of assuming it was Dury himself who sent them into England.

25   Moriaen to Hartlib, 12 March 1640, HP 37/60A.

26   Ibid.

27   Ibid. - 'so hatt das kind einen vnrechten nahmen bekommen vnd sind das dan so schröckliche sachen? ist doch niemand dabej verkurzet, Ich kan mir fast nicht einbilden das die Bischoffe dißfals beÿ einigen verständigen Politico beÿfall ihres vnzeitigen eÿfers (die materiam betreffend) finden werden'.

28   Dury to Hartlib, 31 March 1640, HP 2/2/10A.

29   Sic, probably a scribal error.

30   Dury to Warwick (scribal copy), 1 May 1640, HP 6/4/46A.

31   Dury to Hartlib, 18 Sept. 1642, HP 2/9/24A, n.d. but obviously slightly earlier, HP 2/9/17A, and 16 Oct. 1642, HP 2/9/34B.

32   Dury to Hartlib, 23 Oct. 1642, HP 2/9/39B; it is quite obvious from the context of earlier letters that this 'Epistolical Dissertation' is the Answer to the Lutherans.

33   Moriaen to Hartlib, 30 October 1642, HP 37/115A.

34   Dury to Hartlib, 31 Aug. 1646, HP 3/3/32A. For the 'somethinge extraordinarie' Dury had in mind, see below.

35   HP 37/3A-B and 37/167A.

36   Moriaen to Hartlib, July 1650, HP 37/164A.

37   Serrarius to Dury, in An Information concerning the Present State of the Jewish Nation in Europe and Judea, by Dury and/or Henry Jessey (London, 1658), 13; cit. Van Der Wall, Serrarius, 182.

38   See Van Der Wall, 'The Amsterdam Millenarian Petrus Serrarius (1600-1669) and the Anglo-Dutch Circle of Philo-Judaists', Jewish-Christian Relations in the Seventeenth Century, ed. J. Van Den Berg and E.G.E. Van Der Wall (Dordrecht, Boston and London, 1988), 73-94, 90-4, and Gershom Scholem, Sabbatai Sevi, The Mystical Messiah 1626-76 (London, 1973).

39   An Information, 2; cit. Van Der Wall, 'The Amsterdam Millenarian Petrus Serrarius', 80.

40   Richard Popkin, 'Hartlib, Dury and the Jews', SHUR, 118-36, esp. 132; and see ibid., 130-2 for a fuller account of Shapira's visit and relations with Dury's circle. Shapira had come to Amsterdam intending to raise money from the Jewish community, but had been turned down by them, providing the Christians with an opportunity to outdo them in charity.

41   Moriaen to Van Assche, 9 May 1643, UBA N65g, and see Van Der Wall, Serrarius, 159-60.

42   See Popkin, 'Hartlib, Dury and the Jews', 125-7.

43   Ibid., 126.

44   See Webster, Great Instauration, 222-4.

45   See Popkin, 'Hartlib, Dury and the Jews', SHUR, 118-36, esp. 123-4, and 'Some Aspects of Jewish-Christian Theological Interchanges in Holland and England 1640-70', Jewish-Christian Relations in the Seventeenth Century ed. J. Van Den Berg and

E.G.E. Van der Wall (Dordrecht, Boston and London, 1988), 3-32.

46 Cf. Van Der Wall, 'Three letters by Menasseh ben Israel to John Durie', *Nederlands Archief voor Kerkgeschiedenis* 65 (1985), 46-62. For a succinct account of Menasseh's (unsuccessful) mission, see *Worthington Diary* I, 78, n.1.

47 7 Oct. 1650, HP 37/159B.

48 HP 37/153A and 159B.

49 HP 4/3/2A.

50 Dury, 'Epistolicall Discourse' to Thomas Thorowgood, *Jewes in America* (London, 1650), cit. E.G.E. Van Der Wall, 'Johann Stephan Rittangel's Stay in the Dutch Republic (1641-1642)', in J. Van Den Berg and E.G.E. Van Der Wall, eds., *Jewish-Christian Relations in the Seventeenth Century* (Dordrecht, Boston and London, 1988), 119-34, 120.

51 Moriaen to Hartlib, 19 April 1639, HP 37/21B.

52 'seine Gegner selbst haben ihm nie solches vorgeworfen' - *Jöcher-Adelung* VII, 30-2.

53 See Chapter Four, section 5.

54 Dury and/or Hartlib?, *Englands Thankfulnesse, or An Humble Remembrance presented to the Committee for Religion in the High Court of Parliament* (London, 1642): for full title, see *HDC*, 90.

55 'das Er von dem herrn durch nicht vbersendung seiner sachen nun wiederumb wie dorten werde auffgehalten werden' - Moriaen to Hartlib, 22 May 1642, HP 37/109A.

56 Moriaen to Hartlib, 10 Feb. and 27 March 1642, HP 37/102A and 106A.

57 Hartlib to Worthington, 12 Dec. 1655, *Worthington Diary* I, 79. See J. Van Den Berg, 'Proto-Protestants? The Image of the Karaites as a Mirror of the Catholic-Protestant Controversy in the Seventeenth Century', *Jewish-Christian Relations in the Seventeenth Century*, ed. J. Van Den Berg and E.G.E. Van Der Wall, 33-50.

58 HP 1/33/62A-63B, copy enclosed with a letter from Cyprian Kinner to Hartlib.

59 See *Encyclopædia Judaica* X, 507-8 (under the heading 'Kabbalah').

60 'bin woll versichert das der gleichen secreta Rabinorum sonderlich doctrinam de Triunitate belangend zuevorn niemalen ans liecht kommen sind, vnd trage gleichfals keinen zweyfel man wird seiner arbeit so woll gegen die Anti Trinitarios als Iudæos nuzlich gebrauchen können' - Moriaen to Hartlib, 27 March 1642, HP 37/106A.

61 Letters from Moriaen of 10 Feb. and 3 March 1642, HP 37/102A and 105A.

62 Moriaen to Hartlib, 2 Dec. 1641, HP 37/96A. The fact that Moriaen evidently misread 'Ticcunei' (or perhaps 'Tecunei') as 'Tecuum' suggests his interest in Rittangel's work was more enthusiastic than informed. See Gershom Scholem, *Kabbalah* (Jerusalem, 1974), 218-19 and *passim*.

63 Virtually every mention of Rittangel is accompanied by a complaint. In the letter to Van Assche, 24 June 1642, UBA N65e, Moriaen said that he was prevented by one thing after another from undertaking a visit to his friend, 'vindende alle daegen nieuwe belaetselen als t'ene over is soo is ander voor de deure Rittangelius heeft my dit geheele Iaer geoccupeert met het ouersien van syn Liber Iezirah' ('finding new hindrances daily, as one is past there is another at the door. Rittangel has kept me busy the whole year overseeing his *Liber Jezirah*').

64 'ich [habe] etliche mal mit ihnen essen müssen, vnd dz auch, in præsentz hoher herrschaft, hören müssen: Diß ist der einige Man in den orientalischen Sprachen, den ganz Europa nicht hat!' - HP 1/33/63B.

65 'Er ist auch dermaßen selzam das nichts oder wenig mit Ihm anzuefangen ist' - Moriaen to Hartlib, 24 Oct. 1647, HP 37/123B.

66 Moriaen to Van Assche, November 1644, UBA N65h, and Moriaen to Hartlib, 9

March 1657, HP 42/2/4A.

67 'wolt ich ruhe fur ihm haben' - Moriaen to Hartlib, 9 March 1657, HP 42/2/4A.

68 'allein vmb des süßen honigs willen muß man zue zeiten das stechen der bienen mit geduld verschmerzen' - Moriaen to Hartlib, 27 March 1642, HP 37/106A.

69 Moriaen to Hartlib, 28 March 1641, HP 37/82A

70 Moriaen to Hartlib, 27 March 1642, HP 37/106A.

71 Moriaen to Hartlib, 24 Oct. 1647, HP 37/123B.

72 HP 3/3/32A-33B; Popkin, 'Some Aspects of Jewish-Christian Theological Interchanges', and see also A.K. Offenberg, 'Jacob Jehuda Leon (1602-1675) and his Model of the Temple' (*Jewish-Christian Relations*, 95-115).

73 Dury to Hartlib, 31 Aug. 1646, HP 3/3/33B.

74 Ibid.

75 Ibid.

76 On perverse usage of the word 'Jew' (or in this case 'Jude'), see Victor Klemperer, *LTI* [= *Lingua Tertii Imperii (Language of the Third Reich)*]: *Notizbuch eines Philologen* (Berlin, 1949), a chilling and thought-provoking first-hand account by a German Jewish philologist of the linguistic policies of the Third Reich, which raises many questions that resonate beyond its immediate historical context.

77 Dury to Hartlib, 31 Aug. 1646, HP 3/3/33A-B.

78 Ibid. I do not wish to overstate the point: 'which' was used synonymously with 'who' at this period, and implies no derogation to Leon, but the statement that Boreel 'made use of' him clearly reflects Dury's notion of a hierarchy in the relationship.

79 November 1644, UBA N65h, stating perhaps hyperbolically that the value of the shares had halved, and 27 Feb. 1648, HP 37/131B, in which he reported a loss of 800 guilders.

80 Moriaen to Hartlib, 29 Oct. 1647, HP 37/123A.

81 'Euserlichen ansehen vnd Weltweißheit nach, hab Ich freÿlich (wie die freunde <wohl> vrtheilen) dem Sprichwort nachgethan alijs in serviendo consumor' - Moriaen to Hartlib, 8 April 1650, HP 37/149A.

82 See Chapter Four, section 4.

83 Moriaen to Hartlib, 8 April 1650, HP 37/149A.

84 'dit quaem mij seer beswaerlyck voor [...] well om hem niet te laeten soo hadde al geresolueert hem te helpen' - Moriaen to Van Assche, Nov. 1644, UBA N65h.

85 Moriaen to ?, 7 Feb. 1647, HP 37/118B.

86 Moriaen to Hartlib, 24 Oct. 1647, HP 37/123A-B, reporting 65 guilders repaid and over 200 still outstanding.

87 On Wheeler, see Webster, *Great Instauration*, 372-4. He was an inventor whom Hartlib promoted for a while in the 1640s but who soon lost credit with the circle. After obtaining a twelve-year Dutch patent for a drainage mill in 1639 (Doorman, *Patents for Inventions*, 139), Wheeler fled the Netherlands leaving debts of over £1000, which the state met by selling his patent to a consortium of eight, including William Boswell and Janszonius Blaeu. Wheeler always maintained that he had been cheated, and wrote an impassioned but not very coherent account of the affair, *Mr William Wheelers Case from his Own Relation* (London, 1649), which, however, does little to inspire confidence in his competence or probity.

88 Moriaen to Hartlib, 1 April 1650, HP 37/148A, and 7 Oct. 1650, HP 37/159A.

89 'Ich [muß] beÿ so unträglichen schaden vnd verlust gleichwoll mit allem ernst vnd fleiß dahin bedacht vnd auch damit geschäfftig sein [...] wie Ich vor meinem ende [...] meine sachen in richtigkeit bringen [...] vnd also meine ehre, die nächst meinem

guten gewißen mein höchster schaz auff Erden ist, erhalten vnd retten möge' - Moriaen to Hartlib, 8 April 1650, HP 37/149A.

90 Hartlib to Boyle, 14 Sept. 1658, Boyle, *Works* VI, 114.

91 Hartlib to Boyle, 16 Dec. 1658, Boyle, *Works* VI, 115.

92 The fullest account of him is Inge Keil, 'Technology transfer and scientific specialization: Johann Wiesel, optician of Augsburg and the Hartlib circle', *SHUR*, 268-78, to which the following account is heavily indebted. See also her forthcoming *Augustanus Opticus. Johann Wiesel (1583-1662) und 200 Jahre optisches Handwerk in Augsburg* (Berlin, [1998 or 1999?])

93 Keil, op. cit., 269.

94 Wiesel to Moriaen, 17 Feb. 1650, copy in a letter from Moriaen to [Hartlib?], HP 37/144B.

95 Ibid., 272. On Pell, see below, pp. 113-16.

96 See especially Moriaen to Hartlib, 25 March 1650, HP 37/146B. Hevelius, Blaeu and Sotherby each wanted a telescope, Boyle a microscope and Worsley one of each. On 19 July 1650, Wiesel mentioned four microscopes ordered from him through Moriaen, but by whom is not clear (HP 37/154B).

97 Wiesel to Moriaen, 17 and 30 Dec. 1649, HP 37/144B (copy extracts included in a letter from Moriaen to Hartlib).

98 HP 37/149A, 37/153A, 37/154A.

99 *Eph 51*, HP 28/2/3B.

100 'machet einen floch so groß als ein schildkroten [...] wer solchen durch dießes Instrumentlein schawete müste sich von herzen darvor entsezen' - Wiesel to Moriaen, 17 Feb. 1650, HP 37/144B.

101 'diß mit sonderlichem lust zu schawen' - Wiesel to Moriaen, 17 Dec. 1649, HP 37/144B.

102 Keil, 'Johann Wiesel and the Hartlib circle', 276-8.

103 Moriaen to Hartlib, 18 Jan. 1658, HP 56/2/1A, with mention of the period 'when Herr Clodius lived in my house' ('da H Clodius beÿ mir wohnte').

104 The recommendation itself does not survive, but Moriaen promised to send one on 19 April 1652 (HP 63/14/19B).

105 Reports from him suddenly start appearing in the *Ephemerides* from about April 1651 onward.

106 Boyle to Clodius, 27 Sept. 1653

107 See Webster, *Great Instauration*, 303, and Hartlib to Boyle, 8 May 1654, Boyle, *Works* VI, 86.

108 Kuffler's case is dealt with in detail below. See HP 31/13A for Moriaen's recommendation of Franck, HP 31/18/31A for his recommendation of Stahl, and HP 31/16A for his association with Faber. Faber (1641-78) is briefly mentioned by Thorndike (VII, 233) and Partington (II, 182).

109 See Turnbull, 'Peter Stahl, the first public teacher of chemistry at Oxford', *Annals of Science* IX (1953), 265-70; Webster, 165, and Partington, II, 488.

110 Incomplete copy at HP 18/3/1/1A-8B.

111 See Webster, *Great Instauration*, 304.

112 *Chymical, Medicinal, and Chyrurgical Addresses*, 161.

113 'Remeum werd ich Ihnen fürderlich zusenden, mit den balsamis chirurgicis' - Moriaen to Hartlib, 24 April 1654, HP 31/13A. The 'you' is in the plural, presumably meaning Hartlib and Clodius.

114 Hartlib to Boyle, 8 May 1654, Boyle, *Works* VI, 87.

115 Hartlib to Winthrop, 16 March 1660, HP 7/7/4B.

116 On 6 May, Dury mentioned having been with him in Amsterdam 'last week' (HP 4/3/3A); 16 Oct. is the date of his first surviving letter from Arnhem.

117 The Kuffler brothers moved to the Netherlands from England, where they had also run a dye-works (at Stratford le Bow), just before the outbreak of the Civil War (*NNWB* is incorrect in dating their return c. 1650: Moriaen reported their recent arrival in Amsterdam to Van Assche on 24 June 1642, UBA N65e). By September they were in the Hague (UBA N65f), but had moved to Arnhem at least by 16 Oct. 1646, when Heinrich Appelius wrote to Hartlib about a dyer known as Flensburg whom the Kufflers were supporting at their home there (HP 45/1/27B). On 26 Aug. 1647 Appelius specifically mentioned that they 'dwell & exercise their dying of cloath' at Arnhem (HP 45/1/33A). No patent for the dye-works has survived (cf. G. Doorman, *Patents for Inventions in the Netherlands during the 16th, 17th and 18th Centuries* (abridged trans. Joh. Meijer), The Hague, 1942), but since (according to Moriaen) this was the only dye-works in the province (HP 31/18/1B) they perhaps felt no need of one.

118 Three copies in the Hartlib Papers (HP 53/5A-B, 53/41/4A-5B and 66/18/1A-2B); the document is undated but probably late 1658 (mid-1653 is 'about 5. years since' but Richard Cromwell is Protector).

119 On Comenius's belief that he was invited to England by Parliament, see below, p. 128.

120 A letter from Georg Horn to Hartlib of Sept. 1653, describing a highly skilled dyer specialising in scarlet, well known to Moriaen and planning to visit England to impart his knowledge for a suitable price, surely refers to Kuffler and implies that Hartlib knew little about him (Horn to Hartlib, 15 Sept. 1653, HP 16/2/2A). But Horn may simply have been unaware how well-informed Hartlib was: it was certainly not news to him that Kuffler knew Moriaen and was an expert in scarlet dye.

121 Nine mentions of Kuffler in *Eph 35*, relating to his ovens, optics, medicines, a method of drying malt, and Drebbel's 'weather-glass' (i.e. his perpetual almanac) (HP 29/3/44A, 48B, 52A, 55B, 56A, 56B, 57B, 62A-B, 63B).

122 It is not clear whether the family who set off together with Johann Sibertus included his brother.

123 Petition to Cromwell, HP 66/18/1A. It is not immediately obvious why the change should so adversely have affected Kuffler's prospects. The Council of State which he supposed had invited him was drastically reduced, it is true, to the initially thirteen-strong Protector's Council (later Privy Council), and Major-General Harrison, his supposed champion, no longer featured on it *CSPD* 1653-4, 297-8 (vol. 42), 297-8 (16 Dec. 1653), but it is by no means certain he would have known in such detail of the state of affairs in England. Rumour or sheer uncertainty may well have been enough to put him off.

124 HP 63/14/31B.

125 'Interim wolle der H. diese 2. Inventiones bey Seiner Hochheit dem H. PROTECTORI anbringen, vmb zu vernehmen, wie Ers apprehendire' (Moriaen to Hartlib, 5 Jan. 1655, HP 39/2/21A).

126 HP 39/2/41A.

127 At this juncture, Worsley was Surveyor General of Ireland, though soon to be brought down by his rival William Petty. See below, p. 218 and the literature cited there.

128 HP 39/2/28B.

129 'Nun mein Herr ich bin versichert, daß meine Invention in höherm grad alß H Kufflers stehet, und ehe ich 1000 gl. darauff spendirt, weiß ich gewiß, meine sache demonstrabel zu machen. [...] Ich weiß nicht wie es ist, daß ich das glück habe, die fewer Inventiones ziemlicher massen zuerkündigen [...] Ohne Ruhm zu melden, glaube ich nicht, das einer in Europa einen digerir ofen habe, der lenger, vnd mitt weniger Kohlen könne gehitzet werden, als meiner' - Copy extract by Clodius, 17 Nov. 1654, HP 39/2/25B, probably to Moriaen: it is evident in any case that Moriaen read and responded to this letter.

130 'solte ich [...] eines andern schweiß und arbeit mir zueignen wollen, das seÿ ferne von mir' - 11 Dec. 1654, HP 39/2/24B: though probably addressed to Hartlib the letter was obviously meant for Clodius's eyes too. A similar rebuke of the same date (HP 39/2/24A and 22B) is almost certainly addressed to Clodius personally.

131 HP 39/2/25B.

132 Christine MacLeod, *Inventing the Industrial Revolution: The English patent system, 1660-1800* (Cambridge, 1988), Chapter 1, and see Webster, *Great Instauration*, 343-355 on the resentment earlier aroused by abuses of the patent system and monopolies.

133 On Hartlib's complex attitude to patents, see Greengrass, Leslie and Raylor, 'Introduction' to *SHUR*, 18-21, and Mark Jenner, '"Another *epocha*"? Hartlib, John Lanyon and the improvement of London in the 1650s', *SHUR*, 343-56.

134 L.E. Harris, *The Two Netherlanders* (Cambridge 1961), chapter 17. See also the account of Kuffler's torpedo in Webster, *Great Instauration*, 390-1.

135 'Ich sehe daß werck auch dergestalt an, daß es mehr zu ersparung bluttvergiessens, alß zu vergießung dienen wirdt. Dann wie die Schrifft selbsten vns zu gemüth führet, so gehet niemand so vnbedachtsam zu Feld, oder er überschlägt zuvor seine, vnd des feindes macht, Wie Er dargegen bestehen könne. So nicht; so schicket Er von ferne zu Ihm, vnd bittet vmb Frieden' - Moriaen to ?, 16 July 1655, HP 39/2/38B. The reference is to Luke 14:31-32.

136 Between 3 March, when Moriaen was still trying to secure an invitation (HP 39/2/44A-B), and 20 June, when Kuffler, Hartlib and Ezerell Tonge signed an agreement concerning the promotion of his work to Cromwell (HP 26/49/1A-B; see below).

137 The family was still in the Netherlands when the agreement with Tonge was drawn up in June. An entry in *Eph 56* almost certainly dating from July (the previous entry but one refers to events of 8 July) mentions a medicine known as 'oleum Fraxini' and that 'Dr Ks wife is bringing some along with her'.

138 'Articles tripertite Agreed & Concluded, betwixt Iohn Sivertus Küffeler, Dr. of Physick; Samuel Hartlib Esqr & Ezeral Tonge, Bac of Divinity. this 20th Day of Iune. 1656', HP 26/49/1A.

139 HP 53/41/1A-B, in both Latin and English versions; further copies of the English at HP 53/41/6A and 66/18/2A.

140 'Agreements tripertite', HP 26/49/1A.

141 Webster, *Great Instauration*, 232-42.

142 Ibid., 239-40, and 529-32 for identification of the staff as a whole.

143 Ibid., 242.

144 Moriaen to Hartlib, 2 Feb. 1657, HP 42/2/1B.

145 This is mentioned repeatedly in Moriaen's letters from the first half of 1658: HP 31/18/2B, 31/18/4B-5A, 31/18/15B, 31/18/23A, 31/18/31A..

146 Hartlib to Boyle (quoting Moriaen), 13 May 1658, Boyle, *Works* VI, 108: this letter also mentions Brereton's attendance. Moriaen's own letters from the period are full of remarks in the same vein. Winthrop, who learned about the business later, felt the

same: 'I wish you could prevaile with Dr Keffler to bury that fireworke [...] in oblivion [...] there are menes ynough already knowne to the world of ruin & destruction to mankind' (Winthrop to Hartlib, 25 Aug. 1660, HP 32/1/7B).

147 'so mag Gott kein gefallen an diesem furnehmen haben und den succes deswegen hindern' - Moriaen to Hartlib, 26 May 1658, HP 31/18/27A.

148 'Ich bin mit H Boÿle eines sinnes und will lieber zu einigen furnehmen rathen und gluckwunschen als zue diesem' - Moriaen to Hartlib, 14 June 1658, HP 31.18/29B.

149 On Hartlib's attitude to such subjects, see Timothy Raylor, 'New Light on Milton and Hartlib', *Milton Quarterly* 27 (1993), 19-31, on Hartlib's (and Milton's) promotion of Edmond Felton's 'godly' engine of war.

150 'treffliches arcanum [...] zu verderben des menschlichen geschlechts [...] Es scheint den Engelländern beschert zu seyn durch eine Wunderliche Providentz' - Anon., 8 Aug. 1658, HP 48/6/1A.

151 Hartlib to Boyle, 10 Aug. 1658, Boyle, *Works* VI, 113.

152 Hartlib, testimonial on Kuffler, 26 May 1659, 53/41/3A.

153 Kuffler's petition to Richard Cromwell, HP 66/18/1A-B.

154 Moriaen to Hartlib, 26 April and 14 June 1658, HP 31/18/17B and 31/18/29B.

155 Pepys, *Diary*, ed. Latham and Matthews, III (London, 1970), 45-6.

156 Hartlib to Boyle, 12 April 1659, Boyle, *Works* VI, 119.

157 Ibid., 118.

158 Hartlib to Winthrop, 16 March 1660, HP 7/7/2B.

159 John Evelyn, *Diary*, ed. W. Bray (London, 1879), II, 198. See also Webster, *Great Instauration*, 390.

160 It was a large estate alongside the Rhine, just to the north-west of Arnhem. There is a rather purple description in A.J. Van Der Aa, *Aardrijkskundig Woordenboek der Nederlanden* (Gorinchem, 1844) V, 896-7. It was destroyed in the Second World War.

161 This is abundantly clear from a letter of 26 April 1658 (HP 31/18/17A-18B), in which Moriaen specified the rent (104 Imperials a year) and that he had vouched for it, as also for other debts of Kuffler's.

162 Moriaen to Hartlib, 1 Jan. 1658, 31/18/1A.

163 Ibid., 31/18/1B.

164 'darfur wir Gott vnd EL dankbar sindt' - Moriaen to Hartlib, 10 Dec. 1640, HP 37/71A.

165 'eine sonderliche schickung Gottes vnd gutes zaichen' - Moriaen to Hartlib, 10 Oct. 1641, HP 37/90A.

166 Hartlib to Boyle, 2 Feb. 1658, Boyle, *Works*, VI, 100-101. The published version gives 'Dr Van Mussig', an obvious mistranscription of 'Vnmussig', the pseudonym of the Paracelsian physician Johannes Brun.

167 Ibid., 101.

168 HP 42/2/18B.

169 Van Der Wall, *Serrarius*, 303.

170 Moriaen to Hartlib, 14 June 1658, HP 31/18/29A.

171 Especially Moriaen to Hartlib, 1 Jan. 1658, HP 31/18/1A-3B, but there are examples in almost all the letters from this point on.

172 'Ich werde woll wunderlich geleitet und weiß nicht wohin aber ich will mit blindem gehorsam meinem laidsman folgen, der mags versehen was der in mir sein und werden will des bin Ich zuefrieden' - Moriaen to Hartlib, 19 Feb./1 March 1658, HP 31/18/8A.

173 'nach kindlichem vertrawen in einem blinden gehorsam der mich leitenden hand Gottes' - Moriaen to Hartlib, 5 March 1658, HP 31/18/11B.

174 Simon Schama, *The Embarrassment of Riches: An Interpretation of Dutch Culture in the Golden Age* (Berkely, Los Angeles and London, 1988), 343.

175 Matthew, 19:24; Mark, 10:25; Luke, 18:25.

176 Luke, 16:19-31.

177 Matthew, 25:14-30, the classic Scriptural authority for capitalism: 'Thou oughtest therefore to have put my money to the exchangers, and then at my coming I should have received mine own with usury [...] unto every one that hath shall be given, and he shall have abundance: but from him that hath not shall be taken away even that which he hath' (v.27-29).

178 Ecclesiastes, 11:1.

179 1 Timothy, 6:10.

180 The address appears on a letter from Christian Rave to Moriaen, 12 November 1651, Bodleian MS. Lat. misc. c.17 Fol. 42. I am indebted to Gerald Toomer of Harvard University for pointing this letter out to me. It is the only surviving evidence of his exact address at any point before the move to Arnhem, though it emerges from his own letters that he moved house within Amsterdam at least three times between 1639 and 1641.

181 'Ich habs etwan an mir selbsten wolgehabt' - Moriaen to Hartlib, 5 March 1658, HP 31/18/11B.

182 Details of his alchemical projects are given below, pp. 227-32.

183 *The Embarrassment of Riches*, 309: Schama is referring here specifically to the grand lotteries held in the Netherlands, but it is very much part of his point that any return on an investment involving the risk of loss could be viewed in the same way.

184 'theilen [...] mit seinen gewin proportionalites' - Moriaen to Hartlib, 31 Dec. 1640, HP 31/74A.

185 'sich [...] die Gnade Gottes bei gefährlichen Unternehmungen erkauft' - Blekastad, *Comenius*, 333.

186 Assuming Moriaen's second-hand report to be accurate (to Hartlib, 31 Dec. 1640, HP 37/74A).

187 'kunfftige woche soll und mus ich den leuthen helffen die nun lang auff uns gewartet haben und aus mangel eines kessels nicht haben geholffen werden können' - Moriaen to Hartlib, 25 June 1658, HP 31/18/37A.

188 'umb das einige patienten mit der fallenden Kranckheit [epilepsy] behafftet sich beÿ mir angeben [haben]' - Moriaen to Hartlib, 23 July 1658, HP 31/18/42A.

189 This is obvious from a number of remarks by Joachim Poleman. He asked Hartlib to convey Moriaen's reaction to his (Poleman's) medical ideas (HP 60/4/105A, n.d. but 1659 or 1660), and thanked him for not revealing his (Poleman's) name when passing on his (profoundly negative) assessment of Friedrich Kretschmar to Moriaen (HP 60/4/150B, 17 Oct. 1659). Hartlib in turn reported Moriaen's favourable opinion of Poleman's *Novum Lumen Medicum* (1659) (HP 60/4/183A, 2 Jan. 1660). There is also an alchemical letter, probably from Kretschmar, of 1660, in which Hartlib is urged not to pass on the contents to anyone, especially not to Moriaen (HP 31/23/28A-31B; see below, pp. 203-4 for a fuller account). On 21 April 1661 Moriaen's nephew Isaac de Bra (son of Abraham and Moriaen's sister) sent Hartlib a letter of recommendation from his uncle (now lost but mentioned at HP 27/41/1A).

190 HP 27/44/1A-2B.

191 Dury to Hartlib, 11 March 1661, HP 4/4/5A-B, with instructions to Dorothy Dury to

cash for Hartlib (at a favourable rate) a bill of exchange from Moriaen.

192 Moriaen to Hartlib, 14 Jan. 1659, HP 39/2/79A.

193 Kretschmar to Hartlib, 1 August 1659, HP 26/64/3B, and Poleman to Hartlib, 29 August 1659, HP 60/10/1A, both mention the first visit. Poleman also mentioned his arrival two days before 10 Oct. 1659 (to Hartlib, HP 60/10/2B), and departure before 17 October 1659 (HP 60/4/105A).

194 Kretschmar to Hartlib, 1 Aug. 1659, HP 26/64/3B.

195 Hartlib to Winthrop, 16 March 1660, HP 7/7/3A. Winthrop, who had met Moriaen during a visit to Europe, had asked after him the previous December (Winthrop to Hartlib, 16 Dec. 1659, HP 32/1/4).

196 Hartlib to Boyle, 27 April 1658, Boyle, *Works* VI, 103.

197 Moriaen to Hartlib, 25 June 1658, HP 31/18/37B. Faber (1641-78) was a chemist from Lübeck, possibly a younger relation of the now otherwise unknown Otto Faber who according to *Eph 53* 'is the Man which corresponds with Morian as a true adept. from whom he expects the perfecting of that mystery [the Philosophers' stone]' (HP 28/2/61B). On Albert Otto, see Thorndike VII, 233 and Partington II, 182.

198 Hartlib to Boyle, late April/early May 1659, *Works* VI, 122. On Stahl, see Turnbull, 'Peter Stahl, The First Public Teacher of Chemistry at Oxford', *Annals of Science* 9 (1953), 265-70.

199 Poleman to Hartlib, 19 Sept. 1659, HP 60/4/186A-B.

200 An iatrochemist from Lübeck (1641-78); see Thorndike, VII, 233, and Partington, *History of Chemistry* II, 182.

201 'ein lb. Ludi veri Paracelsi wie derselbe zu Antwerpen, nach Helmonts Anweisungen gefunden wird, vnd ich ihn von Moriano empfangen habe' - Faber to Hartlib, December 1661, HP 39/2/70A-B. The 'ludus Paracelsi' was one of the near-miraculous cure-alls of the Paracelsist chemical physicians.

202 R.C. Winthrop (ed.), *Correspondence of Hartlib, Haak, Oldenburg and others of the founders of the Royal Society with Governor Winthrop of Connecticut 1661-1672* (Boston, 1878), 45; the published edition gives the obvious mistranscription 'Morlaen'.

203 Pamela Barnett seems to me rash to assume that everything recounted in the letter happened in 1669 *Theodore Haak* (The Hague, 1962), 140-1

204 Rave to Moriaen, 12 Nov. 1651, Bodleian MS. Lat. misc. c.17 Fol. 42.

205 I owe all the details about the history of this manuscript to Gerald Toomer, who is writing a monograph on Rave: my warmest thanks to him for his help.

206 His interest in Apollonius was aroused in December 1667, and he had shown Castell the manuscript by 24 June 1648.

CHAPTER THREE

An Intelligencer's Ethos

'Man wird doch auch hiernegst nicht so sehr darauff sehen was fur eine
Persohn einer auff dem Schawplaz dießer weltt agiret sondern wie Er dieselbe
agirt und vertretten habe' ('It will not so much be asked hereafter what role a
person played in the theatre of this world, but how he played and acted it') -
Moriaen to Hartlib, 1 January 1658 (HP 31/18/1A).

Public and Private

Moriaen's correspondence with Hartlib cannot be described as personal or
private. The notion of a 'private' or 'inner' life is a Romantic one which
would have been largely incomprehensible to either man. The very notion of
a private letter to Hartlib, indeed, was virtually a contradiction in terms. His
surviving papers abound in requests to the addressee to show the contents to
no one else, or even to burn the letter after reading it, all faithfully copied out
in the hand of one or other of his scribes. If anything was delivered in
confidence it was necessary to stress the fact, Moriaen's stock phrase being
'sed hæc pereant inter nos' ('but let these [words] perish between us') - not
that Hartlib could be trusted even then to respect such commitments to
secrecy.

This is not to condemn Hartlib as unscrupulous or deceitful. He saw it as
his calling to disseminate information, and must frequently have experienced a
conflict between such private injunctions to secrecy and a sense of duty to
what he perceived as the common good. On the whole, he tended to favour
public over private obligation. He deeply upset Dorothy Dury, for instance,
by publishing her letter to Katherine Ranelagh explaining why she had
decided to marry Dury.[1] George Starkey too was furious when the alchemical
tract *George Riplye's Epistle [...] Unfolded*, which he had confided to
Hartlib, appeared in the *Chymical, Medicinal, and Chyrurgical Addresses*.[2]
Anyone writing to Hartlib was well aware - or at least ought to have been -
that he or she was addressing not an individual but potentially the whole
intellectual community of Europe and even beyond.

Private disburdenment was not, therefore, the purpose of these letters. As
many of Hartlib's correspondents were fond of remarking (often at
paradoxical length), time was a precious commodity loaned by God to be
devoted to the furtherance of His cause, not frittered away on personal
anecdote. The main aim of Hartlib's and Moriaen's correspondence was
either the coordination of projects such as the promotion of Comenius, in
which both men were involved, or the exchange of information; and in either
case the material was intended to be made available to other involved or
interested parties, not necessarily through publication. Among the projects
discussed by the circle, some of the most eagerly pursued were those for
shorthand writing, double or multiple writing machines, and processes for

making copies of letters automatically, to save the time and expense of copying longhand or employing scribes to do so. Hartlib was one of the century's most active promoters of 'scribal publication', the dissemination of tracts and letters in manuscript copy.[3] 'Scribal publication' is a good deal more difficult for later historians to trace and assess than printing, but was at least as important as a means of communicating new ideas and knowledge. The letters Moriaen wrote to Hartlib, and those that reached Hartlib by way of him, were all intended to be fed into this semi-public communication network.

The attitude is exemplified by Moriaen's remark that he had opened, read and made copies of some letters sent him for forwarding, and hoped Hartlib would not object to his taking this liberty.[4] Evidently Hartlib did not, since Moriaen later remarked very much as a matter of course that he had read a letter from Comenius to Hartlib that had passed through his hands.[5] When Worsley complained that Moriaen had not written to him for four months, Moriaen replied that he had not considered it necessary, since he had written to Hartlib and assumed Worsley would have been told all his news.[6] The substantial numbers of his letters that survive as scribal copies or translations prove that copies of these were indeed being passed round by Hartlib to interested friends and acquaintances. He specifically promised Winthrop, for instance, copies of some of Moriaen's letters,[7] and it was probably material from Moriaen that Hartlib referred to when in 1649 he sent Boyle 'the continuation of the respects from Amsterdam'.[8] Poleman acknowledged receipt of an extract from Moriaen and requested more.[9]

There was little room in all this for private opinion or personal anecdote except where it touched directly on more general and public issues. A certain amount slipped through, of course, for these people were not characterless automata, but it had to do so as it were by the back door. The public good could provide the justification for personal anecdote, as in a letter from Hartlib to Boyle about a new medicine, which begins: 'I am so out of love with my tormenting pains, that I have never a good will to mention them, but when they may be an occasion of ushering in some good communication or other, for the ease and health of many.'[10] In fact, Hartlib mentioned his 'tormenting pains' in very nearly every surviving letter of his last years.

Moriaen took exactly the same attitude to the relation of private sorrows and joys. Even the death of his daughter was mentioned only in the guise of an excuse for his failure to have made further progress with the collection for Comenius:

> since my last it has pleased God to visit my only child with sickness and
> finally to call her from this world, which sickness, death and burial and
> the attendant business have kept me at home for some time and prevented
> me from making the progress hoped for.[11]

This is not to suggest he was unaffected by the event, but rather to illustrate how inappropriate he evidently felt it to dwell on so personal a misfortune. In fact, it was surely the delay in the collection that provided the excuse for relating the loss, rather than the loss that excused the delay in the collection.

It is, therefore, singularly difficult to form any clear picture of Moriaen as an individual. As to his physical appearance there is no evidence whatsoever. With regard to his beliefs, he was extremely reluctant to commit himself to an opinion on any but the most concrete of matters. His character and personal qualities can be deduced only from odd stray comments, most of them far from specific, by his various acquaintances, and from reading conjecturally between the lines of his own letters.

There is much of the Reformed ethos of simplicity, moderation and self-control about his habits of thought and what little is known of his behaviour. He had no taste for opulence, either in his prose style or in his own or anyone else's personal habits. He was particularly critical of Kuffler's family (though he obviously had a vested interest in Kufflerian thrift), in which 'no one tries to make matters easier: they expect things to run as smoothly as they were accustomed to when times were easy'.[12] He spoke harshly of people of rank who misused learning for their 'lust and greed'.[13] He specifically commended Comenius's frugality in being prepared to live and work on the relatively modest sum of £100 a year.[14]

Like many of the circle, he was horrified by the immodest dress, loose language and spendthrift habits of Dury's notorious sister (her first name is not known), whose penchant for debt and scandalmongering made her - by their accounts at least - a sore trial to her brother, and still more to his spirited wife Dorothy, who went so far as to threaten to leave Dury if he could not persuade the sister to give up pursuing them around Europe demanding money and spreading gossip.[15] Moriaen's account of her visit to him - undertaken with a view to borrowing money - is a rare instance in his correspondence of graphic physical description, and as such is very revealing, of him at least as much as her. He enumerated in horrified detail her fine items of clothing, down to the materials and colours, and with a sharply puritanical eye singled out the detail of her wearing her hair loose. He was angered and distressed ('geärgert vnd betrubet') by the immodest spectacle.[16]

Only twice in all his surviving letters is there mention of his enjoying a sensual pleasure. One of these is music, the other the admiration of the natural world. A musical instrument he saw and heard in Nürnberg 'could so move me that not a drop of blood remained in its place'.[17] After a particularly hard Dutch winter, he delighted to see the thaw set in and the earth reawaken: 'the lands that have lain so long under water emerge now so green that it is a delight to behold; God make us thankful for his grace'.[18] Beyond these two impeccably pious examples there is not a single mention of the pleasures of the flesh. And its sufferings are given equally short shrift, though there is no doubt Moriaen experienced his full share of them. News of his incipient bladder stone, for instance, was accompanied only by the stoically fatalistic observation that the pain was 'not yet unbearable'.[19] He was also, apparently, afflicted with incurable halitosis: 'Mor. hath a stinking breath not beene able with all his Arts to cure himself of that'[20]

Bad breath notwithstanding, he seems to have been exceptionally well-liked. In a correspondence rich in the abrasive personal attacks so frequently indulged in during the period, it is striking that no one at all has a bad word to say about him, while his friendliness, generosity and trustworthiness excited frequent comment. The Scots scholar William Hamilton found him 'a very learned man, & an humble & cowrteous spirit; & one, whom I much esteeme'.[21] It should be said that when Hamilton wrote this, he had a vested interest in flattering Moriaen, through whom he thought he might be helped to a post at Franeker University.[22] The purpose of his letter was to ask Hartlib for a letter of recommendation to him. But others wrote in similar terms without there being any possibility of an ulterior motive. Comenius's son-in-law Petr Figulus knew him to be 'an honest & good man'.[23] Johannes Brun judged him 'a friendly and upright man, whose company is a pleasure, so far as I can tell'.[24] John Sadler expressly thanked Hartlib for putting him in contact with various friends including 'mr Morian; with whom I am never weary'.[25] Friedrich Kretschmar described him as 'a very respectable, Godfearing and unworldly man, also cheerful and communicative'.[26] Hartlib wrote of him to Winthrop as 'a man of a lovely spirit and a true nathaniel in the main',[27] and Winthrop in turn was delighted to hear good news about 'that honest worthy true Nathaniell as you are pleased rightly to terme him'.[28] Haak's heartfelt lament to the same addressee over the death of 'that dear & worthy frend of ours [...] whom I had so great a Desire to have seen once more' has already been cited.

Even the acerbic Joachim Poleman, whose letters abound in poison-pen-portraits of a wide variety of individuals and who found fault with almost everyone he encountered, accused Moriaen of nothing worse than gullibility, principally on the grounds of his association with Glauber and other pet hates of Poleman:[29]

> It may well be that Herr Moriaen is in possession of more true philosophy than he himself realises, but if such philosophy were a part of Herr Moriaen's own knowledge, it would not be possible for Glauber to dupe him, but it may well be that he has very important pieces of knowledge among the writings he owns.[30]

Coming from Poleman, such mild and morally neutral criticism virtually amounts to a testimonial. Poleman was not alone in seeing Moriaen as credulous: Worsley apparently passed similar judgment, and Moriaen himself - especially after he had lost all his money - did not deny it:

> Mr Worsley judges rightly of me, it is my lack and my failing that I believe too readily and entrust myself to others, and it is this that has ruined me, otherwise I should now stand in need of no one. I have ever striven rather after the innocence of the dove than the cunning of the serpent, which was not given me.[31]

This may ring more than a trifle sanctimonious to modern ears, but there is much evidence to suggest it is no more than the truth.

If he was little criticised by others in the circle, he in turn was singularly slow to chide. Though not afraid to speak his mind, he nearly always did so politely. As will be discussed in more detail, he was forthright in his criticisms of various members of the circle, including Hartlib himself, when he thought such criticism necessary. But his strictures were delivered in very measured, reasonable terms, as friendly admonitions rather than personal attacks. His comments on another man's work could equally well be seen as a characterisation of his own approach. Approving Hübner's harsh but on the whole objective (and certainly never *ad hominem*) criticisms of Comenius's *Didactica Magna*,[32] he asserted, 'it is altogether advisable and necessary that everything be most diligently examined and criticised privately and among friends before it is brought to light and made public'.[33]

It was only those he saw as working actively against the common good who roused his real ire. Given his generally placid and charitable disposition, it is almost startling to find him sharing the blood-lust against Strafford and Laud that gripped England in 1640 and 1641.[34] It would be as well to finish Strafford off quickly, he observed, in a rare excursion into realpolitik, or he would wriggle out of the net and it would have been better not to have tried him in the first place.[35] He saw Laud and Strafford as the men who had caused a schism between the King and his people - separated the head from the body, as Moriaen himself put it with unintentional prescient irony.[36] Laud, moreover, had actively obstructed the collections for the Palatinate, as Hartlib was to testify at the former's trial. Moriaen observed soon after Laud's arrest that he found it hard to believe there were still some in England who believed the Archbishop would be vindicated as a good patriot, the implication being that in Moriaen's eyes he was an obvious traitor.[37] Whether he saw that treachery as lying in Laud's supposed attempt to Romanise the Church of England or in more specific political manoeuvres is uncertain, but he certainly thought it merited the death penalty. Sending Hartlib a cipher by which he might convey politically sensitive information, Moriaen proposed, as a slightly macabre illustration of how it might be used, a sample encodement of the message 'episcopus morietur' ('the bishop is to die').[38]

The other abuse of power that completely outstepped the wide bounds of Moriaen's tolerance was the misapplication of alchemical wisdom. The note of grim satisfaction in a well-merited death is struck again in his bitter remark on the French alchemist Pierre Jean Fabré, 'If Fabré in France is dead, there is one deceiver less in the world'.[39] Fabré is not mentioned elsewhere in Moriaen's correspondence, and quite what he was supposed to have done to deserve such a caustic epitaph remains a mystery. There is little doubt, however, that the charge related to abuse of his art. There is a distinct sense in a great many writers of the group that alchemical enlightenment constituted a divinely-inspired insight into Creation quite as sacrosanct as any understanding of Scripture, so that any wilful misrepresentation or abuse of such knowledge was tantamount to heresy.

The New England alchemist George Starkey (or Stirk) (1628-1665), who introduced himself to Moriaen in May 1651,[40] and corresponded with him for an uncertain period thereafter, became the object of one of Moriaen's harshest denunciations after he lost his credit with the group. When he first reached England in the late 1640s, Starkey made a profound impression on many of the circle, including Boyle, with whom he worked as assistant-cum-collaborator from at least 1651 till 1652. However, a deep disillusionment with Starkey set in in 1654. The alchemist, despite his ability to turn antimony into silver and iron into gold (feats of which Dury was an eye witness[41]), twice found himself in gaol for debt, and Hartlib wrote indignantly to Boyle that 'he is altogether degenerated, and hath, in a manner, undone himself and his family. [...] He hath always concealed his rotten condition from us'.[42] Hartlib was not a man to despise anyone for having run into debt: it was the deceit that angered him, and his unaccustomed vehemence suggests that he bore other grudges too, not specified in the letter. It is typical of him, however, that he did not entirely despair of the American, and concluded the report, with an aptly chemical metaphor, 'When God hath brought you over again [Boyle was in Ireland at the time], we shall leave him altogether to your test, to try whether yet any good metal be left in him or not'.[43]

Reacting probably to comment of this sort from Hartlib, Moriaen denounced the American in no uncertain terms, hinting this time not just at false claims but at positively nefarious use of his undisputed gifts:

> It is a crying shame that the man does not better apply his understanding to good rather than evil, but that is the way of almost all such quick wits; they prefer to devote themselves to vanity rather than to pursue good works, while others who would gladly do so are not gifted with so much understanding.[44]

It is tempting to speculate that among these unfortunate souls whose good intentions are not matched by their gifts, Moriaen had himself in mind. But if to be principled and ungifted was a misfortune, to be gifted and unprincipled was a sin, and the force of this condemnation should not be underestimated. Moriaen was not a man to use the word 'evil' ('böße') lightly, and this passage represents not just disapproval but deep moral outrage.

Perhaps Moriaen's greatest disappointment in this respect was Clodius, a disappointment compounded no doubt by Moriaen's being at least partially responsible for his introduction to the circle and indeed his inclusion in Hartlib's family. Even from the first, the generally favourable impression made by Clodius was not universally shared. John Evelyn later described him, apparently with some justification, as 'a profess'd adeptus, who by the same *methodus mendichandi* [*practice of lying*] and pretence of extraordinary arcana, insinuated himselfe into the acquaintance of his father-in-law'.[45] It was not long after his arrival in England that Clodius's behaviour began to upset and offend his old patron. His high-handed and transparently duplicitous response to the publicity for Kuffler's ovens has already been described. This, however, was only the beginning of Moriaen's disillusionment.

Clodius repeatedly failed to reply to Moriaen's letters, and particularly to his requests for details of medicinal recipes and alchemical processes which Moriaen clearly saw as just return for similar secrets passed on by him to Clodius. This elicited many bitter complaints from the older man. Worst of all, Clodius neglected to put his skill in chemical medicine (of which few seem to have been in any doubt) at the disposal of his ailing father-in-law.[46] Indeed, at the beginning of 1658, he and his family moved out of the Hartlib household altogether. The reasons for this break-up of the family remain unknown, but there is an unmistakeable sense of disillusion in the cryptic account of the move Hartlib sent to Boyle: 'to my very great perplexity, Clodius is again in such a labyrinth, that he will be forced to break his ovens, and to remove to another house, which also is a new kind of undoing of him'.[47] (Whether Mary Hartlib took any consolation in having her kitchen restored to her goes unrecorded.)

Hartlib implied in the same letter that his son-in-law's departure meant he would have no more access to a medicine for the stone which Clodius had been preparing for him according to a recipe sent by Friedrich Kretschmar, which Hartlib considered the best he had ever tried. Again in April or May 1659, Hartlib told Boyle that 'my son [ie. Clodius] might have prepared

Ludus Helmontii for me before this time, but he wants bowels'.[48] Later, he sent a recipe for a 'water against the stone', hoping Boyle would persuade the chemist Peter Stahl to 'make a good quantity for yourself and the poor, and to let me also be partaker of it. Really, Sir, next to the ludus Helmontii I have found it the best medicine. There is no trusting to *Clodius* for it'.[49] Moriaen was furious with Clodius for this neglect of Hartlib. Like Starkey, he was failing to accept the responsibility that a gift from God entailed, and using it for personal advantage instead of rendering it back to the donor through service of his fellow man. The sense of such a responsibility lay at the heart of the ethos of Reformed intelligencers such as Moriaen, and his letters vividly demonstrate how central that ethos was to their perception and projection of themselves.

'Without Partialitie': the Irenic Ideal

There can be no question of Moriaen's piety. The manner of its expression, since he was entirely ungraced by the literary flair of a Böhme or a Bunyan, can at times come across misleadingly as smug or sanctimonious. He was much given - more and more so as he grew older - to long and often repetitious disquisitions on divine providence and the importance of abject submission to the will of God. While these may tax the patience of the modern reader, they were an essential part of a Reformed thinker's mind set, providing genuine comfort in the face of adversity and reassurance that there was a point to all his undertakings, whether successful or not. The same formulae recur over and again, like a litany, particularly with regard to his own and even more so to Hartlib's medical tribulations. It seems likely Hartlib found real solace in such effusions. He thought it worth abstracting a similar burst of pious platitudes from a letter of Poleman and noting it, in his own hand, under the heading 'Pietas Polmaniana'.[50]

Moriaen's orthodoxy in doctrinal terms is, however, much more in doubt, whichever brand of 'orthodoxy' one cares to look for. It is not that he was given to unorthodox pronouncements, rather that he was conspicuously not given to orthodox ones. His pious outbursts remain so firmly within the realm of generalisation, and so thoroughly avoid even the implicit invocation of any particular doctrine, that few of them, taken out of context, could be viewed as evidence of commitment to anything more specific than monotheism, let alone to any Christian sect.

I do not wish to suggest that the Enlightenment deism of figures such as Voltaire had sprung fully-fledged into being a century early in the mind of this unassuming amateur natural philosopher. Moriaen undoubtedly regarded himself as a Christian, and the almost complete lack of reference in his letters either to Christ himself or to Christianity as a world-view merely reflects the fact that he took them as so self-evident as not to be worth mentioning. What is significant, and is in striking contrast to the majority of writers of his period, is his discreet but steadfast eschewal of assent to any particular understanding of the nature of Christ and his teaching. Though it was the ostensible view of all in the Evangelical camp that the whole truth was contained in the Scriptures and no other foundation was required for true faith, in practice, most found themselves repeatedly obliged to clarify or elaborate on the pronouncements of Christ for the benefit of less 'spiritual men' who had managed to misinterpret them - whether at the most refined theological level or simply in respect of day-to-day behaviour. The distinctive feature of Moriaen's writing is that he quotes the Bible, or at least refers to God and His word, in virtually every surviving letter, but without a single trace of exegesis.

If he was recognisably the product of a Calvinist upbringing, it is clear that, at least by the beginning of his surviving correspondence (for it would be rash to assume his opinions were consistent throughout his life), he troubled himself little about the finer points of Calvinist doctrine. Two of Moriaen's closest friends in the ministry, Justinus Van Assche and Petrus Serrarius, were excommunicated for their unorthodoxy, Serrarius temporarily, Van Assche, it seems, permanently. There is not the least sign that Moriaen thought any the less of either of them for this. When Serrarius applied to be accepted back into the fold at the beginning of 1637, Moriaen wrote to Van Assche, 'I wish Mr Serrarius a better success than I can well hope for, partiality being all too great nowadays'.[51] As is evident from the terms of this gloomy (as things turned out, unduly gloomy) prognostication, Moriaen thought not that Serrarius was too intransigent to deserve readmission, but that the Church was too intransigent to readmit him.

The fact that Moriaen was for several years a minister of the Reformed Church - and not just occupying a comfortable living, but undergoing constant personal danger for what can have been at best a paltry material reward - should not be seen in any sense as evidence of wholehearted assent to the finer points of that Church's teaching. Of the hundreds of 'enthusiasts' whose supposedly extravagant and misguided opinions caused so many headaches for both the Lutheran and the Calvinist authorities of Germany as well as the Anglican ones in this country, a great many were ordained ministers. I do not mean to suggest that Moriaen was himself such an 'enthusiastic' preacher: on the contrary, all the evidence suggests he had no doctrinal tub whatsoever to thump. My point is merely that the fact of his ministerial calling gives no more than a very broad indication of what his beliefs were. And I would suggest that, in later life at least, he distanced himself from all doctrinal details, including those his ostensible church deemed fundamental, to a degree that amounts to unorthodoxy by default.

Neither Calvin's name nor any derivation of it is mentioned in his extant writings (with one exception, where he is quoting someone else).[52] But this does not in itself reflect any rejection of Calvin's views. On the contrary, Calvin had never set himself up as the founder of a sect (any more than Luther), and would himself have thoroughly disapproved of the term 'Calvinist'. Insofar as Moriaen was of the Reformed faith, it was not in its respect for but on the contrary its rejection of any merely human authority in matters of religion.

This is precisely the charge laid against the Lutherans among whom he had grown up in the one surviving letter in which Moriaen commented on the validity of any particular church's teaching. His remarks on Lutheranism confirm that he disapproved not so much of this sect in particular as of sectarianism per se. The great fault of Lutherans, in his eyes, was that implicit in their name: that they had set up an individual human being as arbiter of matters beyond human jurisdiction, ascribing to him an authority he had never claimed for himself, and 'taken this mans every utterance for pure Gospel'.[53] He cited the faithful noting down of Luther's *Table Talk* in all its notorious vulgarity as a prime example of this inappropriate (if not positively idolatrous) excess of respect for an individual human authority. But Moriaen characteristically went out of his way to absolve Luther himself of the errors committed in his name: 'the blame for which, however, is not so much to be laid on Luther as on those who unthinkingly take his every word for pure holy writ'.[54] Luther had only aspired to be the translator and broadcaster of the sacred word, or a commentator upon it, not its author. Though Moriaen was fairly disparaging about the *Table Talk* itself, he maintained a discreet silence with regard to his views on Luther's more serious theological work - or, for that matter, anyone else's.

Van Der Wall summarises well the attitude of Serrarius and intimates such as Moriaen and Van Assche: 'Impartial, catholic, universal: these are the key words by which they expressed their ideal of Christianity'.[55] ('Impartial', at least in its modern sense, is less than satisfactory as a translation of either the Dutch 'onpartijdig' or the German 'unparteilich' (older German 'unparteiisch'), but there is no modern English word that will do. There is a sense not only of disinterested standing back from overt espousal of any camp, but also of disapproval of the existence of such camps in the first place. This is the sense of 'impartial' as it was used by Dury and other irenicists and the one in which it will be used here in characterising Moriaen's ideas.) 'Unparteiisch' was one of Moriaen's highest commendations of a group or an individual, and its opposite, 'parteiisch', by the same token one of his sternest criticisms.

His one initial objection to Bisterfeld was, 'He is still rather too much given over to partiality'.[56] Hugely impressed by the writings of Hübner, he declared: 'this bespeaks a penetrating and profoundly understanding spirit, and, which to me is the most important, one free from partiality and thirsting only after truth',[57] and again in almost the same words, 'I already sense remarkable gifts in this man, and, which delights me above all, a free and impartial spirit'.[58] He similarly recommended the (unnamed) bearer of one early letter as 'an upright and impartial lover of truth whose company is a pleasure'.[59] It was perhaps part of the appeal of Comenius that he belonged to a church (the Unitas Fratrum - 'Unity of Brethren', also known, inaccurately, as the Bohemian Brethren[60]) that acknowledged neither Luther nor Calvin as its founder but respected both, while its acknowledged father figure Jan Hus was in turn respected by the adherents of both main branches of Western European Evangelicism. One of the things that most distressed Moriaen about Comenius was, conversely, his addiction to doctrinal debate and personal polemic. Even the refutation of as unorthodox a figure as Felgenhauer seemed to Moriaen counter-productive, liable to alienate in advance a portion of the potential audience for Pansophy, the universal wisdom to which all humankind might acquiesce: 'this takes up much of his time and renders him partial in the eyes of many'.[61] Advising in similar terms against Comenius's becoming embroiled in controversy with opponents of Pansophy, Moriaen urged a course which Comenius certainly never followed, but which does provide quite a good description of Moriaen's own approach in his correspondence:

> My advice, in my simplicity, would be that, given such diversity of sects
> and opinions, one should keep oneself disinterested and impartial as far and
> for as long as possible, keeping to generalities and not entering into
> particulars.[62]

This conscious and conspicuous standing back from controversy about
doctrinal niceties is a consistent feature of Moriaen's approach to religion from
his earliest surviving letters to his last. Like Dury, he was convinced that the
'incidentals' of faith were of little significance, provided a community could
be formed on the basis of 'fundamentals'. Dury too had a marked liking for
the word 'impartial' (or, as he more often wrote, 'unpartiall').[63] So thorough
was Moriaen's eschewal of comment on potentially divisive 'incidentals' that
it is virtually impossible to deduce what he did regard as fundamental, beyond
the idea that there is one Supreme Being whose will is discernible in the Bible
and the natural world, and that it behooves mankind to acquiesce unreservedly
in that will.

Very revealing of his attitudes is his reaction to the report that his and
Hartlib's mutual friend Johannes Brun (better known by his pseudonym
'Unmüssig', i.e. 'diligent') had fallen prey to atheism, the spectre that so
haunted the experimental scientists of the seventeenth century. Brun was a
Paracelsian physician who, after an itinerant youth during which he was for a
time employed (and, he claimed, cheated) by Prince Rakóczi of
Transylvania,[64] and also spent some time in Turkey, joined the influx of
European projectors and scientists to England from 1648 on. He bore a
recommendation from Rulice and soon made friends with Hartlib:[65] he
appears with considerable frequency as a source of information and
commentary on medical and chemical matters in the *Ephemerides* of 1648
onwards. He later moved to Ireland, which is where he allegedly fell into
atheism.[66]

Moriaen's first response to the news was appropriate horror - 'it fairly
staggered me'[67] - but he immediately followed this by making the crucial
semantic distinction so rarely formulated at the period: was this atheism in the
strict sense - that is to say a rejection of the existence of any god of any kind -
or denial of the 'correct' understanding of such a being?

The looseness with which the term 'atheism' was so widely used at the
time should not lead us to underrate the seriousness with which the charge
was laid. If 'atheism' tended not to mean knowing no god but having a false
impression of God, that did not make it any less worrying and dangerous an
error.[68] For the majority of believers, of whatever brand, to misunderstand
God's nature was tantamount to denying His existence, if not worse. To
most people at this period, the idea that there was no divinity at all was such
manifest nonsense that it barely called for refutation. A distorted image,
however, was likely to be far more seductive to those insufficiently strong in
the faith (whichever faith). Hence, the vast majority of attacks on 'atheism'
address not denials but misconceptions of God. Such misconceptions could
refer to any number of the divine attributes: to the Trinity, to God's
providential scheme and activity in the world, to his nature while on earth in
person, to transubstantiation or consubstantiation at communion, and so on ad
infinitum.

Moriaen explicitly distanced himself from this etymological inexactitude in a manner that has important implications for an assessment of his own views. He wanted to know of the charge against Brun 'whether it is atheism in the strict sense or a rejection of Holy Scripture'.[69] A clear distinction is drawn here between the rejection of god as a concept and the rejection of a particular conception of God. While it is not stated in so many words that the latter error is less serious than the former, the implication is barely veiled. The sentence almost demands to be read '... or *only* a rejection ...'.

This is followed by a suggestion for guiding Brun back onto the true path: 'Herr Boreel customarily argues against atheists by the light of Nature, and convinces them by it both that there is a God and that Scripture is his word'.[70] But if this is a recommendation of Adam Boreel's philosophy - and it can hardly be seen as anything else - Moriaen was selecting an authority peculiarly unacceptable to any established church of the day. Boreel, who has already been encountered in the context of his studies of Judaism, was the founder of the Collegiants, a group which was virtually by definition unorthodox. The Collegiant position was that any human mediation between God's word and mankind was a corruption of it. They accepted no church and recognised no form of preaching beyond the unadorned reading of the Bible. God, they maintained, had already said what he meant and did not need mortals to clarify it. To attempt to explain his message was to pervert it.[71]

Indeed, if Moriaen's account of Boreel's attitude is accurate, his views were even more radical than this. It was generally accepted as a given, within all the Evangelical camps, that Scripture is true. There remained endless scope for dispute on how to interpret it, but that fundamental point was taken as read. This is the starting point, for instance, of Dury's *Analysis Demonstrativa*.[72] Dury's aim in this work was to establish a method of Scriptural analysis that would be acceptable to all sides, so that having applied it, all sides might concur on the unambiguous interpretation it would yield. Though there is much discussion in the tract of undeniable first principles on which the edifice of interpretation can be founded, the initial assumption that what Scripture is found to mean once it has been interpreted aright must necessarily be true is taken as so self-evident that it is not even mentioned. Here, however, we have Boreel (as reported by Moriaen) considering that this tenet itself needs to be proven - as does God's very existence. Particularly interesting is that he is said to have set out to do so 'by the light of nature'. This supplies an interesting counterpart to Descartes' more famous crisis of faith. Descartes' solution to mounting uncertainty about the nature of knowledge was to take his own intellect as the given, and to found his whole inductive logic on the first principle of *cogito ergo sum*. Those hailing from the Evangelical wing who fell prey to similar doubts tended to rely less on their rational faculties for reassurance, and to depend rather on the evidence of their senses, as illuminated by a blend of personal spiritual enlightenment with practical observation.

Regrettably, Moriaen made no attempt to explain how Boreel purported to demonstrate the existence of God and the divine provenance of the Scriptures 'by the light of Nature'. But such a strategy represents a bold assertion of the primacy of enlightened observation and demonstration over doctrine and faith. For there was developing at this period an unsettling sense that these two camps were in opposition. Thomas Browne regarded such conflict as an opportunity for salutary exercise in subjugating reason and sense perception to faith: 'thus I teach my haggard and unreclaimed reason to stoope unto the lure of faith [...] this I think is no vulgar part of faith to believe a thing not only above, but contrary to reason, and against the arguments of our proper senses'.[73] Boreel's approach, to be sure, denies such a conflict: on the contrary, faith, reason and the senses are portrayed as pointing all to the same conclusion. But it is not Scripture that confirms the accuracy of observation, it is observation that confirms the validity of Scripture. This shift in priorities was viewed with alarm by more conservative thinkers, and with good reason. For if 'haggard and unreclaimed reason' refused to stoop, what would happen when human faculties misguidedly pointed to a conclusion that, instead of confirming Scripture, flatly contradicted the divinely vouchsafed truths?

Moriaen, however, seems to have had no such difficulties. He was himself throughout his life a tireless investigator of nature and an equally tireless quoter of Scripture. The latter habit was of course second nature to a trained Protestant preacher, though the Scriptural references became if anything more numerous as the years went by and the days of his active service in the Church receded into the past. But nowhere in his surviving correspondence - not even when he was commenting on specifically theological tracts - is there any remark whatsoever about any given Scriptural interpretation. One almost gains the impression that Moriaen did not bother his head unduly about the precise meaning of God's word, that being assured in general terms of the covenant between his Creator and himself and of the duties it imposed on and reassurances it offered him, he was content to go through this life at least suspending judgment on the finer details.

This apparent indifference to doctrinal issues may of course merely have been a stance adopted in the interests of avoiding discord and of promoting his ideal of a Church unity based on tolerance and latitudinarianism. There can be no knowing what inner debates he kept to himself. But the fact that he advocated the use of non-Christian texts as supporting evidence of religious belief, and that he saw the validity of Scripture as being endorsed by empirical evidence rather than vice versa, strongly suggests an anti-literalist stance, an acceptance that the sacred texts were true according to the spirit rather than the letter, and a willingness to modify the understanding of them on the basis of non-Scriptural evidence.

Given his milieu, it is particularly stiking that he never commented, so far as the surviving letters reveal, on the millenarian speculations and prophecies that were so eagerly discussed in Hartlib's circle and that have been depicted (I think correctly) as an important motive force driving its three great proposed reforms: Comenius's of education, Dury's of the church and Hartlib's of knowledge. But without overtly espousing such notions, he did, just occasionally, himself strike a revelatory note reminiscent of the millenarians and chiliasts with whom he was so familiar. The apocalyptic flavour of his comments on the gathering political crisis in England at the beginning of the 1640s has already been noted. In an alchemical letter to Van Assche, he directly related the Paracelsian prophecy of an unveiling to all men of the hidden secrets of Nature to the visions of Revelation: 'we expect, according to His will, not only a new Heaven but also a new earth in which redemption shall dwell'.[74] In other letters too he spoke explicitly of anticipating a 'Dawn of Wisdom'.[75] The nearest he came to an overtly millenial statement was in his comments on the plans Hartlib was promoting in the 1650s for a universal language that would undo the curse of Babel:[76]

> it is to be hoped that the time has come, or is not far off, when not only
> shall we be able to write to and understand one another in a common
> script, but shall learn to acknowledge, praise and glorify God with one
> voice, in the day of the revelation of the Son of Man.[77]

One of Moriaen's favourite platitudes was 'time will reveal all' ('die zeit wird alles offenbahren') - neatly encapsulating both the confident expectation that all *will* be revealed and the modest acceptance that it has *not* been revealed yet. While this is generally used with regard to relatively mundane matters rather than to God's broader purposes, a man of his background and training could hardly use the word 'reveal' without at least half-conscious reference to the last book of the Bible.[78] This suggests again a willingness to dispense with certainties about specific details, to suspend judgment on exactly how and when the prophecy would be fulfilled until the event itself should reveal it.

Comenius was explicit about the millenarian impulse behind his work, as was Dury (though he became more sceptical about the subject after Christ's expected reappearance in the 1650s failed to occur). Moriaen's friend Serrarius was an utterly committed chiliast. Hartlib is frequently assumed to have shared such views, though in fact concrete evidence of Hartlib's personal opinions is almost as scanty as that of Moriaen's. He certainly took a lively interest in the discussion, and encouraged or sponsored publication of the apocalyptic speculations of John Stoughton, Joseph Mede and Francis Potter ('the 666. divine', as Hartlib called him with probably unintentional humour[79]), but this should not be taken as wholehearted assent to their opinions.[80] It is not justifiable to assume that Hartlib unqualifiedly agreed with whatever he had a hand in printing or publishing: his aim was to promote discussion rather than to promote any one school of thought. It is nonetheless clear that these men moved in circles where millenarianism was a burning issue, and if Hartlib's acquaintance with Stoughton and Potter, or Moriaen's with Serrarius, is no proof that they accepted their views, it is clear they did not object to them and virtually inconceivable that they were wholly untouched by them.

Uncertain as Moriaen's private views on pretty well any specific point of Christian doctrine must remain, what does emerge quite unequivocally from his correspondence is that he did not wish to impose those views on anyone else. He repeatedly stressed his advocacy of freedom of conscience, and as has already been noted it was precisely that freedom that most appealed to him about the United Provinces.

His comments on the views of Paul Felgenhauer, for instance, are strikingly non-committal. Though Felgenhauer disagreed violently with Boreel, and accused him of Socinianism,[81] their attitudes to organised religion were in many respects very similar. Felgenhauer too rejected every form of established church. He was particularly scathing about the Lutheran faith in which he had grown up as the son of a pastor, but his scorn was spread liberally across the whole spectrum of Christian confessionalisation. Felgenhauer, like Böhme, maintained that Christ had come to save the entire human race, Jews, Moslems and heathens not excepted, let alone Christians of any specific denomination. His views on the nature of Christ were perhaps the most notorious element in what was one of the century's more notorious unorthodoxies. He vehemently denied the doctrine that Christ had literally become human, for Christ was God, and it was inconceivable that the Creator should become a creature. Christ was indeed the word of God made flesh, but this was a spiritual flesh wholly distinct from the perishable flesh inhabited by mortals. By the same token, the Lutheran idea of consubstantiation at Communion was as absurd, in Felgenhauer's eyes, as the Catholic notion of transubstantiation. Christ, as a partaker of the divine nature, could not possibly be constituted in perishable matter, be it wafers, bread or human flesh. He had taken on human form but never human substance.

The fact that, in what was effectively a semi-public account of such a heresy, Moriaen made not the slightest attempt to distance himself from it is in itself a statement of sorts, especially given that he knew very well the account was likely to be copied out and distributed. His reports state merely the opinion Felgenhauer held and the fact that he had been arrested for it.[82] There would be no justification for reading this as agreement with or support for Felgenhauer's views, but it can surely be seen as a tacit declaration that the man was entitled to his opinion. Moriaen had earlier been very keen to obtain a copy of Comenius's refutation of Felgenhauer, which he received in late 1640 and subsequently passed on to Hartlib,[83] but here again he gave not the least hint as to which side of the controversy he favoured, or indeed as to whether his own mind was made up on the subject. His only comment on Comenius's work was that he was sorry to see him engaging publicly in polemics.[84]

He had been more explicit in condemning the prescriptive attitude of the Hamburg school authorities to Joachim Jungius's *Logica Hamburgensis*.[85] Jungius was rector of Hamburg gymnasium, a linguist and natural scientist of considerable distinction, and an innovative educationalist who took a keen interest in the pansophic project of Comenius backed by Hartlib and Moriaen. The *Logica Hamburgensis* was commissioned as a standard up-to-date school text on logical method, but while still in preparation it fell foul of the authorities for being altogether too up-to-date in its criticisms of and diversions from Aristotle. It was not, to be sure, suspected of being anywhere near as controversial as Felgenhauer's work; but on the other hand, it was a commissioned text-book for use in schools, and the school authorities did not want to see their wards steered too far from the traditional educational ethos that still regarded Aristotle (or medieval and Renaissance interpretations of him) as the highest authority in secular matters.

Exactly how much of the text Jungius reworked to comply with their specifications cannot now be ascertained, but one of Jungius's students put it about that the work was called *Logica Hamburgensis* because it represented Hamburg's idea of logic, not that of Jungius.[86] Moriaen's letters lend weight to this by retailing exactly the same story, with another acquaintance of Jungius, Johannes Tanckmar, as the source: '[Jungius] says of his *Logic*, "It is not my *Logic* but the Hamburg schoolmen's," for they have prescribed to him how they wish to have it'.[87] Moriaen deemed it 'a crying shame both for him and for us that Herr Jungius, because of the intransigence of those among whom he lives, must rein in his spirit and cannot express it freely'.[88] It appears there was talk of Jungius's obtaining a university post at Amsterdam, and Moriaen was extremely keen for him to take this up, that he might have liberty to apply his brain as he saw fit.[89] In the event, however, nothing came of the idea.

Worse still, in Moriaen's eyes, was the attitude of the Unitas Fratrum to the controversy engendered when Hieronim Broniewski, a lay elder of the Unity, denounced Comenius's pansophic work as an unseemly blend of divine and human wisdom. Comenius was called before Synods of the Unity in August 1638 and March 1639 to defend his stance, and though the outcome was far from being a vindication of Broniewski, it still entailed much more of a circumscription of Comenius's activities than Moriaen thought reasonable. Though he was given official sanction to proceed with his pansophic studies, this was with the rider that he should publish nothing without first submitting it to the Synod and receiving their approval. Moriaen was immediately concerned that Comenius would be driven, like Jungius (he drew the comparison explicitly), to commit himself to a doctrinal camp, compromising the treasured ideal of impartiality: 'the freedom to write the truth as he perceives it with his own heart and soul is thereby taken from him; he will be forced to commit himself to a party and by that token be the less acceptable to any other'.[90]

He seems to have been in no doubt that Hartlib would view the situation similarly: indeed, he went on to suggest that Hartlib was providing a means of side-stepping this censorship by receiving copies of Comenius's work without the Synod's knowledge, thus ensuring the survival of the original, undoctored versions: 'the best of it is that you [Hartlib] receive his things before they fall into the hands of the censors; if they will then not permit them, the right thing may be still be done'.[91] Whether Comenius was aware of such machinations to protect his work from the supervision of his own church is unfortunately not known, though it is certain that Hartlib did not, in the event, publish anything the Synod had censored. Indeed, the only thing they did forbid Comenius to publish was the book of prophecies *Lux in tenebris*, about which Hartlib and Moriaen themselves had considerable misgivings, and in this instance Comenius went against both the orders of his superiors and the advice of his friends, and had the thing published at his own expense anyway. But it is striking to find Hartlib being presented in this fashion as guarantor of Comenius's freedom of speech, protecting him and his work, in effect, from his own confessional allegiance.

Most unequivocal of all such statements was Moriaen's reaction to a report of the arrest in England of a number of anabaptists. As usual, he gave no indication as to whether his sympathy for the detainees extended to their opinions or merely to their right to hold them, but he observed most forthrightly that that right was inalienable, and that the English Parliament was being hypocritical by condemning religious compulsion on the one hand (in such manifestations, presumably, as the Laudianisation of the Church of England and the Catholicisation of the Palatinate) while exercising it on the other against these hapless anabaptists. It was an action

which becomes them most ill who condemn compulsion of conscience in others. It were well done to encourage the release of these people at once, if they have indeed been apprehended only for their beliefs and are not otherwise criminal.[92]

This is, surely, a broad hint that Hartlib should use his contacts in Parliament to sue for the prisoners' release.

It was this steadfast refusal to make any concessions to partisanship or sectarianism that led, if not exactly to a falling out, at least to a marked difference of opinion and cooling of relations with Dury, with regard to the strategies to be adopted in the quest for church unity. Where Moriaen parted company with Dury was in that the latter, seeing 'incidentals' as unimportant, was prepared ostensibly to espouse (or reject) any of them at any given time in order to win round a given candidate to the cause of reconciliation. Rather than pick and mix, Moriaen consistently distanced himself from the lot.

Dury's idea was to draw up, as it were, a new and more inclusive Formula of Concord, an elucidation of the fundamental truths of Christianity to which all the Evangelical churches would be willing to subscribe. Having achieved this, he would persuade them all to agree publicly that freedom of conscience on all other issues should be granted, and that no one should criticise anyone else for holding a different view on such incidentals. To this end, he engaged for half a century in what was effectively a form of shuttle diplomacy, devoting a quite extraordinary amount of time, money and energy to travelling around England, Germany, the Netherlands and Scandinavia, conducting negotiations with the ruling bodies of the assorted Protestant groups and attempting to present each side's views to the others in as favourable a light as possible. As one of his less well-disposed chroniclers puts it, 'His powers of boredom had wearied a continent'.[93] To Moriaen's suggestion that he would do better to settle down in one place and devote himself to private study, Dury retorted without a trace of irony that he quite agreed and had every intention of settling in Bremen at the first opportunity, but needed first to conclude a few outstanding negotiations in Lübeck, Helmstadt, Rostock, Hamburg, Denmark, England and Holland.[94]

Dury's somewhat uncritical biographer remarks with supreme understatement that his 'method of presenting his cause varied from time to time'.[95] His devoted scribe and future brother-in-law Heinrich Appelius meant to compliment him by writing that he 'imitated Paul labouring to become all things to all men, that hy might in any respect gett et gaine men to the trueth'.[96] But a good many others profoundly mistrusted him (as many at the time had mistrusted Paul) for precisely this reason. To the Puritan William Prynne he was a 'time-serving Proteus and ambidexter divine',[97] while Caspar Heinrich Starck's staunchly Lutheran *Lübeckische Kirchen-Geschichte* is no less scathing of this 'ill-starred peacemaker and as it were Apostolic Nuntio of the Reformed' and his 'irenical, or rather ironical counsels'.[98] His conscious policy throughout his 'irenical' projects of presenting whatever face he thought a given interlocutor would find most appealing, in order to alienate none of them, more often than not had precisely the opposite effect and alienated them all. Moriaen himself became quite exasperated with Dury, not indeed because he thought him a hypocrite, but because he saw how counter-productive his strategies were.

Not only did Moriaen consider that Dury was wasting time, energy and money that might be devoted to more useful causes on his endless diplomatic journeys, he also felt that Dury's personal involvement in the endeavour was positively detrimental to the aim of reconciliation. Some account has already been given of the very low esteem in which Dury was held on both sides of the doctrinal divide. Moriaen repeatedly stressed how poor Dury's reputation was in the Netherlands, on account, presumably, of his extensive and very public contacts with Anglicans and Lutherans: 'most people here disapprove of his project and are suspicious of his person'.[99] After Moriaen had repeated this point three times in less than a month, Hartlib apparently objected to this assessment of his friend, for a little later Moriaen carefully dissociated himself from these condemnations of Dury and assured Hartlib, 'Nor do I neglect to redeem his honour and defend his good name as often as the occasion arises'.[100] Nonetheless, while protesting his own confidence in Dury's personal integrity, he continued to cast doubt on the feasibility of his pacification work and to express his disappointment that Dury would not accept some settled post and devote himself to private scholarly activity for the furtherance of Pansophy.

Dury has been celebrated as an 'Advocate of Christian Reunion'.[101] But as Anthony Milton points out in his shrewd and precise analysis of the 'politics of irenicism', virtually everyone in Christendom was an advocate of Christian reunion: 'most thinkers of this period accepted that religious unity was a good idea, in the same way that they believed sin was a bad idea'.[102] The devil, of course, was in the detail. Dury had no great difficulty in persuading Protestants to agree, in principle, to agree, but the question of what to agree about was somewhat thornier. Milton observes, with regard to English Puritans, that 'those divines who were most enthusiastic for union with the Lutherans on the level of theory were most likely to be those least capable of achieving it in practice'.[103] Moriaen made exactly the same point, though in more general terms: 'once one comes down to details and the conditions for reconciliation, there will be far more to be done, and those who seemed most favourable in general terms may well turn out to be the most unwilling'.[104]

It is this letter that provides Moriaen's fullest and most considered criticism of Dury's approach. Negotiation, Moriaen pointed out, had so far served rather to exacerbate than to diminish mutual resentments over contentious details. At least during the earlier part of his correspondence with Hartlib, Moriaen staked his hopes for reconciliation on Comenius's notion of Pansophy, a new way of looking at the world that would teach humanity to put aside all dogma and see everything afresh, unblinkered by received ideas. If Pansophy could not achieve this, declared Moriaen in almost so many words, God would have to do it himself: 'if people can be convinced by this means, reconciliation will follow of its own accord; if not, we must wait on a higher power'.[105]

Hartlib passed this detailed and apposite analysis on to Dury, who replied somewhat huffily and at equal length, but without in fact addressing Moriaen's main point.[106] The gist of his response is a tautology: once people have been persuaded to commit themselves not to argue about incidentals, they will find themselves bound by their own word not to argue about incidentals. He gave no straight answer to the question of how people were to be persuaded to agree on the definition of an incidental. Dury was very prickly, and for good reason, about charges that he was behaving like a mere diplomat, a political negotiator interfering with the balance of temporal power: he 'declared his passionate determination to avoid "worldly wisdome" precisely because it was a constant temptation for him.'[107] This aspect of

Dury's character comes to the fore in his high-handed dismissal of the objections to his schemes made by Moriaen and others:

> they do imagine a thing which is more humane and politic then I aime at therefore theire doubts are to *them* true difficultyes, but to mee none; because I walke not in *the* sphere wherein theire apprehension of *the* matter doth stand.[108]

Later, Moriaen lost faith in Pansophy, or at least in the prospect of Comenius's providing an adequate formulation of it, and looked rather to the experimental investigation of Nature for a frame of reference on which humanity might agree to build afresh a new and unifying religious vision of the world. Dury features with significantly less frequency in his later letters, and in mid-1657 Moriaen remarked that he had lost touch with him altogether.[109] Moriaen's attitude to the irenical scheme, however, remained unchanged. He commented on it a last time at the beginning of 1658 by damning it with faint praise: so long as Dury kept up his efforts, he wrote, the lovers of truth and peace would at least be able to say no stone had been left unturned.[110]

This disagreement with Dury over the strategies to be adopted in the promotion of ecumenicism goes to the heart of Moriaen's ideological outlook. Dury's mistake, as Moriaen saw it, was to attack the symptoms of discord instead of the cause. Dury wanted to negotiate about details, about outward forms and ceremonies, to achieve compromise between the different sects on the externals of religion, and thus by paring back such externals to demonstrate that all these branches grew from the same stem. Moriaen, though never so overtly radical as Boreel or Felgenhauer, shared their desire to go back further, to set aside all sectarianism and begin again from the root. Whether or not he shared the millenarian and chiliastic views of many of his friends and associates, he certainly anticipated, and believed he was contributing to, a new and more fundamental Reformation. The time for quibbling over niceties was over: what was needed now was to look at the whole Creation afresh, to learn a new and truer reading of Scripture, of Nature and of Mankind itself.

> In sum, the Dawn of Wisdom will hopefully soon break, for all things in all places point so promisingly towards it. God grant that the Sun of Justice may create a new day, enlightening in sanctity the whole pitch dark world.[111]

He spent his whole life watching for the dawn.

Notes

1 *HDC*, 248; Dorothy Dury to Hartlib, n.d., HP 3/2/143A-144B. The publication has not survived.

2 William Newman, 'Prophecy and Alchemy: The Origin of Eiranæus Philalethes', *Ambix* 37 (part 3, Nov. 1990), 97-115, esp.101-2.

3 See Mark Greengrass, 'Samuel Hartlib and Scribal Publication', *Acta Comeniana* 12

4   (1997), 89-104

5   Moriaen to Hartlib, 20 Oct. 1639, HP 37/44A.

   Moriaen to Hartlib, 23 Jan. 1640, HP 37/53B.

6   Moriaen to Worsley, 27 Jan. 1651, HP 9/16/1A.

7   Hartlib to Winthrop, 16 March 1660, HP 7/7/3A.

8   Hartlib to Boyle, 24 July 1649, Boyle, *Works* VI, 78. The first mention of Moriaen in their surviving correspondence occurs on 9 May 1648 (ibid., 77).

9   Poleman to Hartlib, 5 Dec. 1659, HP 60/4/159A; cf. Chapter Five, section 3.

10   Hartlib to Boyle, c. June/July 1658, Boyle, *Works* VI, 111.

11   'zeithero meinem Iungst*en* hatt es Gott gefallen mein ainiges Kindt mit kranckheit zue besuch*en* vnd endlich von dieser welt abzuefordern, welche kranckheit tod vnd begräbnus vnd was demselb*en* anhängig mich eine zeit hero zue hauß gehalten, vnd an gewunschter fortsezung gehindert hatt' - Moriaen to Hartlib, 12 Aug. 1639, HP 37/36B-37A.

12   'niemand sich behelffen sondern vollauff haben will wie mans beÿ guten zeiden gewohnet hatt' - Moriaen to Hartlib, 24 Aug. 1657, HP 42/2/18B.

13   Moriaen to ?, 31 Jan. 1651, HP 63/14/4A.

14   Moriaen to Hartlib, 1 Sept. 1639, HP 37/39A.

15   *HDC*, 244-9, and see especially Dorothy Dury's letters to Hartlib of 1644-45 (just before and after her marriage), HP 21/5/18A, 21/5/22A, 3/2/144A.

16   Moriaen to Hartlib, 5 April 1640, HP 37/62A.

17   'konde mich so bewegen das nicht ein bluts-tropfe an seinem ortt bliebe' - Moriaen to ?, 17 Oct. 1653, HP 63/14/22A.

18   'die Bethaw diese lange zeit ganz under waßer gelegen kombt nun wied*er* so grun herfur das ein lust anzuesehe*n* ist Gott mach uns danckbar für seine genade' - Moriaen to Hartlib, 2 April 1658, HP 31/18/15A.

19   'noch nicht unerträglich' - Moriaen to Hartlib, 25 June 1658, HP 31/18/37A.

20   *Eph 48*, HP 31/22/29B

21   Hamilton to Hartlib, 16/26 Nov. 1650 MP 9/11/27A.

22   Hamilton had become friendly with Dury and Hartlib in 1647 and not long afterwards added his signature to their pact with Comenius committing themselves to mutual support both moral and financial in their efforts for church unity and the reform of learning (HP 7/109/1A-2B, transc. *HDC*, 458-460). Ten years later he fell out with them and was released from it (HP 9/11/31A-34B). See *HDC*, 262-3, 287-9. He had left England to avoid complying with the 1650 Act of Allegiance and was seeking employment in the Netherlands.

23   Figulus to Hartlib, 2 Nov. 1658, HP 9/17/43A, transc. in Blekastad, *Figulus Letters*, 235.

24   'ein freundlicher vnd aufrichtiger Man [...] deßen man wohl genießen kan so viel ich vermercke' - Brun to Hartlib, 13 June 1649, HP 39/2/9A.

25   Sadler to Hartlib, n.d., HP 46/9/23A.

26   'ein sehr stattlicher gottliebender, welthassender, erfahrner, auch lustiger und conversabler mann' - Kretschmar to Hartlib, 1 Aug. 1659, HP 26/64/4A.

27   Hartlib to John Winthrop, 16 March 1660, HP 7/7/3A.

28   Winthrop to Hartlib, 25 Oct. 1660, HP 32/1/9A.

29   See below, pp. 203-5..

30   'Daß Her Morian mehr rechte philosophie beÿ sich habe, als er selber wiße, solches kan gar wol sein [...]; so aber Her Morian solche philosophi in seiner

eigenthümblichen Scients hatte, so würde er vom Glaubero nicht können bethöret werden; aber es mag wol seÿn, daß er magk sehr wichtige wißenschafften in Scriptis haben' - Poleman to Hartlib, 19 Sept. 1659, HP 60/4/101A.

31   'H Worslej urtheilt recht von mir dz ist mein mangel und fehler dz ich so leicht glaübe und des besten mich zue anderen versehen thue und das hatt mich umb das meinige gebracht sonst würde Ich izund niemands nötig haben. Ich habe der einfalt der dauben mich allezeit mehr beflissen als der Schlangen klugheit die mir nicht gegeben ist' - Moriaen to Hartlib, 14 June 1658, HP 31/18/29B; cf. Matthew 10:16.

32   See Kvacala, 'Über die Schicksale der *Didactica Magna*', *MCG* 8 (1899), 129-44.

33   'es ist durch auch [*sic, for* durchaus] rathsam vnd nötig das alles inter amicos privatim auffs fleisigste examinirt vnd censurirt werde, che mans vnder die leuthe vnd ans liecht kommen laße' - Moriaen to Hartlib, 5 Dec. 1639, HP 37/49A.

34   For a full account of this, see Anthony Fletcher, *The Outbreak of the English Civil War* (revised edition London, 1984), 6-17.

35   Moriaen to Hartlib, 18 April 1641, HP 37/85A.

36   'Nun müßen wir mit großen betrubnus vernehmen das das haubt vnd der leib getrennet werden' - Moriaen to Hartlib, 27 Jan. 1642, HP 37/101A.

37   Moriaen to Hartlib, 31 Dec. 1640, HP 37/74A.

38   Moriaen to Hartlib, 2 Dec. 1641, HP 37/96A.

39   'Wan Faber in Frankreich todes verfahren so ist ein betrieger weniger in der Welt' - Moriaen to Hartlib, 24 April 1654, HP 31/13A. Fabré was physician to Louis XIII, and according to Partington wrote 'a large number of little-esteemed works' (Partington II, 181), his speciality being alchemical interpretation of Classical myths. See also the equally dismissive notice in Thorndike VII, 194-5, and for a more sympathetic account, Bernard Joly, *La rationalité de l'alchimie au XVII siècle* (Paris, 1992). Moriaen was misinformed about his death: Erasmus Rasch wrote of visiting him on his sick-bed two years later (HP 42/9/1B). Rasch was equally unimpressed by his iatrochemical abilities, remarking that his illness was proof in itself of their limitations.

40   Starkey to Moriaen, 30 May 1651, HP 17/7/1A-2B.

41   *Eph 51*, HP 28/2/18A.

42   Hartlib to Boyle, 28 Feb. 1654, Boyle, *Works* VI, 79-80.

43   Ibid., 80.

44   'Es ist schade und Iammer dz der Mensch sein verstandt nicht beßer anlegt zum guten lieber als zuem bößen aber das ist fast aller solchen geschwinden ingenien artt das sie sich lieber auff Ejtelkeit legen als dem guten obligen andere die es gern thun wollen sindt mit solchem verstand nicht begabt' - Moriaen to Hartlib, 1 Jan. 1658, HP 31/18/3A.

45   Evelyn to W. Wotton, 12 Sept. 1703, *The Diary of John Evelyn*, ed. William Bray (London, 1879) IV, 33.

46   See esp. Moriaen to Hartlib, 24 May 1658, HP 31/18/25A.

47   Hartlib to Boyle, 7 Jan. 1658, Boyle, *Works* VI, 99.

48   Ibid., 122.

49   Ibid., 134, 26 Nov. 1659.

50   Poleman to Hartlib, 19 Sept. 1659, HP 60/4/69B.

51   Mr Serrarius wensch ick een betere uytcoomste als ick wel hopen can door dien de partyligheyt hedens tags te seer groot is' - Moriaen to Van Assche, 17 Jan. 1637, UBA N65d.

52   HP 63/14/6B.

53 'so gar alles was nur von diesem Man kommen ist fur lauter Euangelium gehalten' -
Moriaen to Hartlib, 7 Oct. 1650, HP 37/159A.

54 'daran aber nicht so sehr Luthero [... die Schuld] zuezueschreiben, sondern den Ienigen
welche unbesonnenerweiß darfur gehalten es seÿe lauter heiligthum was von ihme
außgehe' - ibid.

55 'Onpartijdig, katholiek, universeel: dat zijn de sleutelwoorden, waarmee het ideale
christendom door hen wordt aangeduid' - Van der Wall, *Serrarius*, 119.

56 'Er ist dem partheÿlichen wesen noch etwas zue sehr ergeben' - Moriaen to Hartlib,
13 Dec. 1638, HP 37/2B. The *ADB* comments on Bisterfeld's conversion from
strong opposition to the Puritan party in Transylvania to ardent support for it (*ADB*
II, 683).

57 'das zeugt von einem tieffsinnichen vnd grundlich verständigen vnd was beÿ mir das
maiste ist, von parteÿligkeit befreÿten vnd der warheit allein begierigen gaist' -
Moriaen to Hartlib, 7 March 1639, HP 37/11A.

58 'Ich spühre in diesem Mann schon sonderlichen gaben, vnd welches mir vor allem
liebet ein freÿ vnd vnparteÿisch gemuth' - Moriaen to Hartlib, 14 April 1639, HP
37/18A.

59 'ein auffrichtig vnd vnparteÿischer der warheit liebhaber mit dem woll vmbzuegehen
ist' - Moriaen to Hartlib, 2 Oct. 1639, HP 37/42A.

60 The church was not nationally exclusive and included Moravians, Poles and others.
Comenius himself was not Bohemian but Moravian.

61 'das nimbt ihm viel zeit weg vnd macht Ihn beÿ vielen parteijsch' - Moriaen to
Hartlib, 11 Oct. 1640, HP 37/68A.

62 Mein einfältiger Rath were das beÿ so verschiedenen sinnen vnd secten [...] man [...]
so lang vnd viel müglich sich indifferent vnd vnparteijsch halten, in generalibus
bleiben vnd sich ad particularia nicht begeben soll - Moriaen to Hartlib, 31 March
1639, HP 37/15B-16A.

63 The heading for this sub-section is borrowed from Dury's self-justificatory tract *A
Peace-maker without Partialitie and Hypocrisie* (London, 1648).

64 *Eph 48*, HP 31/22/12B.

65 *Eph 48*, HP 31/22/9A.

66 See Webster *Great Instauration*, 302, and several mentions in Hartlib's letters to
Boyle (Boyle, *Works* VI, 81, 85, 87, 94, 96, where his pseudonym is consistently
mistranscribed 'Van Mussig').

67 'es hatt mir halb davon geschwindelt' - Moriaen to Hartlib, 30 Nov. 1657, HP
42/2/26B.

68 See Michael Hunter, 'Science and heterodoxy: An early modern problem
reconsidered', *Reappraisals of the Scientific Revolution*, 367-96.

69 'ob es nun atheismus stricte dictus oder eine verwerffung der Heiligen Schrifft seÿe' -
Moriaen to Hartlib, 30 Nov. 1657, HP 42/2/26B

70 'H Boreel pflegt sonsten ex lumina Naturæ contra Atheos zue disputirn und dieselbe
zue convincirn beides das ein Gott und das die Schrifft sein Wortt seÿe' - ibid.

71 On Boreel and the Collegiant movement, see Walter Schneider, *Adam Boreel: Sein
Leben und seine Schriften* (Giessen, 1911).

72 See below, pp. 118-20 for a fuller discussion of this work.

73 Browne, *Religio Medici* (1643), *Works of Sir Thomas Browne*, ed. Geoffrey Keynes
(London, 1928, new edition 1964) I, 19.

74 'wir verwachten ommers naer syn belofde neffens den nieuwen hemel oock een
nieuwen aerde daer rechtveerdigheit in wonen sal' - Moriaen to Van Assche, 23 Sept.

1642, UBA N65f, fol. 1v. Cf. Revelation 21:1.

75   HP 37/34A, quoted at the end of this chapter, and HP 9/16/5A, the epigraph to Chapter Seven.

76   See James Knowlson, *Universal Language Schemes in England and France 1600-1800* (Toronto and Buffalo, 1975), Vivian Salmon, *The Works of Francis Lodwick: A Study of his Writings in the Intellectual Context of the Seventeenth Century* (Longman, 'throughout the world', 1972), and Comenius, *Panglottia* (trans. A.M.O. Dobbie, Shipton on Stour, 1989).

77   'die zeit wird verhoffentlich gekommen oder Ia nicht fern sein das wir nicht allein aus einem Charactere uns undereinander werden berichten und verstehen können sondern auch das wir mit einem mund Gott werden bekennen loben und preißen lernen, am tage der offenbahrung des Sohns des Menschen' - Moriaen to Hartlib, 19 Oct. 1657, HP 42/2/25A.

78   This is particularly pertinent to a German speaker, as the German words for 'reveal' and 'Revelation' - 'offenbaren' and 'Offenbarung' - are even more obviously cognate than the English.

79   *Eph 52*, HP 28/2/43A.

80   See John Stoughton, *Felicitas Ultimi Sæculi: Epistola In Qua, Inter Alia, Calamitosus ævi præsentis status serio deploratur, certa felicioris posthac spes ostenditur, & ad promovendum publicum Ecclesiæ et Rei literariæ bonum omnes excitantur* (London, 1640), Francis Potter, *An Interpretation of the Number 666* (Oxford, 1642), and Joseph Mede, *The Key of the Revelation, searched and demonstrated out of the Naturall and proper Characters of the Vision* (London, 1643).

81   Felgenhauer attacked Boreel on these grounds in his *Refutatio Paralogismorum Socinianorum* (Amsterdam, 1656), and the now lost *Perspicillum theologicum sive Examen eorum qui theologi videri et audiri volunt, cum responsione ad librum illum qui inscribitur Ad legem et ad testimonium cujus Autor est Adamus Borelius latine* (date uncertain: Boreel's *Ad legem et testimonium*, a sort of Collegiant manifesto, appeared in 1645). See Wolters, 'Paul Felgenhauers Leben und Wirken' part I, 68.

82   The arrest occurred in 1657; why Felgenhauer suddenly attracted attention at this time for a doctrine he had been preaching publicly for decades remains uncertain. In the event, the sentence was commuted to banishment from Braunschweig-Lüneburg, and the destruction of his books was ordered. Felgenhauer was as surprised as anyone that he was released from prison after only a year, for he had (not unreasonably) expected to remain there until his death. See Wolters, op. cit. part I, 68-70.

83   This consisted of two letters to Daniel Stolzius, dated 6 May 1639 and 28 June 1640 (*KK II*, 17-33 and 36-65); it circulated in manuscript (as Moriaen's correspondence demonstrates) but was not published until 1662 as *A Dextris et Sinistris* (Amsterdam, 1662).

84   Moriaen to Hartlib, 11 Oct. 1640, HP 37/68A.

85   Published Hamburg 1638. See G.F. Guhrauer, *Joachim Jungius und sein Zeitalter* (Stuttgart and Tübingen, 1850), 110-11.

86   Guhrauer, *Jungius*, 111. The remarks of this student, Vincenz Placcius, are recorded in Moller, *Cimbria litterata* III, 348.

87   'sagt von seiner Logica [...] Es ist nicht meine sondern Hamburgensium Logica dan sie haben Ihme furgeschrieben wie Sie es haben wollen' - Moriaen to Hartlib, 23 June 1639, HP 37/29A.

88   'Das nun H Iungius wegen unbändigkeit der Ienigen under welchen er lebet, seinen gaist dempfen müßen vnd nicht freÿ herauß gehen dürffen das ist zue Iammern für Ihn vnd vnß' - Moriaen to Hartlib, 13 Dec. 1638, HP 37/1A.

89 Moriaen to Hartlib, 20 Oct. and 3 Nov. 1639, HP 37/44B and 37/46A.

90 'die Libertet nach seinem herz vnd gemuth zue schreiben wie Ers in der Warheit befindet ist Ihme damit schon genommen, wird sich auff eine parteÿ legen müßen vnd beÿ allen andern desto weniger gelten' - Moriaen to Hartlib, 23 June 1639, HP 37/29A.

91 'das beste ist das der herr die sachen von Ihme bekombt ehe Sie den Censoribus in die hände kommen[;] wollen sie es dan nicht zuelaßen so kan gleichwoll geschehen was recht ist' - ibid.

92 'welches denen sehr vbel anstehet welche den gewißens zwang an andern improbirn Man würde woll thun wan man vnder der hand dieser leuthe erledigung beförderte wehren sie anderst allein vmb ihrer bekandtnus willen verhafftet vnd sonsten keine vbeltheter sind' - Moriaen to Hartlib, 21 Jan. 1641, HP 37/77A.

93 J.C. Whitebrook, 'Dr John Stoughton the Elder', *Transactions of the Congregational Historical Society* VII (1913-15), 89-107 and 177-87, esp.183.

94 Dury to Hartlib, 26 April 1639, HP 9/1/82A. The letter is largely given over to answering Moriaen's to Hartlib, 14 April 1639, HP 37/18A-20B. This use of Hartlib as intermediary in what is essentially an exchange between Dury and Moriaen is characteristic of the operation of the network, and the fact that a copy of a letter could reach Dury in Hamburg from Hartlib in London within twelve days of Moriaen's writing the original in Amsterdam is testimony to their efficiency.

95 J. Minton Batten, *John Dury: Advocate of Christian Reunion* (Chicago, 1944), 94.

96 Appelius to Hartlib, 23 August 1650, HP 45/1/42A; cf. 1 Corinthians 9:22-3.

97 William Prynne, *The time-serving Proteus, and ambidexter divine, uncased to the world* (London 1650).

98 'unglücklichen Friedemacher/ und gleichsam Nuntio Apostolico der Reformirten' ... 'concilia irenica, oder besser ironica' - Caspar Heinrich Starck, *Lübeckishe Kirchen-Geschichte* (Lübeck, 1724), 860-1.

99 'ist sein furnehmen an diesem ortt von den maisten improbirt vnd seine persohn verdächtig' - Moriaen to Hartlib, 19 April 1639, HP 37/21A.

100 'Ich laße auch nicht seine ehr zue retten vnd guten nahmen zue verthätigen so offt es nur gelegenheit gibt' - Moriaen to Hartlib, 30 June 1639, HP 37/31A..

101 J. Minton Batten, *John Dury: Advocate of Christian Reunion* (Chicago, 1944).

102 Anthony Milton, '"The Unchanged Peacemaker"? John Dury and the politics of irenicism in England 1628-43', *SHUR*, 95-117, esp.96.

103 Ibid., 101.

104 'wan man aber einst auff die particularia vnd Conditiones concordiæ kommen solte da wird man noch viel mehr zue thun vnd woll die Ienige am vnwilligsten finden die sich zuevorn in generalibus am besten angelaßen haben' - Moriaen to Hartlib, 14 April 1639, HP 37/19A.

105 'kan die vberzeugung dardurch gefunden werden so wird die Concordia sich auch woll finden wo nicht so muß alles von höherer hand erwartet werden' - ibid., HP 37/19B.

106 Dury to Hartlib, 26 April 1639, HP 9/1/80B-83B.

107 Anthony Milton, '"The Unchanged Peacemaker"?', p.116.

108 Dury to Hartlib, 26 April 1639, HP 9/1/82B.

109 Moriaen to Hartlib, 20 July 1657, HP 42/2/12A.

110 'zum wenigsten kan ein solches den friedhäßigen undt unverständig eyfferigen alle entschuldigung benehmen die friedliebenden aber trösten das sie an ihnen, nichts haben erwinden laßen' - Moriaen to Hartlib, 18 Jan. 1658, HP 56/2/1B-2A.

111 'In Summa Aurora Sapientiæ wird verhoffentlichen bald anbrechen mußen weil sich

alles an allen orthen so fein darzu schicket *Gott* gebe dz Sol Iustitiæ den folgenden tag machen v*nd* die gantze stockfinstere Weld dermal einst seliglich erleuchten möge' - Moriaen to ?, 21 July 1639, HP 37/34A. 'Aurora Sapientiæ' is the title of one of Felgenhauer's tracts (Magdeburg, 1628).

PART TWO

Universal Wisdom

CHAPTER FOUR

Panaceas of the Soul: Comenius and the Dream of Universal Knowledge

'The Pansophical Vndertaking is of mighty importance. For what can bee almost greater then to have All knowledge. If it were with the addition to have All love also it were perfection' - Joachim Hübner, cited in *Ephemerides* 1639, HP 30/4/12A.

Origins of the Pansophic Project

From Moriaen's first surviving letter to Hartlib, it is evident that when he arrived in Amsterdam he already had a deep - indeed, a missionary - commitment to his friend's project to fund and publicise Pansophy, the vision of universal wisdom being worked out by the Moravian theologian and pedagogue Jan Amos Komensky, or Comenius.[1] This scheme was the main preoccupation of both men in the first few years of their correspondence. Moriaen repeatedly expressed his commitment to it in fervent and explicitly religious terms: it was 'the labour I have taken upon myself at Gods behest and which I can now make my sole occupation for the common good. I have as it were set myself aside for it and devoted myself to it'.[2] Their expectations were spectacularly high. Moriaen approvingly quoted back to Hartlib the latter's conviction that 'nothing more useful has ever been offered to the world than this very work, since through it the schools, and by their means the Church, the State and the world can and should be reformed'.[3] Before a detailed account is given of the project and Moriaen's involvement in it, some analysis is called for of what it was that was being promoted, and how it came to be seen as of such epochal significance.

Born in 1592, Comenius studied at the Reformed academy of Herborn, before spending a year at the more traditional University of Heidelberg.[4] Heidelberg was also Moriaen's university, though it is not known whether his time there overlapped with Comenius's. Herborn was among the many higher educational establishments founded in the late sixteenth century by Reformed German princes in which a new educational ethos was being forged.[5] In most cases of the 'conversion' of small German states to the Reformed religion there was a signal lack of enthusiasm for the new faith among the general populace, and the leaders bent on persuading them saw education - through school, academy and pulpit - as a powerful tool for doing so. As the confessional divisions within Protestantism widened and took on clearer definition, such rulers benefited from an influx of Reformed preachers and educationalists evicted for their beliefs from their posts in Lutheran territories within the Empire, as well as the exodus from Switzerland, the Netherlands and England.[6] A further stimulus to Protestant educational reformers of all stripes was provided by the undisputed success of the Jesuit colleges, with their relatively traditional curricula, founded in the latter half of the sixteenth century.[7] As J.A. Pöhmer observed to Hartlib, 'I am often astounded at the fatal diligence of the Jesuits: had they pursued the study of nature as thoroughly as the compulsion of conscience they might have done much good'.[8] Deploring the lack of support for Hartlib's educational projects, Dury observed bitterly that 'If he was among the Iesuites, they would find him both worke & meanes to follow it out, but wee [ie. the Protestants] are dead in things of such a nature'.[9]

The Reformed educational tradition - or, one should perhaps say, new departure - played a crucial role in shaping the thought of Comenius, as of Hartlib and Dury (both educated in Elblag (Elbing), the Eastern outpost of the Second Reformation).[10] Particularly significant in moulding the thought of the Pansophists was the influence of one of Comenius's teachers at Herborn, the encyclopedist Johann Heinrich Alsted. It should be emphasised that an encyclopedia, in Alsted's terms, was not merely a comprehensive list of facts and references (or at least was not supposed to be): it was, as the word implies, a unified whole, and a major part of Alsted's project was to work out the arrangement of his compendium of knowledge in a logical, coherent and harmonious fashion such that the student could proceed through the work in sequence, progressing always from the known to the unknown and from the general to the particular. It was not merely a reference source, it was a text book of universal learning. Comenius worked as Alsted's amanuensis while in Herborn, and the master composed a Greek poem lauding his student's love of universal wisdom.[11]

Such knowledge was not only to be compendious, it was above all to be 'useful'. 'Useful knowledge' became something of a catchphrase for the Hartlib circle and other 'Second Reformation' thinkers. It should not be misinterpreted as mere utilitarianism. For knowledge to be 'useful' or 'practical' did not simply mean that it would enable people to move around faster or increase crops or build better bridges - though all such things could be useful, provided they were directed to the right ends. It meant above all that it would have an application in the ethical and religious ordering of daily life. What increasingly came to be seen as the empty, abstract, semantic disputations of the scholastic tradition were to be replaced by knowledge that was of practical relevance to the behaviour and beliefs of the individual. 'Practical divinity' in particular, an especial enthusiasm of both Alsted and Hartlib, might not grow more turnips, but was emphatically regarded as 'useful'. 'Usefulness' lay not in the private gain of one individual at the expense of another, but in the mutual profit derived from enhanced social interaction, a profit which in turn redounded to the glory of the Creator whose last and perhaps most important commandment to his creatures was that they should love one another as themselves.

But it should be stressed that if the growing vogue for a curriculum grounded in the practical rather than the theoretical can be described as an important and characteristic feature of the 'Second Reformation' ethos, it was certainly not denominationally exclusive. Like Alsted before him, Comenius drew on a very disparate range of sources, some of them on the face of it mutually exclusive: on Aristotelians as well as Ramists, hermetic mystics as well as rationalists, and thinkers of every shade of Christian, or indeed non-Christian, confessional allegiance.[12] After the loss of his library in the sack of

Leszno in 1656, he himself singled out, as the authors whose works he most needed to recover in order to proceed with his work, Francis Bacon, Juan Luís Vives and Tomasso Campanella[13] - an Anglican and two Catholics. Nor was it only among the Reformed that he found acceptance. One of his warmest admirers in Germany was the Lutheran pastor Johann Valentin Andreæ. Andreæ's depiction of an ideal educational system, which occupies over a quarter of his Utopian novel *Christianopolis*,[14] foreshadows many of Comenius's educational ideas, such as universal infant education irrespective of gender or social status, appreciation of the fact that learning begins at birth if not before, the encouragement of enquiry rather than the inculcation of received wisdom, teaching in the vernacular rather than Latin, and the imparting of ideas through images and demonstrations rather than merely through words. Similar ideas are to be found in Campanella's *Civitas Solis*, debatably the inspiration for *Christianopolis*.[15] A number of German thinkers, particularly in Protestant territories, were pursuing reforms of the same sort. Among these was Elias Bodinus, whose influence Comenius later acknowledged, and whom Moriaen visited, together with Alsted's son-in-law Johann Heinrich Bisterfeld, in order to assess the spectacular claims he made for his image-based 'Art of Memory'.[16] Another such was Wolfgang Ratke or Ratich, whose method earned him an encomium from the great natural philosopher and pedagogue Joachim Jungius (another devout Lutheran).[17] A collection of didactic writings assembled by Ratke, including the report on his own method drawn up by Jungius and his friend Helvich, bore the epigraph 'Per inductionem et experimentum omnia' ('All things by induction and experiment').[18] This in turn is a phrase forcefully reminiscent of the terms used in Bacon's great manifesto for educational reform, *The Advancement of Learning* (1605). In all these works, the stress was on ways of making education practical, relevant to daily life, and compendious. Pansophy was not the product of any particular denominational allegiance, though it is true that the particular circumstances of the Reformed German principalities provided the most fruitful ground for putting such ideas into practice (or at least trying to), while elsewhere they tended to remain at the level of theory, manifesto or Utopian fiction.

The reformation of educational theory was crucial to the very notion of Pansophy. Universal knowledge could be attained only by an education that was itself universal, in the fullest sense of the word, teaching 'all things to all people in all ways'.[19] Just as Bacon's *Advancement of Learning* was intended as a trail-blazer for the 'Instauratio Magna', the reformation of all science and knowledge, and just as Alsted's (supposedly) all-encompassing *Encyclopædia* grew out of a practical teaching course,[20] so all Comenius's educational work was conceived as so many steps on the path to the ultimate synthesis of Pansophy. Hartlib, significantly, had his *Prodromus Pansophiæ* (1639) translated as *A Reformation of Schooles* (1642).

It was as a pedagogue rather than a Pansophist that Comenius first came to the attention of the European intelligentsia. He achieved considerable international fame through his educational writings, principally the *Janua linguarum reserata* (*The Gateway of Languages Unlocked*) (1631) long before he became popularly associated with the notion of Pansophy. At this time, Comenius was living in exile in the Polish town of Leszno, he and his co-religionists in the Unitas Fratrum (Unity of Brethren) having been driven out of their native Bohemia and Moravia by the occupying forces of Emperor Ferdinand II. Here, Comenius took charge of teaching Latin and music at the Unity's 'Gymnasium Illustre', and the *Janua Linguarum* came about as a direct result of his teaching activity, in response to the paucity of teaching material and the unimaginativeness of the teaching methods he encountered at the Gymnasium. From the outset, the work was designed as more than merely a language course. It aimed to exemplify the principle that language education should be an integral part of the broader curriculum rather than a separate discipline, and that the teaching of words should be - and could best be - effected *through* the teaching of 'things', not alongside it. Instead of memorising irrelevant and uncomprehended phrases and grammatical rules, pupils might far more readily and far more profitably absorb new structures and terminology - either in their own language or in another - in the context of following an intrinsically interesting and useful course. And this course was to be - true to the ideals Comenius had imbibed at Herborn - practical, ethical, and encyclopedic.[21]

Others at the school were highly impressed with Comenius's tentative first draft and persuaded him to publish it on the Unity's press. In a remarkably short time, the work achieved a colossal international success, appearing the same year in German, French and English versions.[22] Comenius, to his own mild alarm, suddenly found himself a celebrated figure among the educationalists of Europe, bombarded with congratulations, eager enquiries and expressions of interest.[23]

Encouraged as well as intimidated by this surge of interest, he found himself contemplating an extension of his project to make it still more practical and compendious. As he later described his reaction:

> I came to this point in my thoughts: if it seemed good that the words of a language should be learnt through the guidance of things, it were better that things themselves should be taught through the guidance of words already known. That is, that, when by the help of my *Janua Linguarum* youth had learnt to distinguish things from outside, it should thence become accustomed to explore that which is within things, and to comprehend what each thing is in its essence.[24]

Herein lay the germ of his 'Pansophy': 'a general book [...] exhibiting in it all necessary things so that all shameful ignorance would be excluded'.[25] Such a work would be called, on the model of the *Janua Linguarum*, the *Janua Rerum* or Gateway of Things. Like Alsted before him, he found what had initially been intended merely as a school book developing under its own momentum into a vision of universal learning.

It was the *Janua Linguarum* that brought Comenius to Hartlib's attention, and in about 1632 he began to correspond with and subsidise the Moravian.[26] Hartlib was greatly enthused by the idea of the *Janua Rerum*. He urged Comenius to send him a plan of the proposed work, and was rewarded, in 1637, with a rough draft outline in manuscript.

Hartlib had moved to England almost a decade earlier, in 1628, full of zeal to further the educational plans of the secret quasi-Rosicrucian society 'Antilia' he had been involved with in Elblag, which sought nothing less than the reformation of the world. Quite how it intended to bring this about, or whether indeed it had any clearly formulated programme for doing so, will probably never be known, but it is clear that it proposed to start by reforming education, and that Hartlib's mission lay partly at least in this field. Johann Fridwald, Hartlib's main contact in Antilia, wrote to him shortly before his departure 'as regards Antilia, it has been decided that the teaching of children [*or* boys] is to be made a priority and laid as the foundation stone of the endeavour'.[27] J.A. Pöhmer, another leading figure in the society, hoped to speak to Hartlib in person about the subject before the latter left for England, 'since you are to do something extraordinary in this field'[28] Shortly after his arrival in England, Hartlib founded an academy in Chichester 'for the Education of the Gentry of this Nation, to advance Piety, Learning, Morality, and other Exercises of Industry, not usual then in common schools'. This was surely his first attempt at accomplishing his pedagogic mission, and the school's almost immediate failure must have been a bitter disappointment to him.[29] Comenius's programme provided a fresh opportunity to make a contribution in his appointed field, not this time as an instigator, but in the role he was to excel in throughout his subsequent career, as a promoter and populariser of other people's schemes. He took it upon himself to act as catalyst in the development of Comenius's ideas, not only in intellectual but in strictly practical terms.

Perhaps his most important contribution was to publish the manuscript Comenius had sent him as the *Conatuum Comenianorum Præludia* (Oxford, 1637). He published it, or so he claimed in the preface, because it had aroused so much interest that he had not had scribes enough to produce the requisite copies. Typically enough, it had not occurred to him to ask Comenius's permission to do this, and it was a considerable shock for the Moravian when he suddenly received an unsolicited copy of a book by himself which he was quite unaware had gone to press. As he told Hartlib in the above-mentioned letter of January 1638, the printing had been undertaken without his knowledge, let alone consent: had he been asked, he would never have allowed the work to appear in this imperfect form. At the same time, however, he was evidently flattered and encouraged: he thanked Hartlib for his interest and support, and observed that if his Pansophy ever came to light, it would be due to Hartlib's incitement. And since the work was out, the best thing he could do was to rework it and have it republished in a more satisfactory form as the *Prodromus pansophiæ*, also published by Hartlib but this time with Comenius's authorisation, in 1639. Hartlib having thus set the wheels in motion, Comenius was to spend the rest of his life labouring to produce the book of universal wisdom he had proposed in this sketch. Hartlib for his part, together with like-minded friends such as Dury, Haak, Hübner and Moriaen, devoted himself single-mindedly throughout the 1630s to raising funds for Comenius, to disseminating his work, and above all to his great goal of attracting Comenius himself to England to supervise the 'great instauration' of learning he believed was about to take place there.

The Notion of Pansophy: Beyond Bacon and Alsted

Comenius repeatedly cited Francis Bacon as an exemplar and an inspiration to him. As has been mentioned, Bacon was one of the three authors he most wished to recover after the loss of his library in 1656. Just before his visit to England in 1641,[30] he wrote to Hartlib in passionate terms that this was the time for the great Lord Verulam's [ie. Bacon's] plans to be put into effect, and even suggested that Hartlib adapt Bacon's supplication to James I in Book II of *De Augmentis Scientiarum* to be addressed to Charles I.[31] Hugh Trevor-Roper, indeed, goes so far as to see Bacon as the primary influence on the thought of all the 'Three Foreigners' (Hartlib, Dury and Comenius), though he also maintains they completely misunderstood their hero.[32] He avuncularly describes the thought of the Hartlibians (or Comenians) as 'vulgar Baconianism':[33] a somewhat frantic, disordered assembling of scraps of knowledge, with a lowbrow Puritan emphasis on practical utility and a constant worry that the job might not be finished in time for the Apocalypse:

> Bacon's great philosophical synthesis had been fragmented: his 'experiments of light' had been transformed into inflamed apocalyptic speculations, his 'experiments of fruit' into the uncontrolled elaboration of gadgets. Still, it was Baconianism of a kind, and the men of the country party took it seriously.[34]

This is not the place to venture an analysis of the full range of Bacon's multi-faceted thought and the even more various interpretations that have been put upon it. But it should be pointed out that the fact that many of the Hartlib circle took a lively interest in Bacon does not mean they followed him (or their conception of him) slavishly or uncritically. In Moriaen's case, there is no firm evidence he had read Bacon at all, and nothing to suggest he set much store by him if he had. The only mention of him in all the surviving letters is a less than ecstatic reaction to a catalogue Hartlib had sent him of Bacon's extant manuscripts: 'there will doubtless be many excellent things among the writings left by Verulam'.[35] Furthermore, I would suggest that there are elements in the pansophic programme that are not so much misunderstandings of Bacon's views as conscious adaptation of or even reaction against them.

What is particularly relevant here is that in at least one important respect Baconian inductivism was recognised as the antithesis of pansophic universality. Inductivism, by definition, proceeds from the particular to the general, requiring long and diligent labour in what Bacon called the 'inclosures of particularity'[36] before proceeding to establish more general axioms. It is true that, in speaking of the ultimate goal of his preliminary *Natural Histories*, Bacon made promises as grandly universal as any of the claims of Pansophy:

> let such a history be once provided and well set forth, and let there be added to it such auxiliary and light-giving experiments as in the very course of interpretation will present themselves or will have to be found out; and the investigation of nature and of all sciences will be the work of a few years.[37]

Yet after all the enthusiasm of his descriptions of data-collection and experimentation, the 'investigation of nature and of all sciences' in 'a few years' sounds here oddly perfunctory, almost an anti-climax. Bacon is more convincing when presenting his method as a quest never to be concluded, 'an endless progress or proficience'.[38] Aubrey's story that Bacon caught his death of cold while trying to refrigerate a chicken is a fitting tribute to the man's devotion to experimental minutiae.[39] In any case, for the purposes of the comparison I am drawing here, it is irrelevant whether Bacon saw the achievement of such an overarching synthesis as a grand culmination of his programme or as a distant and not very interesting prospect. In either case, his agenda for the foreseeable future involved a slow, meticulous and cautious progress through particularities that was wholly at odds with the intellectual climate of the 1630s.

Among Hartlib's papers is an anonymous catalogue of natural creatures and phenomena, set out in what is clearly supposed to be a typological sequence, preparatory no doubt to something approaching a Baconian Natural History, and bearing the appealingly self-deprecatory title, 'An imperfect Enumeration of natural thinges'.[40] No 'Natural History', however well conducted, could aspire to higher status. There will always be more to know, and any inductively established rule can only be accounted a hypothesis not yet disproven: once an exception to it is discovered it loses its validity, or at least its universality. Bacon, it has been argued, was more optimistic than this, and genuinely did expect his method to attain ultimately to a standard of absolute verification.[41] This claim, however, met with considerable scepticism from many of the thinkers under discussion here, to whom inductivism seemed a highly unsatisfactory tool for uncovering ultimate, absolute and universal truths. Comenius, for instance, specifically remarked in the *Prodromus* that Bacon's proposals, though laudable, were inadequate for the project he had in mind. Bacon's inductive method

> requireth the continuall industry of many men, and ages, and so is not onely laborious, but seemeth also to be uncertaine in the event and successe thereof [...] it is of no great use, or advantage towards our designe of Pansophy, because [...] it is onely intended for the discovery of the secrets of Nature, but wee drive and aime at the whole universality of things.[42]

Inductivism (by this analysis at least) starts at the bottom, in the realm of raw data, and works its way up tentatively and speculatively to more general rules that can never be more than provisional. This will seem to some an over-simplification of Bacon's ideas, to others a valid critique of their ability to deliver what they promised. In either case, it was the view Comenius took, and that is the point at issue here. What Pansophy set out to do was to discern *from the outset* a pattern whereby the lineaments of infinity might be conceptualised, and to grasp (insofar as human capacity permitted) the principles according to which the universe is ordered. This of course presupposes a conviction that the universe *is* ordered, and my contention is that the mounting (though still largely unformulated) sense that the explosion of information and technology was beginning to undermine that conviction, or that article of faith, was the challenge that made the reassurance of Pansophy seem so urgently necessary. The question raised by much reading of pansophic texts is: if these people are so confident of universal harmony and order, why do they reaffirm it so insistently?

The amount of knowledge available to the scholar was increasing at an unprecedented rate, thanks to the rapid advances in the technology both of scientific investigation itself and of its dissemination in print. Acceptance of the Copernican-Galilean model of the universe did away with the notion of a bounded, and hence potentially knowable, sub-lunary sphere. (Comenius himself throughout his life stubbornly refused to accept the evidence for heliocentrism.) Meanwhile, exploration and microscopy were revealing a hitherto unimagined wealth of subjects for investigation and a hitherto unimagined complexity in what had previously seemed simple and comprehensible organisms. Above all, the enormous increase in the output of literature was making it, for the first time in history, impossible for an educated and tolerably wealthy individual to keep broadly abreast of the current state of knowledge on all subjects in the known world. It was the consequent rise of specialisation, and the increasingly clear demarcations drawn perforce between different branches of knowledge, that led to this sense of losing a grip on the totality, coherence and fundamental unity of Creation. As Comenius put it in the *Prodromus*,

> Good God! what vast volumes are compiled almost of every matter, which if they were laid together, would raise such heapes, that many millions of years would be required to peruse them? [...] Hence comes that (so commonly used) parcelling and tearing of learning into peeces, that men making their choyce of this, or that Art, or Science, take no care so much, as to looke into any of the rest.
> Who knowes not that this is so? and who sees not, that this distribution, and sharing of Arts, and Sciences, proceeds from this supposition, That it is not possible for the wit of one man to attaine the knowledge of them all?[43]

J.V. Andreæ, an acknowledged inspiration to and keen supporter of Comenius, was similarly distressed by the sheer quantity of information humankind was confronted with, and lamented (to cite another Hartlib-sponsored translation):

> Now in the worlds weaknesse, most humane affairs are committed to Learning, the masse whereof is become infinite, which fills not the world so much with truth as falsehood, not so much with solidity as curiosity.[44]

There was, for some Pansophists at least, altogether too much 'curiosity' in the inductive method championed by Bacon: too much emphasis on data and not enough on the broader and nobler vistas promised by their conception of 'right method'. He was, as it were, looking through the wrong end of the newly-invented telescope. Bacon had emphasised that no detail should be omitted from the Natural Histories, specifically prescribing the inclusion of

> things the most ordinary, such as it might be thought superfluous to record in writing [...] things mean, illiberal, filthy [...] things trifling and childish [...] and lastly, things which seem over subtle, because they are in themselves of no use.[45]

At least one proponent of 'vulgar Baconianism' found this concern for 'things mean, illiberal, filthy' too vulgar to take: 'To mangle tyrannise etc over the Creatures for to trie experiments or to bee imploied so filthily about them as to weigh pisse etc as Verul. prescribes is a meere drudgery curiosity and Impiety and no necessity for it'.[46] The same commentator, who I strongly suspect is Hübner,[47] pursued this criticism of Bacon's excessive zeal for detail:

> It is sufficient if wee had a true History out of every country of the meere outward shapes operations etc. and so of all Mechanical things and their several manners of working [...] This would not require a sæculum as Verul. projects but within 10. years come to a very great perfection if it were set down by every Country.[48]

There is a suggestion of urgency, or at least of hurry, in this which points up another important ingredient in the positively missionary fervour with which Pansophy was preached, and that is the idea of preparing the way of the Lord. It is important to avoid over-generalisation. Not all Pansophists were millenarians and not all millenarians were Pansophists. Comenius, like Alsted, certainly did hold millennarian views, but that does not mean everyone who supported his overall programme agreed with him on this particular point. As has already been argued, it is not possible to determine what stance either Hartlib or Moriaen took on this subject, and the same can be said of Hübner. It was not, however, necessary to accept any particular exegesis of Biblical prophecy to share a widespread sense that some sort of culmination of human history impended - especially not for men whose homeland was experiencing what was at the time the most destructive war in European history. It was a political and intellectual atmosphere that provided a constant reminder to all readers of Scripture to guard against the error of the foolish virgins of Matthew 25, who were not prepared for the moment of the Bridegroom's arrival, and were shut out from the wedding.[49] The likes of Moriaen and Hübner may not have been committed chiliasts, but the intensely religious terms in which they discussed Pansophy strongly suggest that they viewed it as an essential part of the required preparation. We cannot be sure, and cannot be sure they were sure, what exactly they were preparing for or when exactly they expected it to happen. But we can be fairly sure they thought such preparation incumbent upon them as a matter of some urgency.

A 'sæculum', therefore, could seem an uncomfortably long time. Bacon's choice of a motto from Daniel - 'many shall run to and fro, and knowledge shall be increased'[50] - carried an unmistakeably apocalyptic resonance, for this increase of knowledge was to take place in 'the last days'. Comenius in the *Prodromus* refers twice to the same citation, pointing up the millenarian implications.[51] For those convinced that the last days were already upon them, or might well be, the leisurely time spans envisaged by Bacon for the accomplishment of his research programme were simply not available.

The mere amassing of knowledge, then, was only part of the task in hand: more fundamental, and far more urgent than the inductive method allowed for, was the arrangement of it in such a fashion that the parts might contribute to the comprehension of a whole that was more than their sum. Hence the obsession with 'right order', 'true Logick' and so forth.[52] The aim of Pansophy, however much its proponents might disagree about the means, was to discern the divine pattern governing Creation, to gain access to the heavenly architect's blueprint.

Again, this runs directly counter to the spirit of Bacon, who, with regard to the study of 'the book of God's word' (the Bible) and 'the book of God's works' (Nature), exhorted men to beware that 'they do not unwisely mingle these things together'.[53] Indeed, this was precisely the objection to the *Præludia* made by Hieronim Broniewski, a lay elder of the Unitas Fratrum, against which Comenius had to defend himself before the synod of the Brethren in 1638 and 39.[54] But for the pansophists, the dangerous presumption of too many thinkers was precisely to leave God out. Comenius's objection to the *Pansophia* of Peter Lauremberg (Rostock, 1633) was that it 'contained nothing appertaining to divine wisdom or the mysteries of salvation' and was consequently 'unworthy of so sublime a title'.[55] The gravest defect of contemporary education identified in the *Prodromus* was that studies were 'not sufficiently subordinate to the scope of eternity'.[56] The agriculturalist Gabriel Plattes, whose works abound in strictly utilitarian self-help schemes for the common man,[57] was anonymously criticised because he was 'too confident for the improvement of those secondary meanes as if men should be the lesse beholden to God and so inclines to Atheisme'.[58] It was an error that was becoming alarmingly common:

> The greatest philosophers should address them*selves* more to God in prayers and in a holy life and so they should finde out m*ore* the secrets of Nature then ever they have done.
> Eg. wee see it in Cartes glasses [ie. Descartes' parabolic lenses] though his demonstrations bee never so punctual yet it will not doe the reason is be*cause* that God is so little regarded in this matter as if humane wit were able to accomplish all. And it may bee an obvious smal matter is only wanting w*hich* God hides of purpose from his and other eys.[59]

Another important diversion from Bacon, which I suspect may well be a conscious modification of his portrayal of the world, is that to his 'book of God's word' and 'book of God's works', which between them comprehend the whole of knowledge could we but learn to read them aright, Comenius added the book of Man's mind.[60] As he was fond of pointing out, Man was made in God's image. Man is a microcosm, not only of the universe but of God himself. The universe is comprehensible to the individual because the individual mind contains it, and contains God's knowledge of it, in miniature:

> [Man] being the last accomplishment of the creation, and the most absolute Image of his Creator, containing in himself onely the perfections of all other things, why should he not at last habituate himselfe to the contemplation of himselfe, and all things else?[61]

The slightly hysterical insistence on order, pattern and universality in the writings of the pansophists represents the microcosm-macrocosm theory in its death throes.

In Hübner's memorably surreal simile,

> Truths or thi*ng*s being known out of their due order are like to an Elephant's Snout or proboscis. The vse of them cannot bee so evidently

and fully bee [*sic*] perceived as when they are linked together which the
Pan*sophia* will best performe.[62]

The sense of this, I take it, is that a stray and unrelated piece of data is as
redundant and absurd as this 'proboscis' must have appeared to Europeans
seeing an elephant for the first time, but that just as the trunk turns out to be
not only useful but absolutely integral once the organic context of the elephant
is grasped, so 'due order' will illuminate the interdependence and mutual
relevance of all fragments of knowledge. Comenius was to make almost
exactly the same point, albeit more prosaically, when defining what he called
the 'syncretic' method of analysis:

> to understand things in isolation, as men generally do, is a minor part of
> [the learning process], but to understand the harmony of things and the
> proportions of all the related parts is the vital factor which brings pure and
> all-pervading light to men's minds.[63]

The key was method. This quotation is strongly reminiscent of the
encyclopedic ideas of Keckermann and Alsted. But it was becoming
increasingly apparent to the younger generation that Alsted had not gone
nearly far enough in the methodising of his compendium. And Comenius,
much as he respected his former teacher, surely had him among others in
mind when he complained

> that as yet in all the bookes that ever I saw, I could never find any thing
> answerable unto the amplitude of things; or which would fetch in the
> whole universality of them within its compasse: whatsoever some
> *Encyclopædias*, or *Syntaxes*, or books of *Pansophy*, have pretended to in
> their titles.[64]

What was needed, but had never been attempted, was a method that would so

> square and proportion the universall principles of things, that they might
> be the certain limits to bound in that every-way-streaming variety of
> things: that so invincible, and unchangeable *Truth* might discover its
> universall, and proportionate harmony in all things.[65]

One anonymous German correspondent of Hartlib actually cited Alsted as an
exemplar of *un*methodical writing, incidentally providing a vivid description
of the sense of distress and confusion induced by lacking a predetermined
sense of order:

> there are many things that one does not know where to put. And so is
> obliged to leave them buried in the dung of many scattered useless
> aphorisms, or with Alsted to submit I know not what idiotic *farragoes of
> arts* and *particulars of systems* to the usual misbegotten arrangement, as
> the confusion of his *Encyclopædia* ought sufficiently to have shown
> him.[66]

'Farragoes of arts' is a sarcastic reference to the seventh and last book of
Alsted's *Encyclopædia* (1630), entitled 'Farragines disciplinarum' (lit.

111

'Farragoes of Disciplines')[67], to which Alsted consigned all those disciplines - from alchemy to 'tabacologia' (the study of tobacco) - which he could not fit into his scheme anywhere else. The writer would have agreed with Howard Hotson, who argues that this represents a disintegration of Alsted's entire system.[68] Hotson well summarises the growing disillusion with Alsted and the encyclopedic tradition among 'the generation of English natural philosophers which reached maturity in the mid-seventeenth century',[69] though as this quotation suggests the trend was by no means exclusive to England.

Another commentator, writing in favour of the notion of Pansophy (though not in this instance with particular reference to Comenius), observed that a work might contain the greatest confusion that had ever been seen in writing, but nonetheless, provided the author treated his proposed subjects solidly and thoroughly, 'we shall think him worth more than a thousand Alsteds with all their supposed methods'.[70] Hübner too provides a good example of this growing disillusion: many of Alsted's works, he complained, had 'no direction or reality of notions in them but I know not what at random scribled'.[71]

Ironically, this can now seem a very apt description of much of Hartlib's papers, particularly the *Ephemerides* in which the remark is recorded. There is an unresolved dichotomy between a genuine appreciation of the multifariousness of raw fact and a passionate need to discern the divine order that would reveal its coherence. Hartlib collected stray facts with tireless zeal, and can often seem less than meticulous in applying Bacon's precept that 'whatever is admitted must be drawn from grave and credible history and trustworthy reports'.[72] But he was generally assiduous in noting his sources, thus providing himself with a means of verification when it came (as it never did) to assembling his database in due order. Maddening as it may be to come across six consecutive entries attributed to 'id.' when the entry preceding them is not attributed to anyone at all, it would be unjust to assume that Hartlib himself would not have known whom he meant. His 'vulgar Baconianism' was not nearly as silly, and certainly not as trivial, as it often looks in the shipwrecked form in which it has come down to us. His papers are the fittingly incomplete record of a desperate last-ditch attempt to reconcile the widening scope of seventeenth-century factual knowledge with faith in a symmetrical, harmonious and comprehensible universe.

'To Leave No Problem Unsolved': The New Mathematics as a Model for Pansophy

The bullfinch, if J.S. Kuffler's report in the *Ephemerides* of 1656 is to be believed, is

> One of the most Musical birds and that is most susceptible to bee taught any kind of melodies or songs [...] as Mr Morian hath found by experience who hims*elf* hath taught him *Psalms etc etc* for wh*i*ch hee hath beene famed over all Amsterd*am*.[73]

However much this report owes to the inventor's fertile imagination, it is a telling and rather attractive image of the idea of Moriaen built up by his correspondents in England. And it is certainly not inconceivable that Moriaen *tried* to teach a bullfinch psalm tunes, and possibly believed he was making progress with the project. To persuade a bird to apply its God-given voice to explicitly divine melodies would have provided a splendid example of the divine spark latent in all created things, and of the potential for humankind to apply its divinely-appointed dominion over Nature to the specific end of glorifying God.

Music was regarded at this period as a branch of mathematics - which is emphatically not to say it was seen as a merely abstract or intellectual process. On the contrary, the divine spark discernible in music extended throughout its parent discipline, offering unique insights into the lineaments of Creation. In the idealised pansophic educational programme of J.V. Andreæ's *Christianopolis*, the mathematical part of the course, described in chapters 61 to 63, begins with arithmetic - for whoever does not know arithmetic knows nothing; proceeds to geometry - which teaches us to understand 'the pettiness of our little body in the narrow confines of the grave and the tiny ball of this little earth'; and concludes with the 'secret numbers', comprehensible only by revelation, which provide an insight into the means by which God has measured the universe. From this course, the Christianopolitans proceed directly to music (chapters 64-66), which is depicted as a form of spiritual sustenance.

Moriaen's love of music figures in miniature, like a microcosm, his love of mathematics, and the expansion in the purview of mathematics taking place at the time in turn figures the expansion of learning in general that he and Hartlib anticipated. It was harmony that fascinated him in mathematics, as in music, the abstract beauty of numerical patterns - though in his eyes these patterns were not abstract, they were applicable in all fields of learning, including those that would today be considered the least 'scientific', and were simply easier to discern in this area than in others. Mathematics provided the reassurance that there was an ordered harmony to the universe, for 'in this errant and deceitful world, there is hardly anything sure and certain left us besides mathematics'.[74]

The music of the spheres might no longer literally be believed in, since the spheres in question had turned out not to exist, but their metaphorical charge - the concept of universal harmony - was redeemable by mathematics. Moriaen was captivated by the idea that an infinite number of problems can be solved by a single verified principle, and saw in this the model for all subjects after the pansophic reformation of learning. He observed with specific regard to mathematical works sent him by Hartlib that

> All my life I have been eager beyond measure for such things, but now even more so, since through them I can picture forth the possibility of Pansophy to myself and others. By this means I have already silenced many gainsayers and convinced many doubters.[75]

It was this passion that informed his interest in and sustained support for the leading mathematician among the pansophists, John Pell.

During his own lifetime, Pell (1611-85) enjoyed colossal esteem as a mathematician. As a young man he was a schoolmaster in Sussex, probably for a while at Hartlib's academy in Chichester. In due course, Hartlib persuaded Pell to follow him to London, and he became, along with Dury, Haak and Hübner, an intimate of the pansophic group centred on Hartlib. His friends were eager to advance him, but Pell was temperamentally incapable of making any effort for his own promotion or of bringing any project to a conclusion. Or as Aubrey more kindly put it, he was 'naturally averse from suing or stooping much for what he was worthy of', 'no Courtier' and 'a most shiftless man as to worldly affaires'.[76]

From as early as 1639, Moriaen was active in seeking opportunities in the Netherlands for the mathematician, who numbered Dutch among the many languages he was fluent in. His efforts on Pell's behalf earned him the one mention in print that can ever have caught the eye of non-specialists: a passing reference by Haak preserved in Aubrey's *Brief Life* of the mathematician:

> [Pell] communicated to his friends his excellent *Idea Matheseos* in half a sheet of paper, which got him a great deal of repute, both at home and abroad, but no other special advantage, till Mr John Morian, a very learned and expert Gentleman, gave me [Haak] notice that Hortensius, Mathematical Professor at Amsterdam, was deceased, wishing that our friend Mr Pell might succeed.[77]

The reason the post became vacant was not in fact that Hortensius[78] had died, but that he had been called to Leiden University, though in the event he did die almost immediately after his move. Moriaen recommended Pell as an 'Architectus Pansophiæ' and an ideal replacement for Hortensius to the burgomasters Cunrad and Bourg, and to the English resident at The Hague, William Boswell. Through Hartlib, Moriaen urged tirelessly - and fruitlessly - that Pell should produce concrete evidence of his talents to lend weight to these recommendations. It is a sign of the slight regard in which mathematics was held by traditional academics and the majority of students that the Athenæum's authorities seriously considered letting the post lapse after Hortensius's departure, since his lectures had been so poorly attended,[79] and it was indeed left vacant for four years. But in 1643, despite Pell's continuing failure to publish anything, Moriaen's persistent lobbying at last bore fruit. At Moriaen's suggestion, Pell took the gamble of moving to Amsterdam in order to recommend himself in person, and was duly offered a probationary year. This he completed with considerable success: the celebrated scholar G.J. Vossius personally congratulated Moriaen on his recommendation.[80] Pell remained in Amsterdam until 1646, when he was invited by the Stadholder Frederik Henrijk to the newly-founded academy at Breda.

Moriaen was one of Pell's first contacts in Amsterdam, and helped the shiftless mathematician to settle in to his new surroundings, taking it on himself to find him lodgings and, no doubt, introducing him to new friends and showing him round the city.[81] The two men remained in close contact during Pell's nine years in the Netherlands (he finally returned to England in 1652 and subsequently became a diplomat under Cromwell, thanks this time to a recommendation from Haak), and were friends for the rest of Moriaen's life. Moriaen deplored the poor remuneration he received for his teaching work, and always hoped he might distinguish himself sufficiently in print to attract a patron who would allow him to devote his time entirely to mathematical research and Pansophy.

This was a vain hope. Pell published hardly anything at all besides the *Idea* mentioned by Aubrey, which is not in itself a mathematical work, and which, furthermore, was brought out not on Pell's initiative but on Hartlib's. As his biographer in the *DNB* severely remarks, 'Pell's mathematical performance entirely failed to justify his reputation'.[82] But in the late 1630s and early 1640s, Pell was seen as one of Pansophy's rising stars, and after Comenius himself, it was he, Dury and Hübner who were most often cited in Hartlib's publicity material as worthy recipients of sponsorship and likely producers of genuinely pansophical work. His *Idea of Mathematics* was distributed by Hartlib alongside Dury's writings on exegetical and Hübner's on political method as an exemplar of and advertisement for the vision of universal learning adumbrated in Comenius's *Prœludia* and *Prodromus*.

Pell's *Idea*, which Hartlib published in 1638,[83] can fairly be described as an 'idea' in the modern sense of an innovative suggestion, since it consists of a set of concrete proposals for a state-sponsored programme to improve mathematical education and research. But the word 'idea' would have been understood at the time in a rather more elevated and philosophical sense, akin to Comenius's 'præcognita'.[84] It meant the prior conception of the nature of a discipline in broad and abstract terms, the conceptual framework that was to be fleshed out with more specific knowledge. For in the course of suggesting means toward the advancement of learning in this particular field, Pell also depicted an ambitious and distinctly pansophic ideal of what mathematics could and should become. His work argues for three main developments: first, the compilation of a comprehensive mathematical encyclopedia and bibliography; second, the foundation at state expense of a universal mathematical public library-cum-museum containing 'all those bookes, and one instrument of every sort that hath beene invented',[85] to foster interest in the uninitiated and provide research facilities for the expert; and finally the writing of three new text books comprehending the whole of mathematical theory. It is the proposal for the third text book that strikes the truly pansophic note, as this is to deal not only with past and present mathematical problems but all conceivable problems whatsoever, being

> An instruction, shewing how any Mathematician that will take the paines, may prepare himselfe, so, as that he may, though he be utterly destitute of bookes or instruments, resolve any Mathematicall Probleme as exactly as if he had a complete *Library* by him.[86]

This work was distributed around Europe by Hartlib and Haak: the latter sent a copy, together with the *Prodromus*, to Mersenne, who passed it on to Descartes. Both thought the design a worthy one, but balked at the scale of it. What struck them as unfeasible was not, interestingly, the final pansophic vision of universal method (which Pell himself foresaw would 'perhaps seeme utterly impossible to most'[87]), but the enormous size and expense of the proposed library. Mersenne, however, after making contact with Pell personally, was won round by his arguments and became a wholehearted advocate of the plan.[88] Moriaen received a copy soon after the work's publication in 1638, and it excited him as much as anything Hartlib sent him. This, he thought, was the sort of concrete evidence needed to convince people that workable pansophic schemes could be and were being produced. He was zealous in distributing copies of the tract, and specifically requested other works of a mathematical bent, including those of Thomas Harriott and William Oughtred, for the same purpose of promoting Pansophy.

It was the universal validity of mathematical principle that made it illustrative of Pansophy. The notion that mathematical principle is universally and abstractly valid was itself a relative novelty at the time. Jacob Klein suggests in an illuminating study that the very concept of number was undergoing a radical transformation at precisely this period.[89] Numbers were coming to be seen as concepts in their own right, rather than merely as a means of measuring or counting determinate objects. This he sees as the crucial shift in conceptualisation that made possible the development of modern symbolic algebra. Those who see an infant stage of algebra in the ancient Greek mathematicians are, according to Klein, reading the Greeks anachronistically, according to their own intentionality (that is, 'the mode in which our thought, and also our words, signify or intend their objects'[90]). Euclidean presentation

> is *not* symbolic. It always intends *determinate* numbers or units of measurement, and it does this *without any detour through a 'general notion' or a concept of a 'general magnitude'*. [...] It does *not* identify the object represented with the means of its representation, and it does *not* replace the real determinateness of an object with a *possibility* of making it determinate, such as would be expressed by a sign which, instead of *illustrating* a determinate object, would *signify* possible determinacy.[91]

Modern mathematics, by contrast, which Klein sees as originating with Vieta, Stevin and Descartes, 'turns its attention first and last to *method as such. It determines its objects by reflecting on the way in which these objects become accessible through a general method'*.[92] Consequently, the focus of mathematical investigation shifts from the solution of given problems to the consideration of how, in the abstract sense, problems are solved: from the ontological to the epistemological. The concept of indeterminate number which makes such a shift of intentionality possible is seen by Klein as first being given conscious, formulated expression in the work of one of Pell's heroes, the earliest of Klein's three founders of modern mathematics, François Viète, or Vieta (1540-1603). It was just such a shift of intentionality that Pell and Moriaen anticipated in the impending establishment of a new, pansophic epistemology.

Pell was not alone in seeing Vieta as an epochal figure in the field. Marin Mersenne, one of the foremost mathematicians of France, who corresponded regularly with Haak and Pell in 1639 and 1640, was eager for a single-volume edition of Vieta to be brought out, and commissioned Abraham and Bonaventura Elsevier of Leiden to print it.[93] In 1639 they published an appeal for manuscripts to complete their planned edition.[94] Pell, in his usual fashion, took note of this appeal but did nothing about it. Three years later, he wrote to Hartlib that he had supposed the whole project forgotten 'till Mr Morian's letters to you told us, not only that they [the Elseviers] still continue in the same mind, but also they looked upon me, desiring to know how able or willing I am to further that design of theirs.[95] This is typical of Moriaen's frequent attempts to chivy Pell into producing something, both for his own and the common good. Pell, however, advised that he could 'hear of nothing of Vieta's in manuscript in England but such pieces as are already printed' and, equally typically, recommended other mathematicians who might be able to provide notes.[96]

Jungius's closest friend and colleague at the Hamburg Gymnasium, the mathematics professor Johann Adolf Tassius, was another correspondent who followed enthusiastically the progress of the pansophic project, and he too received a copy of Pell's *Idea* from Hartlib.[97] Whether he knew the work was by Pell is uncertain (it was published anonymously), but he was certainly as convinced as anyone else of Pell's credentials. He too hoped to see Pell contribute to the Vieta edition, and likewise stressed the transcendent importance of method. His comments are preserved in a report from Dury, who wrote that Tassius

> entreated Mr Pell to elaborate the Analyticall Method which Vieta hath begun to shew but hath not perfected. For if wee have (sayth hee & it is true in all Sciences) The true principles once of Theory & the Method of proceeding from principles to find Conclusions infallibly & sufficiently made knowne wee neede noe more for the resolution of all questions that can bee propounded of what kind soever they bee. For Questions & Cases in all Sciences are infinite but the Rules to find out truth in every thing are few.[98]

This perceived centrality of Vieta and the enthusiasm for him shared by both Pell and Moriaen is important to my argument here because Vieta exemplifies with particular clarity how the new mathematics, the new focus not on individual problems but on method as such, could be seen as a model for Pansophy. To quote Klein one last time:

> In Vieta's 'general analytic' this symbolic concept of number appears for the first time [...] The condition for this whole development is the transformation of the ancient concept of *arithmos* and its transfer into a new conceptual dimension. The thoroughgoing modification of the means and aims of ancient science which this involves is best characterized by a phrase [...] in which Vieta expresses the ultimate problem, *the* problem proper, of his 'analytical art': 'Analytical art appropriates to itself by right the proud *problem of problems*, which is: TO LEAVE NO PROBLEM UNSOLVED' ('fastuosum problema problemarum ars Analytice [...] iure sibi adrobat, Quod est, NULLUM NON PROBLEMA SOLVERE').[99]

This is precisely the ultimate goal proclaimed (a little less portentously) in Pell's *Idea*: to 'resolve any Mathematicall Probleme'. It was cited too - verbatim this time - by Moriaen, soon after receiving a copy of the *Idea*, when enquiring how far Pell's method extended: 'I should be glad to know whether Mr Pell's logic extends as far as Vieta's *nullum non problema solvere*'.[100] That is to say, was Pell himself capable of putting his *Idea* into practice? If he was, then surely it would be possible - and this is where the leap of faith comes in - to apply analogous means to attain the same end in all other branches of knowledge. It would be possible, as Dury insisted in a letter to Cheney Culpeper, to produce a treatise showing 'the universall method of ordering the thoughts, to finde out by our own industry any truth as yet unknown, and to resolve any question which may be proposed in nature as the object of a rationall meditation'.[101]

Again, the contrast with Bacon is instructive. Revelling in the concrete and the specific, Bacon clearly thought mathematics rather a bore:

> For it being in the nature of the mind of man, to the extreme prejudice of knowledge, to delight in the spacious liberty of generalities, as in a champagne region, and not in the inclosures of particularity; the Mathematics of all other knowledge were the goodliest fields to satisfy that appetite.[102]

But to Moriaen, Dury and Tassius (assuming Dury quoted him accurately), mathematics was not a matter of 'spacious generalities', it was a paradigm of 'right method' such as might be applied in any subject, theology not excepted. This application of 'method' and the extent to which it was novel, even revolutionary, in the mathematics of the period, is exemplified in Moriaen's mild boast about his own abilities as a mathematics teacher: in a fifteen minute lesson, he claimed, he could teach anyone tolerably competent in addition and multiplication to calculate any power of any number, the secret being that he did not attempt to teach by rote but from first principles.[103] This can only mean that traditional teachers were wasting an extraordinary amount of time on making their students learn powers by rote, like basic multiplication tables - little wonder that 'hardly anyone advanced far beyond the cube'[104] - and that Moriaen's breakthrough was to advise them to calculate powers instead of memorising them. Like many bright ideas, it is staggeringly obvious once it has been seen, yet Moriaen claimed to have caused widespread astonishment with the success of his 'method'. The moral was that the application of proper method would produce results both far more easily and far more reliably than the uttermost exertions of memory. Pansophy similarly aimed not to cram the totality of knowledge into a single head, but to establish a method, a *way* of looking at the universe, which would enable the student to draw infinite conclusions from the natural symmetry of all things, just as a mathematician using only the basic principles of multiplication can extend a pattern of numbers into infinity:

> I say, we would have such a booke compiled, which alone, instead of all, should be the Spense, and Storehouse of Universall Learning [...] by reading whereof, Wisdome should of its own accord, spring up in mens minds, by reason of the cleare, distinct and perpetuall coherence of all things [...] that so all things which may be known (whether Naturall, Morall, or Artificiall, or even Metaphysicall) may be delivered like unto Mathematical demonstrations, with such evidence and certainty, that there may be no roome left for any doubt to arise.[105]

Dury too, seeking an epistemological tool with which to produce a foolproof method of Scriptural analysis, turned to mathematics as a paradigm. This he described in his *Analysis Demonstrativa*, which Hartlib sent Moriaen in manuscript in March 1639.[106] This method Dury explicitly compared to the infallible procedures of mathematics: it too is 'Methodus [...] demonstrandi rem quamlibet a priori cognito' ('a method of demonstrating any thing from a prior knowledge'), and

> the end of this Method which I vse is to apprehend it [the wisdom of Scripture] demonstratively that is infallibly./ Soe that a man shal be able to demonstrat every thinge which he doth apprehend to be certainly true a priori noto et infallibili [from things previously and infallibly known] till he come to the first principle of infallibility which noe man can deny, for that by a continuall orderly concatenation of apprehentions the vnderstandinge is ledd by infallible degrees from one intellectuall obiect to another till it gather them all vp together in one summe soe that it can all at once apprehend the whole, and all the parts thereof distinctly & conionctly in theire severall relations each to other and each to the makeinge vp of the whole, and I can not compare the manner of proceedinge better then to an arithmeticall addition or multiplication wherein one summe beinge added to another maketh vp the third and many summes or numbers beinge added into one, make vp a greate totall summe, soe it is in this method of apprehendinge intellectuall obiects one obiect is added to another to make vp a third which is common to both and many obiects are reckoned or summed vp together to make a totall summe and generall conclusion of some intellectuall matters[.][107]

Just as Vieta and Pell maintained that the application of right method to mathematics would leave no problem unsolved, so Dury thought the same could be done for the exegesis of Scripture. It seems these musings had their genesis as the resolution of a personal crisis of faith at least four years earlier, at a time when Dury almost despaired of resolving the inherent ambiguities of natural language: 'Dury himself,' wrote Hartlib in 1635, could at one time

> finde no certainties almost in any thing, though hee was able to discourse as largely of any thing as any other. Yet solidly and demonstratively hee knew nothing, till hee betooke himself to the Scriptures and lighted upon the infallible way of interpreting them.[108]

Dury apparently claimed to have confuted Descartes' scepticism with this method: though the French philosopher denied the possibility of such certain knowledge, Dury stuck to his guns and Descartes, 'being brought to many absurdities, left of'.[109] This is almost certainly the germ of the idea that later developed into the *Analysis Demonstrativa,* but the ideas and the language used in this later work bear the clear imprint of the Comenian *Præludia* Hartlib had just published when Dury wrote the *Analysis.* The mathematical analogy provided Dury with the assurance he needed that a merely human language could be interpreted with absolute and universal certainty, at least so long as it had the guarantee unique to Scripture of an originally divine inspiration. And he pushed the analogy rather further than Comenius had done. Though he foresaw the obvious objection that natural language does not correlate directly to extra-linguistic reality in the same way that mathematical language does, he denied it - not, significantly, by argument, but by an assertion of faith in method:

> But here you will say howe can this be done aswell and demonstratively in obiects intellectuall as in arithmeticall numbers? I will answere you that the one can be done aswell as the other yf the right obiects be represented to the minde, and yf the right method of summinge vp the same, be made vse of. For I in this businesse must doe as Mathematicians in theire demonstrative sciences vse to doe, I must take a postulatum to be given or granted vnto me, vpon which the whole grounde of these demonstrations will rest, Nowe this Postulatum is a thinge which I suppose noe rationall man will denye, vizt that yf the vnderstandinge can apprehend truely the simple axiomes of a discourse, and that yf those simple axiomes truely apprehended, be rightly ioyned together, that the compound which resulteth from the same in *the* vnderstandinge cannot be false; vpon this one Postulatum (which yf neede were might be proved by a Mathematicall demonstration of lynes and figures) relyeth the whole demonstrability of this Analyticall Method.[110]

Dury's method of breaking Scripture down into simple unambiguous axioms, and then recomposing it by 'right method' to arrive infallibly at the text's true meaning met with Moriaen's warm approval, despite his habitual scepticism about Dury's irenical projects. What especially appealed to him in this work was no doubt the eschewal, so unusual in Dury, of consideration of particular doctrines as they had been elaborated, and the return instead to first principles and to a single true method that would transcend all doctrine. And he wholeheartedly agreed that mathematical principle could be applied to religion, despite the scepticism of misguided rationalists such as Descartes:

> for many will believe only what they can see, and although they cannot but believe when shown a mathematical certainty, yet will they not believe that such a method can be discovered and practised in religious knowledge, and especially in theology; such a one is M. Descartes.[111]

It has to be said that mathematical concision is not one of the merits of Dury's system. I have quoted it at some length here to illustrate the insistent, almost defensive iteration of the mathematical analogy. Dury wanted to represent the literal sense of Scripture as a series of equations with incontrovertible solutions, and though he did go on to say that there is also a deeper sense accessible only to 'the Spirituall man who hath received vnderstanding to discerne Spirituall things Spiritually',[112] that spiritual sense can only be discerned through a precise and unambiguous grasp of the literal.

The attraction of such a view was that if assent could be 'compelled' by 'mathematical' demonstration of the single unambiguous true meaning of Scripture, religious disputation could be done away with at a stroke. It is a strikingly passive form of analysis:

> the only Prudency to be vsed in this Method is to bringe a mans vnderstandinge to a spirituall Captivitie vnder the sense of the Letter [...] Soe that the vnderstandinge is ledd and becometh wholly passive[:] as an eye that seeketh somethinge is meerely passive in respect of the obiects that it reflecteth vpon, soe must the vnderstandinge be in respect of the words of sacred scripture.[113]

This distinctly echoes the mathematical analogies of the *Præludia*, and foreshadows the passive assent to mathematical demonstration recommended by Comenius in *Panaugia* (Universal Light), the second part of the *Consultatio*:

> The ways of light have been so well designed by God's skill that there is nothing vague about them.
> They have been made to conform to such unchanging laws that everything about them can be proved with mathematical certainty.
>   By the same theory the intellectual light of wisdom can rightly be governed by unchanging laws of method so that in the process of teaching and learning nothing is left vague and uncertain but everything operates with mathematical precision.[114]
>   If you use your eyes, you will see the same thing as I do and there can be no difference between us.[115]

Such was the vision: the laws of method would teach people to see, and once they had learned to see they would realise they were all looking at the same thing. Comenius too repeatedly stressed the irenical nature of his Pansophy, which he predicted would lead to the healing of all schism within Christianity and the conversion of the infidels.[116]

All academic and doctrinal disputes would fall away, the Aristotelian would lie down with the Ramist, the Galenist with the Paracelsian, the Lutheran with the Calvinist, the Jew with the Christian; all would assent to the self-evident truth as meekly and dispassionately as they could all assent to a demonstrable mathematical equation. In fact, as Dury and Moriaen were well aware, people did not always assent meekly to mathematical demonstrations but that, presumably, only meant that at least one of the disputants had not fully grasped the right method. All that was lacking was a proper, incontrovertible exposition of that method, and doubt and division would be at an end, the earth would be filled with the knowledge of the Lord[117] and the stage set for the Second Coming. First, however, that method had to be definitively worked out and mankind in its wilful blindness persuaded to consider it impartially. It was a task Comenius compared to nothing less than the construction of the Tabernacle of the Ark of the Covenant in the wilderness.[118] Moriaen adapted this image to apply it to himself. He cast himself not as one of the craftsmen who actually fashioned the sanctuary, but as someone called to the humbler yet no less necessary task of gathering the material resources necessary for it: 'not only Bezaleel and Aholiab are required for the holy work, but also those who fetch what is needed for the labour'.[119]

The Collection in the Netherlands

It is not known whether Moriaen and Hartlib were already in touch when the latter set himself up as a champion of Pansophy, or whether it was the quest for people through whom to distribute copies of the *Præludia* that first inspired Hartlib to contact Moriaen (perhaps on the recommendation of Dury or Haak). In either case, it is evident from the earliest of Moriaen's surviving letters to Hartlib (13 December 1638) that he had been fairly bombarded with enquiries and publicity relating to the project. The warmth of his response must have been gratifying. Together with Johann Rulice (Rulitius), who was a preacher in the English Church at Amsterdam when Moriaen arrived and moved shortly afterwards to the German,[120] Moriaen soon became the principal agent in the Netherlands for the Hartlib network and all its multifarious activities, particularly the collection for Comenius.

His previous experience of relief work for the Palatine exiles, and the contacts he had made during his previous career, must have made him an ideal candidate for such a role. His years in Frankfurt and Cologne had given him access to the largely clandestine information network of the German Reformed Church, and in the early years of his correspondence with Hartlib, references recur to largely unspecified sources of information in those cities, notably to an agent ('Comißarius') in Frankfurt, and one Budæus in Cologne, through whom he distributed literature sent him by Hartlib.[121] Between May and September of 1641, he and Odilia spent some three months in Cologne and Frankfurt, but no account whatsoever is given of their activities there.

This collection had been Hartlib's principal occupation since the early 1630s - well before the appearance of the *Prœludia*. Its goals, as has been said, were to relieve Comenius's personal circumstances, to publish his works, to supply him with amanuenses and to enable him to visit England. Hartlib also supplied material for the project: in 1633, Comenius thanked him, through his then collaborator Jan Jonston, for promising to send manuscript copies of (unspecified) works by Bacon.[122] In 1634, a Bohemian student and Austin Friars protegé in London, Jan Sictor, complained to the Austin Friars consistory that Hartlib was organising a private collection for Bohemian exiles.[123] Quite what Sictor had against this is unclear. Perhaps, since he specifically remarked that there were Bohemians who could organise such collections better, this is an example of the rivalry which Grell suggests existed between the different refugee groups,[124] or perhaps he doubted the probity of such privately administered relief work. As Grell remarks, 'Hartlib's claim that he was only obtaining a few pounds for the publication of a work by Comenius hardly sounds credible', though it should be added we only have Sictor's word for it that Hartlib did make such a claim.[125] It is probably true that Hartlib's collection was for ends related directly to Comenius rather than the exiles in general, but it is doubtful whether the sums involved were as small as Hartlib apparently suggested and certain that his ambitions extended beyond the publication of one book (presumably, as Turnbull suggests, the *Prœludia*[126]).

Similar efforts by Hartlib on behalf of Comenius personally and the promotion of his work continued until 1641 and are partially documented among his surviving papers,[127] but the extent of the contribution from the Netherlands and Germany (apart from the spectacular case of the De Geer family), and the network through which it was organised have hitherto been underestimated.

In 1639 Moriaen approached the newly-arrived Reformed minister in The Hague, Caspar Streso. As a student in England, Streso had benefited from the charity of Austin Friars, and he was later commissioned to distribute donations from the church to the exiles in Anhalt.[128] Streso was initially sceptical of the pansophic project, suspecting the cause was tainted with Socinianism, but Moriaen won him round and established him as the prinicipal organiser of the collection in The Hague. Moriaen was keen to cast the net as far afield as Danzig and approach his friend Georg Sommer, who was preacher there, though this suggestion does not seem to have been followed up. He hoped to persuade the diplomat Bisterfeld to encourage his master, Prince Gÿorgÿ Rakóczi of Transylvania, to contribute, though there is no evidence he did so. Moriaen himself repeatedly tried (though again with little success) to coax contributions from the Dutch West and East India companies. A visit from two diplomats from Cologne (to whom Moriaen had presumably been recommended by old colleagues or friends there) provided another opportunity to publicise the cause.[129] As has been mentioned, Moriaen in 1639 arranged publication of a petition entitled *An Exhortation for the Worke of Education Intended by Mr Comenius*, which has since vanished without trace.[130]

The clearest indication of the leading role played by Moriaen and Rulice in the Continental campaign for Comenius is Hartlib's use of them to distribute the Moravian's work. He gave away almost three hundred copies of what he described as 'the new Comenian Booke' - evidently one of the works he had himself commissioned publication of, either the *Præludia*, or more probably (Moriaen's letters suggest), its second edition, the *Prodromus*. Moriaen features twice on Hartlib's list of people to whom he sent this work, first as recipient of five copies, then - doubtless in response to his repeated statements that the more publicity he received the better - as co-recipient, with Rulice, of fifty, the largest single consignment by a considerable margin from the total of almost 300 distributed.[131] Streso was sent five copies by Hartlib and more by Moriaen, who also sent some of his copies to Budæus in Cologne for further distribution.

In more concrete terms, Moriaen could report that by 24 March 1639 he had raised 200 Imperials, which he sent directly to Comenius to cover his immediate needs while waiting for more to come in.[132] This is equivalent to something approaching £50,[133] a substantial sum for a charitable contribution to a single person. Hartlib in the same year passed on £42 7s. 6d. to Comenius from his collection in England.[134] Between them, therefore, Hartlib and Moriaen had raised almost the £100 which an anonymous correspondent whose advice on the funding programme Hartlib had canvassed proposed as adequate annual provision for a reasonably frugal scholar.[135] Hartlib would appear to have passed this suggestion on to both Moriaen and Comenius for comment, since Moriaen was initially confident that 'God willing, we shall indeed find means to provide for two or three collaborators at £100 each'[136] and could later declare himself pleased to hear that Comenius considered either £200 or, at a pinch, precisely this sum, £100 a year, sufficient for his needs.[137] However, the long-term goal was not simply to see Comenius himself tolerably comfortable, but to provide both for him and his family, to employ amanuenses and assistants, and to guarantee the peace and leisure he needed to complete his Pansophy. With this in mind, Moriaen's strategy, like Hartlib's, was to gather in not just one-off contributions, but subscriptions committing the signatories to regular support over a period, the longer the better. This, not surprisingly, proved harder to achieve, but on 14 August 1639, having campaigned for over eight months, he triumphantly reported 'that I have now, God be praised, made a start on the subscription, and can only expect matters to improve. It has been a bitter struggle to reach this point. God be praised it is over, and may He continue to grant his blessing'.[138]

And as Moriaen had anticipated, once the ice had thus been broken, the subscription progressed steadily, if less impressively than he had hoped, for the next three years, until the support of Comenius was single-handedly undertaken by Louis de Geer, easily the biggest catch of Moriaen's (or, indeed, Hartlib's) quest for patronage. By the end of 1640, Moriaen had enlisted regular support from the four Reformed Churches of Amsterdam (the German, Dutch, French and English).[139] Unfortunately, no statistics are available for the sums promised or collected, apart from Moriaen's mention of securing 40 Imperials from the Amsterdam consistory in March 1640,[140] sending a further 50 Imperials in mid-July 1640,[141] and raising £25, earmarked especially for Hübner, by 13 January 1641.[142] Hartlib's accounts also mention that 'Mr Morian sent Libr. 4' in 1641, though this relatively small sum probably represents a personal contribution rather than the proceeds from his collection.[143] He also lent 100 Imperials out of his own pocket for Comenius's family on 23 December 1641.[144] This last piece of generosity turned out, in Moriaen's eyes at least, to be superfluous, as Comenius's plea for funds for his family had also reached de Geer, who had sent 100 Imperials independently. However, the Comeniuses apparently found a use for the full 200, as the debt seems not to have been settled until 1648. In Comenius's letter of 11 September 1647 dismissing his assistant Cyprian Kinner, one of the wide assortment of grounds listed is that he could not afford to pay Kinner on account of his debts, especially to Moriaen, whom he owed 100 Imperials.[145] (An unimpressed Kinner added the marginal note, 'Huh! do you want to take away the salary I have already earned? Settle your debts yourself!'.[146]) Moriaen finally reported receipt of the money on 3 February 1648.[147] Comenius had benefited from an interest-free loan for rather more than six years, which may be one of the reasons why Moriaen became perceptibly cooler towards him during the 1640s.

Comenius was never intended to be the sole beneficiary of the collection. Moriaen was keenly aware - as was Comenius himself - that an enterprise of such magnitude could hardly be accomplished by one man, and that Comenius badly needed competent assistance and informed constructive criticism if he was to produce anything more than alluring sketches of his Temple of Wisdom.[148] It would also, he repeatedly pointed out, take more than alluring sketches to persuade sceptical spirits that such an edifice was feasible at all and that Comenius was capable of supervising its construction. In these respects, his views chimed closely with those of Joachim Hübner, who was at once one of Comenius's greatest admirers and severest critics,[149] and it is little wonder Moriaen had such a high regard for the young man's intelligence and perspicuity, and was keener to see him than anyone engaged as Comenius's assistant. Hübner and Comenius between them, he declared, would convince all doubters of the viability of their reform programme.[150] (As things turned out, Hübner never did take up such a post, since de Geer disapproved of him, probably on account of his outspoken refusal to commit himself to any doctrinal allegiance.) Comenius was viewed as first among equals in the pansophical undertaking, and Moriaen was given to reminding Hartlib that there were other needy scholars too: he was particularly keen to see funds provided for Hübner and, above all, Pell, who he hoped would be a direct beneficiary of the Dutch collection:

> I hope to send something over, for a start, with my next, that Mr Pell may be kept well disposed and not given cause to rein in the mathematical spirit that seems to be native to him and to turn it to another course, perhaps against the promptings of his own heart and spirit.[151]

Indeed, Moriaen stressed so frequently that the proceeds of the collection should not go to Comenius alone that it seems fair to conjecture he thought Hartlib needed persuading, or at least encouraging, on this point. Comenius made for good publicity, partly no doubt because of the fame of his *Janua linguarum* and partly because of his representative role as senior of the exiled Unity of Brethren, a community remarkably adept at arousing the sympathy of other Protestant denominations for the sack of their country and their persecution by the Habsburgs without alienating them through doctrinal quibbles or political partisanship. Yet Moriaen urged in almost so many words that while the contributors might think they were donating money for Comenius personally, the administrators of the collection should discreetly see to it that a more equitable distribution was effected:

> We ought, as far as possible, to gather whatever comes in here and there into a common purse and distribute it according to need, and not let people send their contributions directly to Mr Comenius himself, otherwise we shall not know where we are, and everything being under his name, he would receive everything and others nothing.[152]

What both men were firmly agreed on was that Leszno was not the place for Comenius. His duties as minister to the Brethren were regarded by many of his West European admirers as a distraction from his far more important pansophic work, worthy enough in themselves but not fit to occupy the time and intellectual resources of a Comenius. As Hübner lamented in 1637: 'I am very sorry to hear that Mr Comenius is now so distracted from his pansophic meditations. If he gives the work up there will hardly be found another to hit on such far-reaching thoughts'.[153] There is also a distinct sense that an eye needed to be kept on the Pansophist. As one collaborator noted, though Comenius had a 'searching pate et vni*versal*' and was 'very Expedit et Laborious', he was also 'very Inconstant et sicke et changeable. very credulous et easy to bee *per*suaded and ther*fore* not good to be alone'.[154] He was prone, Moriaen and many others feared, to allow himself to be side-tracked by such subsidiary labours as the writing of school text-books and, worse still, polemic tracts which rendered him partisan in the eyes of his potential audience and thus compromised the universality of his message. This concern was to become an all too familiar refrain among Comenius's supporters as time went on. As late as 1661, Hartlib could complain to John Winthrop that 'Mr Comenius is continualy diverted by particular Controversies of Socinians & others from his main Pansophical Work'.[155] Moriaen's gravest concern as regards the Comenian tendency to wander down blind alleys was aroused by his efforts to invent a *perpetuum mobile*.

This was a subject Comenius had worked on at least as early as 1632, and to which he kept returning obsessively to the very end of his life.[156] Not that Moriaen ruled out the possibility of such a thing or considered it unimportant. On the contrary, his informed interest in the Drebbel-Kuffler *perpetuum mobile* in Pfalz-Neuburg has already been mentioned, and he himself had made a practical study of the same problem. This was presumably during his time in Cologne or Nürnberg, though his letters reveal no more about his experiments than that they were unsuccessful.[157] L.E. Harris, in his account of Drebbel's apparatus, maintains that the term was not, at the time, taken literally, but was used to mean merely something that would keep moving of its own accord for an exceptionally long time.[158] This may be true of Drebbel and the Kufflers, for whom the profit motive was a more important spur to invention than philanthropy or philosophic delight (which is not to deny them a measure of the latter qualities). Their primary concern was to satisfy their customers, a goal which in this case would be achieved by devising a motion that approached more nearly to the eternal than the customers themselves. What Comenius and Moriaen were talking about, however, does indeed appear to have been a mechanism which, barring accidents, would keep moving until the end of time. An equally important distinction drawn by Harris, which he claims was not drawn at the time, is that between a machine which maintains itself in motion entirely of its own accord and one which relies on the application of some external force such as variation in atmospheric pressure (which he believes Drebbel's depended on) or the use of chemical reactions. But again, as Blekastad's account of Comenius's perpetual motion theory makes plain, Comenius did draw such a distinction, and was quite clear that the application of an external, cosmic and inexhaustible force was the only possible solution to the problem:

> He worked on it according to his own theory that no earthly force could power this machine, since all earthly things are transient. By a method not known to us, he aimed to transfer the cosmic 'emanation' or radiance onto three balls of different sizes and different metals, in order to harness 'the power that moves the stars'.[159]

As so often in the schemes of the group - as, indeed, is intrinsic to the very notion of Pansophy - the practical and the metaphysical were inextricably connected.

The *Ephemerides* are full of excited (and often self-promoting) speculations by a wide range of inventors about the uses to which a *perpetuum mobile* could be put, most of them assuming (though obviously not in so many words) that it would not only sustain but impart energy. One of the most imaginative was William Potter, who in 1652 claimed to foresee that

> by it the vse of Horses will be taken away in references to Coaches, wagons etc. The ships shal be driven with any wind as swift as any swift Gale. A Fort shal be caried along the seas and doe all manner of execution [...] Whole Townes shal bee made a floating vpon the seas. Some thousands of swords shal bee wilded by it to cut slash all manner of ways and to destroy whole Armies.

126

All manner of Musical Instruments shal be made most harmonically to
play by it.
By it may be made to flye throughout the aire.[160]

Moriaen, rather more realistically, recognised that, provided the motion
were perfectly regular, it could be used to solve the problem of establishing
longitudes, one of the greatest scientific (and commercial) desiderata of the
day. What was preventing the establishment of exact longitude was the lack
of a sufficiently accurate chronometer with which to establish the relative
timings of given celestial phenomena in different places at sea level. If the
motion was perpetual and regular, there could be no question of its running
down, and hence it would serve as just such an infallible chronometer. But at
least as important to Comenius as any such potential practical application was
the idea of connecting with the harmony of the cosmos and demonstrating the
most basic tenet of all his thought, that humankind is capable of
comprehending the universal (and, significantly, the term *motus universalis*
was used interchangeably with *motus perpetuus*). Though Comenius did not
expressly say so, the implication is surely that since God created the Universe
as, in effect, a gigantic perpetual motion machine, Man should be able to
replicate this in the 'little world'. He explicitly compared his vision of
Pansophy to a *perpetuum mobile* in which every part is connected with and
conducive to the operation of every other.[161] As Blekastad puts it, 'Purely as
confirmation of the correctness of a philosophical system it was of the greatest
importance'.[162] Moriaen, too, believed that if a truly successful demonstration
could be made, it would serve, by analogy, like Vieta's and Pell's universal
algebra, to demonstrate the truth of Pansophy. He was more concerned,
however, about the converse: a public failure would appear to bring the whole
pansophic scheme into disrepute, supplying the likes of Broniewski with
additional ammunition to use against Comenius.[163]

It was not, then, the study of perpetual motion itself that Moriaen thought
misguided. His argument was that such study should be deferred until the
forthcoming reformation of learning had furnished the materials and
experimental conditions needed to undertake it successfully. Just as in the
case of Descartes' parabolic lenses, dreaming up plausible theories was a
pointless activity in the absence of an adequate means of testing them
experimentally. In the meantime, Comenius would be far better employed in
directing his talents to bringing that reformation about. He was, as it were,
trying to display the products of Solomon's House before it had even been
built.

Comenius's Visits to England and the Netherlands

Hartlib finally succeeded in persuading Comenius to move to England in
1641, having spent some five years pestering him to do so.[164] This visit, and
his subsequent move to Sweden at the invitation of Louis de Geer are already
amply documented.[165] None of the extant accounts, however, properly brings
out the fact that the whole business was a protracted saga of
misunderstandings and conflicting agendas. It is almost impossible to
ascertain how far Comenius appreciated the centrality of the role Hartlib was

casting him in. He can hardly have believed, as he later claimed he did, that he was being asked to undertake, 'for the glory of God', a sea voyage of over a thousand miles merely for the sake of a few days' private conversation.[166] But it seems equally unlikely he would have embarked on such a venture without making any provision for his wife and family or for the future administration of his ecclesiastical duties if he had seriously anticipated settling indefinitely in England and overseeing an altogether epochal transformation of education and science, all which is clearly no less than Hartlib expected. I incline to the view that he was responding to what he genuinely believed was a divine summons without having any clear idea what it was a summons to.

On arriving in England in September 1641, he promptly formed the mistaken impression that he had been summoned by order of Parliament. The grounds he later gave for this assumption, of which he was never disabused, were that he had been shown a copy of a sermon preached before Parliament on 17 November the previous year by John Gauden, which concluded with warm praise of Comenius and Dury and exhorted the members

> to consider, whether it were not worthy the name and honour of this State and Church to invite these men to you [... and] to give them all publike aid and encouragement to goe on and perfect so happy works, which tend so much to the advancing of truth and peace.[167]

If it was not Hartlib himself who told Comenius he had been summoned by Parliament, he evidently did nothing to correct the notion. One of the things that particularly impressed Comenius about the sermon was that Parliament had ordered it to be printed: no one seems to have pointed out to him that this was fairly common practice in the case of Parliamentary fast-day sermons. As Comenius himself recalled the business:

> 'Friends,' said I, 'ye have acted with more caution than candour in that ye have concealed these things [the supposed parliamentary summons] from me. Had I been apprised of them beforehand, I know not whether I should have been of such a mind as to suffer myself to be brought forward into a theatre so great [...] But this I beg of you [...]: let us alone among ourselves be known to one another for the few days that we have, for I must be returning.' They answered that my return was impossible this year. For the King was gone into Scotland for the coronation of the Queen: Parliament was adjourned until the King's return [...] For me this was grievous hearing.[168]

Trevor-Roper's assertion that Gauden was probably unfamiliar with Comenius's work, and was merely parroting what Pym and other Parliament men close to Hartlib had told him to say, is less than just.[169] Gauden had been a recipient of the 'new Comenian Booke' and on 3 March 1641 he donated £5 to Hartlib's Comenius fund.[170] A letter from Dury which it seems altogether likely is to Gauden suggests a more than passing acquaintance. Obviously written at the time Dury was preparing to leave Amsterdam for England (c. January 1641), it expresses his thanks that 'of yr owne accord yow were pleased to recommend to the most honorable Court of Parlament my negotiation'. Dury intended to set out for England the moment the weather permitted, for 'My eares do tingle at the Newes which I heare of the Parliament'. Meanwhile, Hartlib would advise the addressee of Dury's recommendations as to what should be 'thought vppon in my worke'.[171] Gauden was certainly not an intimate of the circle, and, as Trevor-Roper points out, there is no evidence of his having any further connection with them after Comenius's arrival. It may well be that Pym or his allies proposed him as preacher and knew more or less what he was going to say. That does not mean, however, that he was mouthing a prepared script on a subject he knew nothing about.

There can be no doubt that Gauden's sermon had an impact. The printed version included a marginal note advising that anyone inclined to undertake the promotion of Dury and Comenius might find 'a faire, easie, and safe way of adresses to them both, opened by the Industry and fidelity of Mr. *Hartlibe* [*sic*], whose house is in Duks-place in *London*'.[172] Cheney Culpeper, who was to become one of Hartlib's firmest allies in Parliament, later told him, 'I often rejoyce in that hower in which (by a meere occasionall readings of Dr Gaudens sermon) Gods prouidence brought me to your acquaintance, & hathe synce & dothe still by it bringe me to the acquaintance of others.[173] But Trevor-Roper's report that as a result of the sermon Hartlib was 'approached' and 'told to invite both Dury and Comenius in the name of "the Parliament of England"' is pure speculation.[174] Hartlib had allies in Parliament who were keen to attract Comenius to these shores, and it may well be that he misrepresented this, deliberately or otherwise, as an official summons, but there is no evidence anyone told him to do so. It is not inconceivable, but neither is it verifiable.

Something must have happened, however, to make Hartlib's oft-repeated invitation take on in June 1641 the extra urgency and sense of divine imperative that proved too much for Comenius to resist. I would suggest that the convening of the Long Parliament in November 1640, followed up by the impeachment of Laud in December and the execution of Strafford the following May, and the apparent prospect of Parliamentary support for educational reform schemes, persuaded the ever-optimistic Hartlib, probably after consultation with Pym and his allies, that the time was ripe to confront Parliament with the appearance of Comenius and Dury in England as a providential *fait accompli*. The best efforts of Hartlib and Moriaen in the way of private subscriptions were falling far short of the projected £500 a year to maintain Comenius and some four assistants plus funds for printing, binding and distributing the products of their labours. Once Parliament saw Comenius and Dury not just as hypothetical worthy causes otherwise engaged in foreign countries, but as a golden opportunity within its grasp, a physical presence in England free of other commitments and ready to set to work at once on a practical programme, it would surely not balk at voting the modest sum necessary for a work so manifestly worthy and beneficial. No matter if Comenius himself was a little confused about the sequence of cause and effect, provided the divinely appointed goal was attained.

This was the purpose of the petition presented by the group immediately after the reconvening of Parliament on 20 October 1641 - that is, at the first possible opportunity after Comenius's arrival.[175] It was hoped in particular that Parliament would fund a complete overhaul of some educational establishment, recasting it as a centre of experimental and pansophic learning, a 'College of Light' such as Comenius set out to describe in the *Via Lucis* (*Way of Light*), written during his visit to England. And for a brief while, until the outbreak of the Irish rebellion and the civil wars put paid to all such notions, it must have seemed the plan would indeed bear fruit. Parliament proposed to earmark the Anglican Chelsea College for just such a project.[176] The plan was doubtless to install Comenius as head of this visionary new establishment, or at least as a prominent member of it. At a stroke, the problem of Comenius's maintenance would be solved, and a major step forward taken in the reformation of schooling that in time would spill over into a reformation of the world.

Moriaen, however, while he fully agreed with Hartlib that a semi-permanent transfer of Comenius to north-west Europe was devoutly to be wished, had very different ideas about what should be done with him once established there. Though an enthusiastic backer of the collection from private individuals, he never held with the idea of thrusting Comenius onto the public stage in an attempt to secure state funding. Throughout the discussions on the subject, he repeatedly stressed that the aim must be for Comenius to be relieved of all distractions and allowed to devote himself to his meditations. As he reported having told Burgomaster Cunrad, 'In my opinion the common good would be better served by his settling in a solitary, out-of-the-way place rather than a populous and much-frequented one'.[177]

But Comenius had his own agenda too, one understandably played down in his biographical accounts, which were composed principally as descriptions or defences of his pansophic work. He was, first and foremost, a minister of the Unity of Brethren and, as Blekastad puts it, 'a member of a church in which "none belongs to himself", its spokesman and senior representative. In these circumstances, his work on Pansophy had to be combined with the greatest responsibility towards the Unity as a whole - or abandoned'.[178] Comenius was given a commission by the elders of the Brethren to go to England to promote a collection for the exiles. This work had originally been assigned to two other members of the Unity, Daniel Vetter and Jan Felin, who in 1641 were engaged on a similar collection in the Netherlands, but Comenius replaced them as the community's ambassador to England. Comenius later implied that this plan was agreed by the elders merely as a pretext to free him from his ecclesiastical duties for his pansophic mission.[179] This does not strike me as very convincing, nor does it accord very well with his simultaneous claim that he only expected to stay in England for a few days. What interest had the Unity in the reformation of Chelsea College in London? But in any case, whether it was a pretext or not, fund-raising was his official mission, and while there was undoubtedly a strong personal appeal for him in the prospect of meeting such fervent admirers as Hartlib, Hübner, Haak and Dury and discussing his work with them, he was also well aware that these were seasoned and effective organisers of charitable collections. Besides the money they had provided for Comenius himself, Hartlib and Haak in particular had been prominent figures in the relief operation for refugees from the Palatinate. It is evident enough now that the success of that operation depended not so much on the organisational skills of any individual fund-raisers as on a royal sanction gained through the political influence of the senior members of the Austin Friars church and the marshalling of public opinion behind the cause of the Palatine Protestants. But whether this was evident in Leszno in 1641 is very much to be doubted.

Just after his arrival in England, Comenius received yet another invitation: to Sweden this time, to live - indefinitely, it would seem - as the guest of Moriaen's old associate Louis de Geer. The motivation behind de Geer's proposal is harder to pinpoint. His offer of accommodation and funding was issued, through Hotton and Rulice, in late summer 1641, probably in September, just as Comenius was on his way to England.[180] The Dutch entrepreneur was then resident in Finspång, near Stockholm, and eager to gather about him a group of learned and pious men, among whom he hoped Comenius would feature.[181] There is no evidence exactly what form and function de Geer envisaged for the group, but such societies were very much in vogue at the time. Patronage of them tended to be the province of the nobility: typical examples are Prince Moritz of Hessen's 'Orden der Temperanz' (Order of Temperance), Prince Ludwig of Anhalt's 'Fruchtbringende Gesellschaft' (Fruit-bearing Society), and Princess Anna Sophia von Schwarzburg-Rudolfstadt's 'Tugendliche Gesellschaft' (Virtuous Society); at the same time that de Geer was casting around for pious and learned company, J.V. Andreæ was doing his utmost to interest Duke August the Younger of Braunschweig-Wolfenbüttel in fulfilling a similar role for his projected 'Societas Christiana'. De Geer, a Swedish citizen since 1627, was ennobled as Baron of Finspång in 1641 for services to Sweden (principally loans of money for the war effort). The inauguration of such a society would have set the seal on his new status, besides constituting another of the good works which, as a devout Calvinist, he was assiduous in performing (throughout his career, ten per cent of his profits were set aside for charity). Moriaen, however, was firmly convinced that de Geer, out of the sheer goodness of his heart and devotion to his God, expected nothing at all from Comenius for himself, not even his conversation: he simply wished to enable him to continue laying the foundations of the reformation envisaged by Moriaen and Hartlib, either in Sweden or elsewhere, as might be deemed best by Comenius himself and his collaborators.

The kindest description that can be given of Hartlib's reply to de Geer, ostensibly at least on Comenius's behalf, is polite prevarication.[182] Its gist is this: delighted as he is by the invitation, Comenius's commitments to the friends in England he has travelled so far to see, together with his obligations to the Moravian exiles whose cause he is to plead there, not to mention his advanced years[183] and need of privacy, compel him to remain where he is for the time being at least. These excuses, especially coming from Hartlib, are not overly convincing.

Hartlib's account of Comenius's situation contrasts strikingly with Comenius's own. Though there can be no doubt of the genuine friendship and affection between the two men, there were certainly times when Comenius felt he was being pushed around by Hartlib. Some years later, upset by a lapse in Hartlib's correspondence, he gave a rather ponderously jesting depiction of himself as a recalcitrant ass and Hartlib as a driver who had given up shouting at the beast because doing so had no effect.[184] If there is a healthy dose of self-mockery in this, it is not exactly complimentary to Hartlib either, and in the years 1637-41, the driver had been shouting his loudest. First, he published the *Præludia* without bothering to ask for

Comenius's authorisation, then (seconded by Moriaen, Hotton and others) he pestered him into setting off for England: if Comenius's account is accurate, one might almost say bullied him into it.[185] Finally, having persuaded him to come, he exposed him at once to the full glare of public attention, in direct contradiction to his express wishes. He later told Hartlib bluntly - and it must have hurt: 'If there be one man who has brought hindrance to the pansophic study, you are he, friend, in not allowing me to do what I had to do in peace, but dragging me forth into so broad a light, and setting me in the midst of such great crowds'.[186] Effectively, Hartlib was telling de Geer that Comenius was not prepared to go through any of the things Hartlib himself had just put him through.

Comenius was highly suggestible to the idea of divine imperatives, terrified of contravening the will of God. It was a side of his character that later became particularly obvious, and particularly damaging to his reputation, in the business of the composition and eventual publication of the prophetic book *Lux in Tenebris*. Comenius had begun collecting the visions of Christoph Kotter and Christina Poniatovská in the 1620s.[187] These were overtly political and explicitly topical prophecies dealing with the restoration of Friedrich V of the Palatinate, the liberation of Bohemia and the overthrow of the Habsburgs. In 1633, a synod of the Unity placed a ban on such controversial material. Nonetheless, despite the fact the ban had not been lifted, Comenius supplemented his collection some twenty years later with a new set of visions in the same vein, this time from another member of the Unity, Mikulás Drabik (Drabicius), who was insistent Comenius should bring them to press. The publication of all three bodies of prophecy, under the title *Lux in Tenebris*, took place in 1657, after a long inner struggle as Comenius debated with himself whether the visions might not be inspired by evil spirits (he had ruled out the possibility of fraud on the grounds that none of the visionaries was educated enough to perpetrate one so convincingly). In the end, Drabik's insistence that the same God who had sent him the visions demanded also that they should be published was more than Comenius's scepticism could withstand. There can be no doubt that there was a political motive to the timing of the publication, which was part of the propaganda drive behind the bid to replace the recently deceased Emperor Ferdinand III, whose only son had narrowly and fortuitously predeceased him, with a Protestant emperor such as Carolus Gustavus of Sweden, or at least an anti-Habsburg such as Louis XIV of France. But this is not to deny a genuine religious impulse to Comenius, for whom religious and political considerations were indivisible. If God chose to act in the world by issuing self-fulfilling prophecies, it was not for Comenius to obstruct him.[188] Wilhelmus Rood goes so far as to say that Drabik 'urged Comenius with threats to publish his visions',[189] but it was God, not Drabik, whom Comenius was afraid to contradict.

The relevance of the *Lux in tenebris* controversy to the much earlier visit to England is that if Drabik can be accused of morally blackmailing Comenius (for whatever motives), Hartlib employed very similar pressures in persuading him to visit this island. That the visit to England has generally received so much better a press than *Lux in tenebris*, both from contemporaries and subsequent commentators, does not alter this fact.

Comenius's own account of the event makes very clear how shrewdly Hartlib played on his sense of divine mission:

> now he invited me to London, now to Amsterdam, or to Hamburg (yea even to Stettin or Danzig, if I wished); he would come there with his friends. But it could not be, because I was now tied to my place by the character of the office I had undertaken.[190] At last in 1641 in the month of July, I received three letters from him (written in the same tenor but dispatched by three different routes), in which he insisted on my coming to him at once, and thus he concluded: 'Come, come, come: it is for the glory of God: deliberate not longer with flesh and blood.' What could I do?[191]

At this stage at least, Hartlib saw Comenius as a lynchpin of the divine purpose he thought was being worked out before his eyes. Throughout his life, he was much taken with the idea that England would be the launching pad of the Third Reformation. For him, Comenius was the right man, England the right place, and 1641 the right time, and having finally, with considerable effort, succeeded in establishing him there, he was extremely reluctant to relinquish him.

Moriaen, thanks perhaps to the perspective lent by distance, seems to have discerned more clearly than Hartlib the way the situation in England was developing, even though it was Hartlib who was his principal informant on the subject. This is not to claim any particular subtlety or insight for Moriaen's political thought. His comments on the developments on the eve of the civil wars follow the standard Puritan line: Strafford, Laud and their supporters are the villains of the piece, who have misguided the King and led him into a factitious quarrel with Parliament based on misunderstandings and misrepresentations. What he foresaw more clearly than Hartlib was just how severe that quarrel would become. He interpreted such matters in distinctly apocalyptic terms:

> We can guess for ourselves how the true-hearted among you must be feeling. We shall be eager above all to hear what the book with seven seals will bring to light, and we suppose that each of the seven seals will signify a particular woe which will be brought down on the head of such or such a one.[192]

But whereas Hartlib in mid-1641 seems to have believed that with Strafford and Laud out of the way and the Long Parliament convened things had taken a decisive turn for the better, Moriaen - though he had initially favoured England as a destination for Comenius - remained sceptical.

Moriaen learned of the invitation to Sweden on 3 October 1641, and wrote to Hartlib the same day endorsing the plan wholeheartedly.[193] The few mild reservations expressed probably sprang from a sense that Hartlib's feelings might be hurt, or his hopes disappointed, by the suggestion that London was not the ideal location after all, for he followed them with a resounding commendation of de Geer, and with more well-judged scepticism about the prospects for funding by the English Parliament. Writing to Comenius himself a week later, he was totally unequivocal in his support for the Swedish plan.[194]

When he discovered what Hartlib's response had been, he made no attempt to disguise his annoyance, declaring roundly that Hartlib had completely misinterpreted the proposal, and heavily implying that he had done so wilfully. 'I wrote plainly', he observed, with unconcealed exasperation, 'that he would be without official obligations or hindrances there, committed only to company, conversation and counsel, with sufficient opportunity to devote himself solely and simply to his studies.[195] Rulice felt the same, and wrote in almost identical terms:

> you have completely misunderstood us: Herr de Geer desires nothing in the world from Mr Comenius but the chance to talk with him from time to time. Mr Comenius is to be well provided for there, with ample opportunity to correspond with others at no expense, and leisure to perfect his meditations.[196]

Moriaen also had personal experience of the generosity de Geer was prepared to bestow on a cause he deemed worthy: as administrator of the Palatine relief project he had seen de Geer contribute over 20,000 Imperials to the cause.[197] Though every bit as convinced as Hartlib that to support Comenius was to undertake missionary work in the cause of world reformation, he was a good deal less optimistic about the potential of England to supply the necessary conditions for this. On 18 November, he again urged acceptance of de Geer's plan, which Hübner (who at this stage was seen as a likely beneficiary of it) by then also approved. He observed in somewhat more down-to-earth fashion this time, 'I cannot see that things in England have yet reached the point I should like to see them at, and I fear that if God does not graciously prevent it there may be bloodied heads'.[198]

By this time, the Irish Rebellion had broken out, and in the end it was political circumstance rather than persuasive argument that determined the outcome. But Hartlib was still receiving donations and hoping for a positive response from Parliament;[199] as late as 23 December Moriaen was still nagging him to come to a decision.[200] By the spring of 1642 even Hartlib must have realised that major state subsidy from England in the near future was a forlorn hope, and Comenius's move to Sweden was settled, though his friends in England continued to insist he should return as soon as circumstances permitted.[201]

En route to Sweden, Comenius spent a month travelling round the Netherlands visiting friends and supporters there (June-July 1642). The event was, however, for Moriaen at least, something of an anti-climax. He would have liked to lodge Comenius himself, but de Geer's son Laurens was on hand to provide much more luxurious accommodation than Moriaen could run to. The crush to see the Pansophist was so great that personal conversation of any depth and intimacy was precluded. Perhaps it was some consolation to Moriaen that all this bore witness to the success of his propaganda drive, but there is no mistaking the sense of let-down in his accounts of their meeting.[202] He was set to work with Budæus (who had evidently joined Moriaen in Amsterdam) examining Comenius's perpetual motion theory, the very part of all the latter's undertakings he had always expressed the greatest scepticism about, and he found it even less satisfactory than he had anticipated. Comenius had almost entirely neglected to provide any experimental demonstration, and Moriaen was openly scathing about the 'derisory models' ('liederliche modellen') he and Budæus were expected to improve on. A few months later, the ailing Budæus was dead, and a somewhat jaundiced Moriaen declared himself heartily sick of perpetual motion, for which he now had 'little time and not much more stomach'.[203] The metaphysical dimension so prominent in his earlier speculations on the subject is conspicuously absent from this letter. In its place is redoubled concern that Comenius would be discredited if his work in the field became known, either through his own publications or through loose talk by his associates. The very thought of the device can only have served to call to Moriaen's mind his dead friend Budæus and his frustrated hopes of Comenius.

The Swedish project too failed utterly to live up to Moriaen's expectations. He had envisaged Comenius settled in comfort and tranquility, free from any distraction other than the stimulating conversation of scholars, secure in de Geer's disinterested munificence, supported by able assistants and labouring diligently at his *Janua Rerum*, not producing sketches of Pansophy any more but the thing itself. In the event, Comenius spent only two months in Sweden, largely taken up with meeting dignitaries such as the effective ruler Chancellor Oxenstierna, the teenage Queen Christina, and Dury's old ally the Lutheran irenicist Johannes Matthiæ, Bishop of Strengnäs.

Oxenstierna came out against de Geer's plan to keep Comenius in Sweden, ostensibly on the grounds that his views on the fundamental goodness of human nature and his particular brand of chiliasm, envisaging a golden age on earth before the Last Judgment, would lead to ructions with the established Lutheran clergy. Instead he suggested Elblag, Hartlib's birthplace, at this time under Swedish occupation, where the climate of religious tolerance would provide a more congenial atmosphere for him to work in.[204] There may have been some truth in this, but Oxenstierna's principal interest was almost certainly in having an informed agent in an area of crucial strategic importance to Sweden. Moriaen's second-hand report of this, summarising a letter from Louis de Geer, and of Oxenstierna's alleged suggestion that the Swedish state should bear some of Comenius's costs, is exceptionally bald and non-committal, in marked contrast to his passionate arguments in favour of the original plan.[205]

The nature of Comenius's undertakings to Oxenstierna remains unknown, but in the event either Oxenstierna changed his mind about state funding or Comenius balked at such an overt commitment to a nation whose intentions in the Baltic were viewed with suspicion, to say the least, by his own exiled brethren there, and it was de Geer who, having reluctantly followed Oxenstierna's advice and given up his plan for a learned society, nonetheless took the whole charge upon himself. He provided Comenius with 1000 Imperials annually, and agreed moreover to donate the same annual sum to the Unity of Brethren.[206] This still only amounts to about half the thousand pounds a year Moriaen had said he could easily spare, but represents a far larger income than Hartlib, and Comenius himself, had considered adequate (though the funding of assistants remained a problem), and also meant that Comenius could claim a measure of success in his official fundraising mission.

Where Moriaen had completely misjudged de Geer, however, was in the matter of the return he expected on his investment. One of the often-invoked advantages of public collections, however troublesome they might be to organise, was that the contributors, not being an organised body, could lay no proprietorial claim to the recipient's work and exercise no control over it: they simply had to trust the organisers' judgment (and honesty) in the use of their money. Private patrons, however generous, were a different matter, and here de Geer turned out to be less exceptional than Moriaen had imagined. His (purely verbal) contract with Comenius, as the latter much later recalled it,[207] committed him to work in the first place on educational materials for Sweden. This was precisely the sort of commitment to sub-pansophic drudgery Hartlib had been so chary of, while Moriaen had strongly insisted no such risk was being run. Why de Geer suddenly became so interested in Swedish educational reform, which had not been mentioned in his original invitation, is not clear: perhaps he felt that if he was not to have his learned society he would distinguish himself in another way in the eyes of his adopted nation; perhaps he had simply never seen Comenius's mission in quite such exalted terms as the Hartlibians. Whatever the reason, the commitment was made.

Moriaen seems to have been completely unaware of this contract. Like many others associated with the business, he was surprised and deeply disappointed to find that Comenius continued to busy himself with schoolbooks. He had always nursed a fear that the high expectations he and his collaborators were raising might not be met: 'We have heaped great praise on him up to now, and raised high hopes in ourselves and others. I devoutly wish our hopes and praise may not be turned to scorn'.[208] During his first year in Elblag, Comenius asked his associates to keep correspondence to a minimum in order that he might not be distracted.[209] Having waited eagerly to see what fruits might be borne of this retirement, Moriaen found his worst suspicions realised:

> I hear that he has only revised his *Janua* and *Vestibulum*, and put them
> into a different form: this is indeed a good work, but it is not what we
> have waited for so long and raised such hopes of in others. I hope there is
> more to it than this, or we should fairly be put to shame that nothing
> should come of it but such schoolbooks.[210]

This marked the end of Moriaen's active involvement in the pansophic project. In part this was because, thanks to the de Geers, the funding problem was substantially solved. But to a much larger extent, it reflected a deep disappointment, a loss of faith on Moriaen's part in Comenius's ability, or perhaps in his willingness, to fulfil the task. The very notion of Pansophy seems to have lost its appeal. Comenius mentioned him in May 1646 as being in a position to send Hartlib copies of his works as they came off the press in Amsterdam,[211] but there is no evidence of his having done so; as will be argued later, there is reason to doubt whether Moriaen was in touch with Hartlib at all at that date. His hopes were raised again somewhat many years later by an encouraging report from Magnus Hesenthaler of Comenius's work on the *Consultatio Catholica*,[212] but the passionate faith of the late 'thirties was gone for good. There is a very striking drop in the number of references to

Comenius from this point on, and as for the word *pansophia*, it never occurs again in the surviving correspondence.

A decade and a half later, in 1656, Comenius finally settled in Amsterdam, under the patronage of Laurens de Geer, and remained there for the rest of his life. Moriaen evinced singularly little response to this event. Though he had by this time left Amsterdam for Arnhem, contact between them would have been made a great deal easier than ever before had they so wished. Moriaen at least manifestly did not. On a visit to Amsterdam at the beginning of 1657, he did indeed briefly meet Comenius on the street, and arranged to spend the whole of the following day with him. He changed his mind, however (or so he later told Hartlib), because a chill was setting in and Odilia was eager to return to Arnhem. Instead of keeping his appointment, he went back home.[213] It should be said that the danger of becoming snowbound was not one to be taken lightly. Nevertheless, for a man in 1657 to cite the weather and his wife's wishes as grounds for breaking an appointment with someone whose cause he had earlier regarded as the defining purpose of his very existence must be seen as a conspicuous snub.

The notion of universal wisdom itself, however, by no means vanished from Moriaen's outlook. His disillusion was not with the ideal itself but with Comenius's particular scheme for realising it. His personal history after 1642 is dominated by a series of attempts to attain by other means the crucial pansophic goals of 'right method' and universal harmony.

Notes

1   The secondary literature on Comenius is enormous. The fullest biographical account is Milada Blekastad's *Comenius: Versuch eines Umrisses von Leben, Werk und Schicksal des Jan Amos Komensky* (Oslo and Prague, 1969), which despite its modest title is a detailed and exhaustive account of his life and work, based heavily and usefully (though at times somewhat uncritically) on Comenius's correspondence and autobiographical writings. Still valuable are the many studies written nearly a century ago by Jan Kvacala, particularly *Die Pädagogische Reform des Comenius in Deutschland bis zum Ausgange des XVII Jahrhunderts* (*Monumenta Germaniæ Pædagogica* XVII (Berlin, 1903) and XXII (Berlin, 1904)). The standard English sources are Turnbull, *HDC* part 3 (342-464), Webster, *Great Instauration* and 'Introduction' to *Samuel Hartlib and the Advancement of Learning* (Cambridge, 1970), and Hugh Trevor-Roper's rather dismissive and anglocentric 'Three Foreigners: The Philosophers of the Puritan Revolution', in *Religion, the Reformation and Social Change* (London, 1967), 237-93 (on Hartlib, Dury and Comenius and their impact in England). Wilhelmus Rood's *Comenius and the Low Countries: Some Aspects of the Life and Work of a Czech Exile in the Seventeenth Century* (Amsterdam, 1970) contains useful material on his stay in the Netherlands and his relations with the de Geer family (discussed later in this chapter). There are vast numbers of articles on more specific aspects of his life, thought and publishing history in the journals *Monatshefte der Comeniusgesellschaft*, *Acta Comeniana* and *Studia Comeniana et Historica*. See also Dagmar Capková, 'Comenius and his Ideals: Escape from the Labyrinth', *SHUR*, 75-92, and, on the background to his thought, Howard Hotson, *Johann Heinrich Alsted: Encyclopedism, Millenarianism and the Second Reformation in Germany* (PhD thesis, Oxford, 1991), summarised in 'Philosophical Pedagogy in Reformed Central Europe between Ramus and Comenius: a survey of the continental background of the "Three Foreigners"', *SHUR*, 29-50.

See also John Sadler: *Comenius* (London, 1969), and Daniel Murphy, *Comenius: A Critical Reassessment of his Life and Work* (Cambridge, 1995). A critical and very stimulating account of Comenius's concept of education in the context of his millenarian Utopianism forms a major strand of James Holstun's *A Rational Millennium: Puritan Utopias of Seventeenth-Century England and America* (New York and Oxford, 1987).

2   'das werck, dz ich nach *Gottes* schickung auf mich genommen vnd nun mehr mein ganzes werck davon mache zum gemeinen besten [...] ich hab mich gleichsam darzu abgesondert vnd devotiret' - Moriaen to ? (probably Hartlib), 16 June 1639, HP 37/25B

3   'der welt nie nichts nuzlichers seÿe angetrag*en* word*en* als eben diß werckh als dardurch die Schulen vnd vermittelst d*er*selben Ecclesia respub*lica* mund*us* reformirt werden sollen vnd können' - Moriaen to Hartlib, 28 Oct. 1641, HP 37/92A.

4   Blekastad, *Comenius*, 23-48. He was at Herborn from 1611-13, at Heidelberg from 1613-14.

5   See Hotson, *Johann Heinrich Alsted*, 23.

6   See Hotson, op. cit., 17-20.

7   See Peter Dear, 'The Church and the New Philosophy', *Science, Culture and Popular Belief in the Renaissance*, ed. Stephen Pumfrey, Paolo L. Rossi and Maurice Slawinski (Manchester and New York, 1991), 119-39, esp.133-4. The curriculum covered (in order) Greek and Latin grammar and rhetoric, logic, ethics, mathematics (including optics and astronomy), physics and metaphysics. The prominent place of mathematics was a novelty, but in other respects this is very close to the standard university curriculum.

8   'Ich wundere mich offtmahl vber der Iesuiten industriam fatalem [...] diese hetten wan sie sich die inquisition der natur so sehr angelegen sein laßen alß den dominium in conscientias, vill guts thun können' - Pöhmer to Hartlib, 25 March 1638, HP 59/10/7A.

9   Dury to ?, 26 Nov. 1635, HP 3/4/37B.

10 As is stressed (and demonstrated) by Hotson, *Alsted, passim*.

11 Reproduced in *KK II*, 234; see Blekastad, *Comenius*, 33-35.

12 Cf. Comenius, *Pansophiæ Prodromus* (London, 1639), translated either by or by command of Hartlib, together with the *Conatuum Pansophicorum Dilucidatio* (London, 1639), as *A Reformation of Schooles* (London, 1642): 'Let even the Gentiles, and Arabians therefore be admitted to furnish us with such ornaments, as they are able for the beauty of this house of God' (p.33).

13 Comenius to [Hartlib?], 3 Aug. 1656, HP 7/99/1A: 'opus erit reparari jacturam eorum Authorum qvi mihi adhuc erunt consulendi [...] Verulamii opera intelligo, & L. Vivis, & Campanellæ omnia, etc'. Vives (1492-1540) was one of the leading humanist scholars of his day and a favourite pupil of Erasmus: he particularly concerned himself with education and foreshadowed many of the ideas of Alsted, Bacon and Comenius, such as pre-school education, education of women, the primacy of sense impressions over intellect, the dignity of the vernacular and above all the importance of rendering learning applicable to life both practically and ethically. See Foster Watson, *Vives on Education* (Cambridge, 1913). Campanella (1568-1639) combined an idiosyncratic Neo-Platonism and a fascination with the Renaissance Art of Memory with impassioned championship of new experimental science. See Luigi Firpo's *Introduction* to Campanella, *La Cité du Soleil* (tr. Arnaud Tripet, Geneva, 1972) for a succinct but incisive account of his life and thought; also Frances Yates, *Giordano Bruno and the Hermetic Tradition* (London, 1964) and *The Art of Memory* (London, 1966), and Paolo Rossi, *Clavis Universalis* (Bologna, 1983). On

Campanella's reception among Comenians, see Martin Mulsow, 'Sociabilitas. Zu einem Kontext der Campanella-Rezeption im 17. Jahrhundert', *Studia Bruniana et Campanelliana* I (1995), 205-32. My thanks to Dr Mulsow for supplying me with an advanced copy of this very detailed and interesting study. On Bacon and Comenius, see below, pp. 105-10..

14 *Reipublicæ Christianopolitanæ descriptio* (Straßburg, 1619). Of the hundred short chapters of this work, ch. 51-78 are devoted exclusively to describing the Christianopolitan education system, while more general educational ideas are discussed throughout. Andreæ translated a work of Vives on poor relief, *De subventione pauperum*, as *Johann Ludwig Vives von Versorgung der Armen* (Durlach, 1627).

15 Campanella, *Civitas Solis* (1623, but written c.1602).

16 HP 37/167A-B and 37/5B-6A. On Bodinus's ideas, see W. Toischer, 'Die Didaktik des Elias Bodinus', *Mitteilungen der Gesellschaft für deutsche Erziehungs- und Schulgeschichte* IX (1899), 209-29 (but Toischer is wrong in his conjecture (p. 217) that Bodinus died soon after 1626; according to Blekastad he died in Prussia in 1651 (*Comenius*, 334)). It was his *Bericht von der Natur- und Vernunfftmessigen Didactica oder Lehr-Kunst* (Hamburg, 1621) that gave Comenius the idea of composing the original Czech version of his *Didactica magna* (*Opera Didactica Omnia* (Amsterdam, 1657) I, 3). The work bears the very proto-Comenian motto 'Omnia faciliora facit Ratio, Ordo et Modus' ('Everything is made easier by Reason, Order and Method').

17 On Ratke, and the reactions to him of both Comenius and Jungius, see G.E. Guhrauer, *Joachim Jungius und sein Zeitalter* (Stuttgart and Tübingen, 1850), 23-43.

18 *Methodus institutionis nova quadruplex* (Leipzig, 1617).

19 *A Reformation of Schooles* 77. Cf. the subtitle of the *Didactica Magna* (Amsterdam, 1657, but written 1637-38): the work claims to exhibit 'Universale Omnes Omnia docendi artificium' ('the universal art of teaching all things to all people').

20 See Hotson, *Alsted*, 91-158 on the genesis of the *Encyclopædia*.

21 See Blekastad, *Comenius*, 170-76 for a fuller account of the genesis and ethos of the *Janua*, which Blekastad describes as being - in the Alstedian sense - 'eine kleine Enzyklopädie' (173). See also Comenius's own account, *Comenius' Självbiografi* (Stockholm 1975), 144-6.

22 Blekastad, *Comenius*, 200-203. As she argues, it was almost certainly the work's efficacy as a pedagogical tool that recommended it to the majority of teachers, rather than its philosophical underpinning.

23 Comenius, *Continuatio admonitionis fraternæ de temperando charitate zelo [...] ad S. Maresium* (Amsterdam, 1670), English translation by Agneta Lunggren in Milada Blekastad (ed.), *Comenius' Självbiografi* (Stockholm, 1975), 145-47. This is Comenius's most important autobiographical work. The section dealing with his visit to England also exists in English translation in R.F. Young, *Comenius in England* (Oxford and London, 1932), 25-51. Despite its somewhat mannered archaism, Young's translation is stylistically far superior to Lunggren's, which it is painfully obvious was never checked by a native speaker. However, Lunggren's is more literal and includes the whole text, and is furnished with excellent notes.

24 *Självbiografi*, 147.

25 *Självbiografi*, 148 (cf. Young, *Comenius in England*, 31). See also *A Reformation of Schooles*, 46-7.

26 See Comenius to Hartlib, 26 Jan. 1638, in O. Odlozilík, *Casopis Matice Moravské* LII (1928), 164; condensed German translation by Blekastad, *Comenius*, 255-6. Comenius mentioned in this letter that he and Hartlib had been in touch for six years.

Their first contact (a letter from Hartlib with a financial contribution) is described in *Självbiografi*, 149, but no exact date is given.

27   'das es in causa Antiliana dahin beschloßen das man institutionem puerorum vorauß treiben vnd alß ein fundament zu diesem legen müste' - Fridwald to Hartlib, 10 Feb. 1628, HP 27/34/1A

28   'weill der H. hierinnen ettwas sonderliches præstiret' - ibid. See also Turnbull, 'John Hall's Letters to Samuel Hartlib', *Review of English Studies* New Series 4 (1953), 221-33.

29   *HDC*, 16-19, 36-9.

30   Described in detail below, pp. 127-34.

31   Comenius to Hartlib, 17 Feb. 1641, in two scribal copies at HP 7/84/1B-3B and 7/84/6A-8A; English summary in *HDC*, 350.

32   Trevor-Roper, 'Three Foreigners', *passim.*

33   Trevor-Roper is very fond of this expression: cf. 'Three Foreigners', 258 and 289; 'Introduction' to Margery Purver, *The Royal Society: Concept and Creation* (London, 1967), xv and xvi.

34   'Three Foreigners', 258. This line of argument is taken furthest by Margery Purver, who sees the Royal Society as having resurrected pure, genuine Baconianism from the fragmented and trivialised form of it propagated by the likes of Hartlib and Haak. She sets out to remove this 'vulgar' stain from the Society's pedigree by denying they had any influence on its genesis at all: see her *The Royal Society: Concept and Creation* (London, 1967), especially Part Two, chapter 4, 'The Royal Society and "Pansophia"', 193-234. See also Webster's devastating essay review of the book, 'The Origins of the Royal Society', *History of Scence* VI (1967), 106-28.

35   'vnder des Verulamij nachgelaßenen schrifften werden ohne zweiffel viel treffliche sachen sein' - Moriaen to Hartlib, 26 May 1639, HP 37/24A.

36   Bacon, *Of the Proficience and Advancement of Learning Human and Divine, Works* ed. James Spelling et al., (London, 1857-74) III, 359.

37   Bacon, *Preparative Towards a Natural and Experimental History (Parasceve), Works* IV, 252.

38   *Advancement of Learning*, 268.

39   Andrew Clark (ed.), *'Brief Lives,' chiefly of Contemporaries, set down by John Aubrey, between the Years 1669 and 1696* (Oxford, 1898), I, 75-6.

40   HP 22/6/2A-5B, undated.

41   See for instance Margery Purver, *The Royal Society: Concept and Creation* (London, 1967), which is very impatient with those who see Bacon as a mere fact-finder, and Lisa Jardine, *Francis Bacon and the Art of Discourse* (Cambridge, 1974).

42   *A Reformation of Schooles*, 35.

43   *A Reformation of Schooles*, 6.

44   Johann Valentin Andreæ (trans. John Hall), *A Modell of a Christian Society*, (original Latin *Societas Christianæ imago*, Tübingen 1620, translation London 1647), reprinted by George Turnbull in *Zeitschrift für deutsche Philologie* 74 (1955), 151-161, 155. The original, preserved in a single printed copy in Wolfenbüttel and two manuscript copies in the Hartlib Papers reads: 'Nam cum hoc Mundi senio omnia propemodum humana, literis concredita sint, qvarum moles in immensum excrevit, & non tàm veritate qvàm falsitate, soliditate qvàm Vanitate Orbem adimplevit' (HP 55/19/5B).

45   *Preparative Towards a Natural and Experimental History, Works*, IV, 258-9. What is under discussion here, it should perhaps be stressed, is the description Bacon gave in

this work of what the Natural Histories *should* be, not the content of the Natural Histories he himself actually produced, which hardly meet his own specifications.

46   *Eph 40*, HP 30/4/54A.

47   Hübner is much the most frequently cited source in the *Ephemerides* of 1639 and 40, something like half the entries being attributed him. The opinion and the blunt, slightly truculent manner of its expression are consistent with Hübner's original writings.

48   *Eph 40*, HP 30/4/54B.

49   Matthew 25:12.

50   Daniel, 12:4, Authorised Version (Bacon cited the Vulgate: 'Multi pertransibunt et augebitur scientia'). Luther, interestingly, gives a completely different reading: 'So werden viel drüber kommen [ie. über diese Schrift] vnd grossen verstand finden' ('Many will come upon it [this writing] and find great understanding in it'): I am advised that the Authorised Version is the more literal (my thanks to the members of Sheffield University's Classical Hebrew Dictionary Project).

51   *A Reformation of Schooles*, 4 and 29. Cf. Popkin, 'The Third Force in 17th Century Philosophy', *Nouvelles de la République des Lettres* (1983), 35-63, esp 43-5, on the importance of this passage for the influential Millenarian William Twisse, whose *Doubting Conscience Resolved* (1652) was written for and published by Hartlib.

52   Cf. Stephen Clucas, 'In Search of the "True Logick": methodological eclecticism among the "Baconian reformers"', *SHUR*, 51-74.

53   *Advancement of Learning, Works*, III, 268.

54   See Blekastad, *Comenius*, 257-260, and Comenius's own somewhat hyperbolical accounts in a letter to Hartlib of autumn 1638, *KK II*, 34-6 and *MPG I*, 139-41 (in both cases misdated August 1639: see Blekastad, *Comenius*, 260, n. 174) and *Självbiografi*, 151. Broniewski's *Annotatiunculæ quædam in præludia Comeniana ad Portam Sapientiæ* are at HP 7/82/1A-4B and are reproduced in *HDC*, 452-7.

55   *Självbiografi*, 148-9 (Young, *Comenius in England*, 32-3).

56   *A Reformation of Schooles*, 6.

57   Especially *A Treatise of Husbandry* (London, 1638) and *A Discovery of Infinite Treasure* (London, 1639), the treasure in question being the inexhaustible wealth of well-husbanded nature. The works are aimed emphatically at the ordinary farmer rather than the large landowner and are very practical (and pragmatic) in tone. Plattes was supported for a time by Hartlib but died in poverty. See *DNB*, 410, and Hartlib's own *Legacie of Husbandry* (London, 1651).

58   *Eph 39*, 30/4/18B; the remark is not attributed but it sounds to me like Hübner again.

59   *Eph 39*, 30/4/26B. This is almost certainly Hübner. On 'Cartes glasses', see above, pp. 22-3.

60   *Conatuum Comenianorum Dilucidatio*: 'My intent was to epitomize those bookes of God, Nature, Scripture and mans Conscience' (*A Reformation of Schooles*, 65); cf. *Panaugia*, trans. A.M.O. Dobbie (Shipton on Stour, 1987) 13; *Pampædia*, trans. A.M.O. Dobbie (Dover, 1986) 130.

61   *A Reformation of Schooles*, 27. Cf. *Panorthosia*, trans. A.M.O. Dobbie (Sheffield, 1993) 25: I say that you must be *Everything* in yourself, as a genuine portion of mankind and a true image of God and Christ. For if every individual Being is an image of the Universe [...] every member of human society ought also to represent human society as a whole, so that [...] one may *be* or *know* or *wish* or *do* what all men are or know or wish or do.'

62   *Eph 39*, HP 30/4/10A. There is again no clear indication that Hübner is being cited, but the style and content overwhelmingly suggest him.

63   Comenius, *Pampædia*, 85.

64   *A Reformation of Schooles*, 15.

65   *A Reformation of Schooles*, 15.

66   'vil sachen weist man nit wo man sie hin referiren soll. Mueß sie also entweder vnter dem koth, vieler Vnnützer zerstrewter Aphorismorum verborgen ligen laßen, oder mitt Alstedio, ich weiß nicht, waß vor narrischen farragines artium et particulas systematum den gemeinen Vngestalten systematibus subjungiren, welches ihme dan allein die confusion seiner Encyclopode [*sic*] gnugsam solt zue verstehen geben haben' - HP 36/4/50A: from a long anonymous tract on combatting atheism, undated but composed c.1638/9.

67   An abridged version of this section appears under the same title in *Acta Comeniana* 12 (1997, 89-99).

68   Hotson, *Alsted*, 156.

69   Ibid., 147.

70   'wollen wir ihn doch viel höher halten, als 1000 Alstedios mit allen ihren vermeinten methodis' - Anon. to [Hartlib?], early 1638, HP 59/10/20B.

71   *Eph 39*, 30/4/2A.

72   *Novum organum*, second book of aphorisms, aphorism 29: *Works*, IV, 169.

73   *Eph 56*, 29/5/89A.

74   'in dieser irrenden vnd verführischen welt [... ist] vnß extra Mathesin fast nichts sichers vnd gewißes vbergelaßen' - Moriaen to Hartlib, 31 Jan. 1639, HP 37/5A.

75   'Ich bin dieser sachen auß der maßen begierig all meine tage gewest nun aber desto mehr weil Ich mir vnd anderen possibilitatem Pansophiæ dardurch einbilden kan, damit Ich berait etliche wiedersprecher stumme vnd zweiffeler glaubig gemacht habe' - Moriaen to Hartlib, 24 March 1639, HP 37/13B.

76   Aubrey, *Brief Lives* II, 127 and 129. The first two comments are from a memo to Aubrey from Haak.

77   Aubrey, *Brief Lives* II, 130. On the 'Idea Matheseos', see below p. 114.

78   Martinus Hortensius (1605-39), mathematics professor at the Amsterdam Athenæum Illustre since 1634. See *NNBW* I, 1160-4.

79   Moriaen to Hartlib, 26 Dec. 1639, HP 37/50A.

80   So at least Moriaen claimed, 2 June 1644, HP 37/117A.

81   Unfortunately, no letters survive from 1643, the year of Pell's move, and only one from the whole period of his stay in Amsterdam. It is clear from this, however, that Moriaen was one of Pell's first contacts, as he came bearing him a letter from Hartlib. This letter also describes how Pell was offered the post, relates the success of his inaugural lecture, and mentions that Moriaen was trying to find permanent accommodation for Pell.

82   *DNB* XLIV, 262.

83   According to the manuscript title page in the Hartlib Papers (HP 14/1/6A), the *Idea* was written in 1634. Turnbull suggests it may have been conceived as early as 1630, when Pell sent Hartlib 'a rude draught of his Method' (*HDC*, 88), though this does not necessarily refer to the *Idea*. For the complete English text and the publication date of 1638, see P.J. Wallis, 'An Early Mathematical Manifesto - John Pell's *Idea of Mathematics*', *Durham Research Journal* 18 (1967), 139-48. Wallis's dating is borne out by Pell's reference in a letter of October 1642 which cannot be to anyone but

Hartlib to 'my letter to you, which you caused to be published just this time four years' (*Correspondance de Mersenne* XI, 311).

84 Comenius derived this term from Alsted's precursor Bartholomæus Keckermann: it refers to Aristotle's assertion that all learning depends on prior knowledge.

85 Pell, *Idea of Mathematics*, ed. P.J. Wallis, in *Durham Research Journal* 18 (1967), 139-48, esp. 143.

86 Ibid., 144.

87 Ibid., 145.

88 Mersenne to Haak, 1 Nov. 1639, *Correspondance de Mersenne* VIII, 580-4; Pell to Mersenne, 21 Nov. 1639 (ibid., 622-630); Mersenne to Pell, 10 Dec. 1639 (ibid., 685-688). See also Wallis's useful summary of the early reception of the *Idea*, *Durham Research Journal* 18 (1967), 145-7.

89 Jacob Klein, *Greek Mathematical Thought and the Origin of Algebra*, trans. Eva Brann, (Cambridge Mass. and London 1968).

90 Ibid., 118.

91 Ibid., 123. In all quotations from him, the italics are Klein's.

92 Ibid., 123.

93 The edition finally appeared in 1646 (see *Correspondance de Mersenne* VII, 33 and 106-9).

94 Facsimile in *Correspondance de Mersenne* VII, facing 109.

95 *Correspondance de Mersenne* XI, 308. The letter is also given in Robert Vaughan, *The Protectorate of Oliver Cromwell* (London, 1839) II, 347-54. The Moriaen letters in question are those of 2 and 9 Oct. 1642, HP 37/112A-114B, in which Moriaen stated that he had recommended Pell to the Elseviers and urged him to contribute to the edition.

96 Ibid., 308-11.

97 Hartlib to Tassius, 10 August 1638, Staats- und Universitätsbibliothek Hamburg, sup. op. 100, fol. 60-63; slightly edited transcript in *KK I*, 32-6. Hartlib said he was sending 'eine andre Idæam Conatuum Mathematico*rum* eines andern Authoris [than J.L. Wolzogen], darvon ich des H. vnparteyliches judicium mit dem ersten erwarte' (63r; *KK I*, 36), which given that this is precisely the period when Hartlib was distributing the *Idea* is almost certainly a reference to it.

98 Dury to Hartlib, 13 September 1639, HP 9/1/95B.

99 Klein, op. cit., 185, quoting Vieta, *In artem analyticen Isagoge* (1591); the capitalisation is Vieta's.

100 'Ich wolte gerne wißen ob sich Mons. Pell*ii* Logistica so weit erstrecke als des Vietæ Nullum non problema soluere' - Moriaen to [Hartlib?], 27 Dec. 1638, HP 37/166A.

101 6 Jan. 1642, Young, *Comenius in England*, 74.

102 Bacon, *Advancement of Learning*, *Works* III, 359-60.

103 Moriaen to Hartlib, 24 March 1639, HP 37/13B.

104 'fast niemand weit vber den Cubum kommen' - ibid.

105 *A Reformation of Schooles*, 25. Similarly on p.51: 'Neither in the delivery of these things, though evidently true, do wee presuppose any thing [...] but we premonstrate rather, that is we deduce one thing out of another continually, from the first principles of Metaphysickes, untill we come to the last, and least differences of Things: and this with such evidence of truth, as the propositions of the Mathematicians have, so that there is a necessity of yeelding to the last as well as to the first, for the continuall, and nowhere interrupted demonstration of their truth.'

106   Moriaen acknowledged receipt on 24 March, HP 37/14A. The *Analysis* consists of a compilation of extracts from letters to Joseph St Amand of November and December 1637 (HP 1/4/19A-22B), and is further elaborated in another letter to him of 26 February 1640 (HP 1/4/1A-8B). Moriaen intended to have it published, but whether he in fact did so remains unclear (see above, p. 39).

107   HP 1/4/20A.

108   *Eph 35*, HP 29/3/14A; transcript in *HDC*, 167. Cf. Popkin, 'The Third Force',40-2. Popkin argues persuasively that it was the millenarian writings of Joseph Mede that first suggested to Dury the way out of his labyrinth.

109   *Eph 35*, HP 29/3/14A.

110   Dury, *Analysis Demonstrativa*, HP 1/4/20A-B.

111   'dan beÿ vielen gehet der glaub nicht außer den augen vnd ob sie woll gleuben müßen dati certitudinem Mathematicam so glauben sie doch nicht das man einen solchen methodum in relig. scientijs sonderlich aber in Theologia finden vnd practisiren könne vnder welchen auch Mr des Cartes ist' - Moriaen to Hartlib, 24 March 1639, HP 37/14A: the remark is made with specific reference to Dury's *Analysis Demonstrativa*.

112   Ibid., HP 1/4/3A.

113   HP 1/4/21B.

114   *Panaugia*, trans. A.M.O. Dobbie (Shipton on Stour, 1987), ch.11, para. 101, p.71.

115   Ibid., ch.15, para. 42, p.99.

116   *Reformation of Schooles*, 26.

117   Isaiah 11:9, a citation also used by Comenius (*Reformation of Schooles*, 26).

118   *Reformation of Schooles*, 24.

119   'zue dem werk des heiligthumbs nicht allein Bezaliel und Aholiab erfordert werden sondern auch die Ienige so herbeÿ schaffen was zur arbeit von nothen ist' - Moriaen to Hartlib, 13 Dec. 1638, HP 37/1B. Bezaleel and Aholiab were the craftsmen selected by God to build the Ark of the Covenant (Exodus 31:1-6).

120   He joined the English church in November 1635 and transferred to the German on 4 Dec. 1639 (Moriaen's letter of the following day, HP 37/49B); cf. O.P. Grell, *Dutch Calvinists*, 181.

121   Blekastad (*Comenius*, 334 and *Unbekannte Briefe*, 18) cautiously suggests this may be the Swedish mathematician Niels Buddaeus (1595-1653), but this cannot be right, since Moriaen's Budæus died on 11 Sept. 1642, as he told Hartlib the following month (HP 37/112A).

122   Jonston to Hartlib, Aug. 1633, HP 44/1/2A. On Jonston, see William Hitchens, Adam Matuszewski and John Young, *The Correspondence of Jan Jonston in the Archive of Samuel Hartlib* (Polish Academy of Sciences, forthcoming).

123   Hessels III, no. 2311.

124   Grell, 203.

125   Grell, 203. Turnbull in his account of the incident takes Hartlib's alleged word for it (*HDC*, 35).

126   *HDC*, 35, n.4.

127   See Mark Greengrass, 'The Financing of a Seventeenth-Century Intellectual: Contributions for Comenius', *Acta Comeniana* XXXV (1996), 71-87 and 141-157.

128   Grell (who spells him Strezzo), 180; Hessels III, nos. 2569 and 2654.

129   Moriaen to Hartlib, 13 Feb. 1640, HP 37/57A.

130   It is not in Wing, nor in Turnbull's list of Hartlib's publications (*HDC*, 88-109), and is mentioned nowhere else in the surviving papers.

131   HP 23/13/1B. I am almost certain the recipient of five copies is 'Morian', but the list is in Hartlib's very worst handwriting. It is certainly 'Morian et Rulit.' who received fifty. Turnbull (*HDC*, 343) thinks it likelier that the work in question is the *Præludia*, but Moriaen's acknowledgement of a number of copies of the *Prodromus* which had been passed on to him by Rulice (12 May 1639, HP 37/23A) would seem rather to suggest the latter. Hartlib's undated list may, however, refer to an earlier consignment of *Præludias* not mentioned in the surviving letters.

132   HP 37/13A.

133   Exchange rates fluctuated, but the pound generally equated to something between 4 and 4 ½ Imperials over the period of Moriaen's and Hartlib's correspondence.

134   HP 26/23/1A-8B; cf. Greengrass, 'Collections for Comenius'.

135   HP 26/23/1A-8B; transcript in Greengrass, 'Collections for Comenius'. The tract is undated but obviously to be placed in the late 1630s. Turnbull gives what seems to me an unduly unsympathetic summary, *HDC*, 347-8.

136   'zue 2 oder 3 collaboratoribus Ieden auff ein hundert lib: geschäzt werden wir wills Gott die mittel woll finden - Moriaen to Hartlib, 7 March 1639, HP 37/11B.

137   Moriaen to Hartlib, 1 Sept. 1639, HP 37/39A.

138   'das Ich Gott lob nun mehr den anfang der vnderschrifft hab. vnd mir nun fort an allein guten succes einbilde. Es ist mir recht saur worden ehe Ichs so weit gebracht hab. Gott lob das es vberwunden ist. der gebe ferner seine genade' - HP 37/38A.

139   This appears from the news that 'diese kirche sich am lezten vnderschrieben hatt' (5 November 1640, HP 37/70A). It is not clear which church he means by 'diese', though he would himself presumably have been most closely involved with the German, of which his friend Rulice was then preacher, but in any case the implication is clearly that all the others had already committed themselves.

140   HP 37/60B.

141   HP 37/66A.

142   HP 37/76A.

143   HP 23/12/2B. This and a record of the £25 for Hübner (HP 23/7B) are, rather surprisingly, the only mentions of Moriaen in Hartlib's surviving accounts.

144   HP 37/97A.

145   HP 1/35/3B.

146   'Hem! vis detrahere mihi salarium jam meritum? [...] Solve tu tua debita ipsemet'

147   HP 37/127A. It is possible, of course, that this represents repayment of a different and later debt not mentioned in the surviving correspondence, but it seems a good deal likelier (given that the sum mentioned is exactly the same) that this was the money Moriaen had forwarded at the end of 1641.

148   Or 'Temple of Christian Pansophy', described in the *Dilucidatio*: *Reformation of Schooles*, 64-84. It is an allegorical account of Comenius's proposed education system based on the structure of the temple in the vision of Ezekiel.

149   There are excellent accounts of the relations between Hübner and Comenius in Kvacala, *MGP II*, 51-9, and 'Über die Schicksale der Didactica Magna', *MCG* 8 (1899), 129-44.

150   Moriaen to Hartlib, 22 Sept. 1639, HP 37/40B.

151   '[Ich] hoffe das mit nechstem zum anfang etwas remittirn werde damit Dn Pell in guter devotion erhalten bleibe vnd nicht vrsach bekomme seinen wie es scheint Ihme angeborenen Mathematischen gaist zue dempfen vnd anderwerts vielleicht auch wieder

sein aigen herz vnd gemuth zue stellen' - Moriaen to Hartlib, 31 Jan. 1639, HP 37/5A.

152 'so müste man so viel müglich ist [...] was hin vnd wieder einkommen möchte in einen gemeinen Beutell samblen vnd nach notturft der sachen ins gemein anwenden. vnd nicht zuelaßen das die leuthe von hauß aus Ihre subsidia H Comenio selbsten zueordnen sonst weiß man nicht woran man ist vnd weil es vnder seinen Nahmen gehet, so würd Er alles bekommen vnd andere nichts' - 26 December 1639, HP 37/50B.

153 'Von H Comenio Vernehme ich sehr Ungerne, dass er so gantz jetzo Von seinen Pansophischen Meditationibus abgerissen ist, wan er dass werk ubergibt, wird schwerlich so bald ein ander wider kommen, der auff solche weütleüffige gedankhen gerathen wirdt' - Hübner to Hartlib, 22 March 1637, *MGP I*, 78.

154 *Eph 34*, HP 29/2/13A: the comment is attributed to Johann Christoph Berger von Berg, himself a Moravian exile, who was cited along with Hartlib as organiser of private charitable collections in the above-mentioned complaint of Jan Sictor to the Austin Friars consistory. See Webster, *Great Instauration*, 218 and 358-9.

155 R.C. Winthrop, *Correspondence of Hartlib, Haak, Oldenburg, and others of the Founders of the Royal Society, with Governor Winthrop of Connecticut, 1661-1672* (Boston, 1878), 10.

156 Kumpera, 219-21; Blekastad, *Comenius*, 657.

157 Moriaen to Hartlib, 31 March 1639, HP 37/15A: 'das Ich aber mehr vermuthe dz es Ihm mißluckhen als geluckhen werde, das geschicht auß aigener erfahrung in einer gleichmäßigen sache'.

158 L.E. Harris, *The Two Netherlanders* (Cambridge, 1961) ch.13 (149-59).

159 'Er arbeitete daran nach seiner eigenen Theorie, dass keine irdische Kraft Antrieb dieser Maschine sein könne, da alles Irdische unbeständig sei. Auf eine uns unbekannte Art wollte er den kosmischen "Dunst" oder die Strahlung auf drei Kugeln von verschiedener Grösse und verschiedenem Metall überführen, um an "die Kraft, welche die Sterne bewegt", anzuknüpfen' - Blekastad, *Comenius*, 303.

160 *Eph 52*, HP 28/2/38B.

161 *Reformation of Schooles*, 24.

162 'Schon als Bestätigung der Richtigkeit eines Weltsystems war es von grösster Wichtigkeit' - Blekastad, *Comenius*, 304.

163 See especially Moriaen to Hartlib, 31 March 1639, HP 37/15A-B.

164 *HDC*, 342.

165 See especially *Självbiografi*, 149-65, *HDC*, 342-70 and Blekastad, *Comenius*, 299-339. Further accounts by Comenius himself are given in English translation in Young, *Comenius in England*.

166 *Självbiografi*, 152 (Young, *Comenius in England*, 41); fuller quotation below, pp. 132-3.

167 John Gauden, *The Love of Truth and Peace: A Sermon Preached before the Honovrable Hovse of Commons Assembled in Parliament Novemb. 29. 1640* (London, 1641), 40-1. Comenius first made the claim publicly in the introduction to *Opera Didactica Omnia* (1657). Again in the dedication of the *Via lucis* (1668) he stated that he had been invited 'by public authority' for discussions on the propagation of the Gospel. He expanded on the account (adding this quotation from the sermon) in the *Continuatio admonitionis fraternæ* (1669) (*Självbiografi*, 152-3; cf. Young, *Comenius in England*, 39-41, 52, 60).

168 *Självbiografi*, 153 (Young, *Comenius in England*, 41).

169 'Three Foreigners', 262.

170 HP 23/13/1A and 23/10A (the donation is also noted at 23/12/2B).
171 HP 6/4/159A. The letter survives only in an undated and unaddressed copy, so it is not certain it is to Gauden, but he is the obvious candidate: cf. *HDC*, 219.
172 *The Love of Truth and Peace*, 43.
173 Culpeper to Hartlib, Dec. 1645, HP 13/110A-B.
174 'Three Foreigners', 262. Trevor-Roper omits to suggest who did the approaching and gives no source for his quotation. It is perhaps a paraphrase of Young's translation of the *Continuatio admonitionis fraternæ*: 'on entering London [...] I learnt at length the truth: I had been summoned by command of Parliament' (Young, *Comenius in England*, 39).
175 *Englands Thankfulnesse, or, an Humble Remembrance Presented to the Committee for Religion in the High Court of Parliament* (London, 1642): extracts in Webster, *Samuel Hartlib and the Advancement of Learning*, 90-7.
176 See Webster, *Great Instauration*, 49, 71, 221; *Självbiografi* 154-5 and n.42; Blekastad, *Comenius*, 313-15.
177 'Meinem bedunckhen nach aber würde es der gemeinen Sache fürderlicher sein wan Er an einem einsamen vnd etwas abgelegenen als volkreichen vnd dem zuelauff vnderworffenen ortt sich enthielte' - Moriaen to Hartlib, 12 May 1639, HP 37/32A.
178 'Mitglied einer Kirche, in der "keiner sich selber angehört", [...] ihr Wortführer und bedeutender Repräsentant. [...] Seine Arbeit an der Pansophie musste unter diesen Umständen mit grösster Verantwortung für die gesamte Unität verbunden sein - oder aufgegeben werden' - *Comenius*, 302, cf. *Självbiografi*, 154.
179 *Självbiografi*, 152 (Young, *Comenius in England*, 39). Comenius did not in fact mention the fundraising mission at all in this work, merely saying the Bishops agreed that he should go and that the co-rector and pro-rector who stood in for him at the school in Leszno in his absence should not know the real reason for his departure, ie. the summons from Hartlib. The official fundraising mission is mentioned in Hessels III, nos. 2607 and 2673. Blekastad, *Comenius*, 302-3, draws the inference.
180 *HDC*, 356; the Latin letter from Hotton on which Turnbull bases his account is at HP 9/7/2A-B. De Geer's letter of invitation (19 Oct. 1641) is reproduced in the appendix to *Comenius' Självbiografi*, 267.
181 Moriaen to Hartlib, 3 Oct. 1641, paraphrased and discussed in *HDC*, 354-6. But note that Moriaen did not report 'that Louis de Geer, being anxious to have good Germans with whom to discuss, has invited Comenius to Sweden' (*HDC*, 354), which would be a very bizarre motive for a Dutchman to invite a Moravian to Sweden. Turnbull has apparently misread 'wackerer' as 'deutscher': Moriaen's words are 'that Mr Louis de Geer is desirous of worthy men with whom he might pursue good conversation, and Mr Comenius has been summoned to Sweden for that purpose' ('das H. Loys de Geer, wackerer leuthe begehrig were mit denen Er gute conversation pflegen möchte, vnd das herr Comenius zue dem ende nacher Schweden beruffen seÿe') (HP 37/88A).
182 Hartlib to de Geer, 4 October 1641, draft version at HP 7/46/1A-2B, English paraphrase in *HDC*, 356-7.
183 Comenius was forty-nine, far from young by seventeenth-century standards, and had led a less than sheltered existence, though he in fact had another twenty-nine years before him.
184 Comenius to Hartlib, 25 May 1646, HP 7/73/1A.
185 See especially *Självbiografi*, 151-2 (Young, *Comenius in England*, 38-9), and see below, pp. 132-3.
186 Comenius's self-quotation from a letter to Hartlib, *Självbiografi*, 157 (Young, *Comenius in England*, 49). Cf. Comenius to Hartlib, 25 May 1646, HP 7/73/1A-

187 6B, and 21 Jan. 1647, Patera, *Jana Amosa Komenského Korrespondence* (Prague, 1892), no. 107 (pp.126-9).
Kotter was a Lutheran by upbringing, a tanner by trade and a Silesian by nationality. He learned to write for the specific purpose of setting his revelations down. Comenius met him in 1625 and translated his visions from German into Czech the same year. Poniatowská, the daughter of a Reformed minister, began experiencing visions in 1627, at the age of seventeen, having been driven, like Comenius, into exile from Bohemia to Leszno. Comenius proceeded to produce a Latin version of both her prophecies and Kotter's.

188 For a detailed account of the circumstances leading up to the publication and its aftermath, see Blekastad, *Comenius*, 573-84. Blekastad tends, however, to play down the extent of the disapproval the work aroused, and takes at face value Comenius's totally unfeasible and indeed (as his correspondence with Hartlib abundantly proves) mendacious claim that the published work was intended only for a few selected and responsible figures.

189 Wilhelmus Rood, *Comenius and the Low Countries*, (Amsterdam, 1970) 170.

190 I.e. the headmastership of the school in Leszno.

191 *Självbiografi*, 151-2 (Young, *Comenius in England*, 38-39).

192 'Wir können an vnß selbst*en* abnehmen wie den guten herzen beÿ Euch zue muth ist [...] fur erst wird vnß angenehm sein zue hören was das Buch mit 7 Siegeln an den tag bring*en* werde vnd mach*en* vnß die gedanck*hen* das ein iedweders der 7 Siegel ein besonder wee bedeuten vnd dem einen od*er* anderen auff den kopff bringen w*erde*' - Moriaen to Hartlib, 10 Dec. 1640, HP 37/71A.

193 HP 37/88A-89B.

194 Moriaen to Comenius, 10 Oct. 1641, HP 37/90A-B.

195 'Ich habe ja deutlich geschrieb*en* das Er [Comenius] da ohne ambtsgeschäffte od*er* hind*er*ung sein soll allein zue geselschafft ansprach vnd Rath mit genugsamer gelegenheit seinen conatibus einzig vnd allein obzueli*egen*' - Moriaen to Hartlib, 28 Oct. 1641, HP 37/92A.

196 'der H hatt uns gantzlich nit recht verstanden: H de Geer begehrt in der welt nichts von H. Comenio nur allein bißweilen mit ihm zu conversiren. [...] H. Comenius solt**ê** alda gutten vnterhalt haben, recht gelegenheit ohn and*er* vnkosten mit andern zu correspondir*en*, vnd otium seine meditati*ones* zu p*er*ficir*en*' - Rulice to Hartlib, 17 Oct. 1641, HP 23/9A-B, summarised in *HDC*, 357.

197 Moriaen to Hartlib, 3 Oct. 1641, HP 37/88B.

198 'Ich sehe die Englische sach*en* noch nicht an dem ortt da Ich sie gern hette, vnd sorge wo es Gott nicht genadigklich verhutet das es noch blutige köpffe kost*en* möchte' - HP 37/94A.

199 *HDC*, 360-61. But compare Dury's letter to de Geer of 19 Dec. 1641, promising that he and Hartlib would petition the Brethren in Leszno to grant Comenius leave to visit Sweden (*Självbiografi*, 268-9). Nevertheless, Dury, who had met with a cool reception from the Lutheran clergy in Sweden, was sceptical of the prospects for Comenius there.

200 HP 37/97A-B.

201 *Självbiografi*, 155 (Young, *Comenius in England*, 48).

202 Moriaen to Hartlib, 3/13 July and 24 July 1642, HP 37/110A-111B.

203 'wenig zeit vnd nicht viel mehr muth' - Moriaen to Hartlib, 2 Oct. 1642, HP 37/112A.

204 Blekastad, *Comenius*, 350; Oxenstierna to de Geer, 14 Sept. 1642 (*Självbiografi*, 271-2).

205 Moriaen to Hartlib, 30 Oct. 1642, HP 37/115A, paraphrased in *HDC*, 367.
206 *Självbiografi*, 164.
207 *Självbiografi*, 164.
208 'Wir haben bißhero viel von Ihme [Comenius] geruhmt vnß selbst*en* vnd andern grose hoffnung gemacht, wolte mir von herzen lieb sein wan wir in vnserem ruhm vnd hoffnung nicht zue schand*en* würden' - Moriaen to [Hartlib?], 5 Dec. 1639, HP 37/49A.
209 Moriaen to Hartlib, 22 Jan. 1643, HP 37/100A.
210 'höre Ich das Er nur seine Ianuam vnd Vestibulum revidirt vnd auff einen andern schlaag gebracht hab*en* soll, welches ob es zwar ein gut w*er*kh sein möchte so ists doch das Ienige nicht darauff man so lang gewartet vnd den leuth*en* hoffnung gemacht/ Ich hoffe Ia es w*er*de was anderes dabej sein sonst müste man sich fast schämen das [...] nun nichts anders als solche schuhl sach*en* herauß kommen solt*en*' - Moriaen to Hartlib, 15 Oct. 1643, HP 37/116A.
211 Comenius to Hartlib, 25 May 1646, HP 7/73/3A.
212 Moriaen to Hartlib, July 1650, HP 37/163A-164B.
213 Moriaen to Hartlib, 2 Feb. 1657, HP 42/2/2A.

CHAPTER FIVE

Curing Creation: Alchemy and Spirituality

'Qui scit in aurum convertere aliud metallum sive cum lucro, sive sine lucro, januam habet apertam in Naturam' ('Whoever knows how to transmute another metal into gold, whether with profit or without, has an open gateway into Nature') - Michael Sendivogius, cited by Heinrich Appelius, letter to Hartlib, 26 August 1647, HP 45/1/34B.

'Ora et Labora': 'Pray and Labour'

The four and a half years following the collapse of the grand design for a pansophic reformation feature a striking gap in Moriaen's surviving correspondence with Hartlib and his associates. Between late 1642 and May 1647, only four letters from him are to be found among Hartlib's papers, in contrast with seventy-seven from the previous four years. This could simply be due to the loss of material from the archive.[1] However, he also disappears almost entirely from the letters of Hartlib's other correspondents.[2] It seems likely, therefore, that this gap does indeed reflect a period of estrangement, or at any rate a cooling of relations, in the wake of the pansophic debacle and Moriaen's rather bitter reaction. If so, however, the rift must have been healed in 1647, and the two remained thenceforth in close contact until Hartlib's death in 1662.

Moriaen, who at the end of the 1630s awaited nothing with more excited anticipation than what he generally referred to as Comenius 'Metaphysica', i.e. the prospective *Janua Rerum*, appears in a markedly different guise in the letters of 1647 on. He could write by 10 February 1648: 'I used, indeed, to be a great lover and defender of metaphysics and metaphysicians, but then when I turned to real and useful knowledge, useless speculations became noisome to me'.[3]

The concept of 'useful knowledge' was discussed in the previous chapter. The whole point of Comenian metaphysics had been, of course, that it should be utterly distinct from what was seen as the empty semantics of the scholastic variety, from what Bacon described as the Schoolmen's 'monstrous disputations and barking questions',[4] and should deal not with ideas or words but with 'things'. As Comenius put it, 'it does not matter which language we speak (whether rude or cultured), since we are all nought but sounding brass and tinkling cymbals so long as words not things (I mean the husks of words, not the kernels of meanings) be in our mouths'.[5] There is an element of deliberate oxymoron in referring to a 'Janua rerum' as a 'metaphysics'. There is also a deliberate ambiguity in the title, literally 'The Gate of Things': is the book the gateway to things, or are the things themselves the gateway? Both senses are intended. 'Metaphysics', the realm beyond the physical, was to be attained not by abstraction, not by bypassing the physical, but on the contrary *through* the physical, through a detailed practical study of nature.

But here, I believe, Moriaen expresses a loss of faith even in Comenius's reformed, pansophic concept of metaphysics, which, whatever its claims, remained in the event bogged down in verbal formulations. He begins to sound a good deal less like Comenius, and a good deal more like Hartlib's new friend Robert Boyle, with his enthusiasm for the new 'philosophical college' in London that 'values no knowledge, but as it hath a tendency to use'.[6] Previously, the 'use' of knowledge had been seen primarily as its relevance to personal morality and social ethics. Here, though that dimension has by no means disappeared, the term becomes something closer to 'application', in the sense of the modern term 'applied science'.

This is not to suggest that there was a sudden sea-change in Moriaen's outlook at some point between 1642 and 1647, that he went to bed one night a mystic Pansophist and woke up a rational empiricist. On the contrary, what seems on the face of it a complete change of tack in the subject matter of the correspondence proves on closer analysis to be a logical development: a change of emphasis rather than a volte face. Though the letters written after this hiatus in the 1640s deal primarily in practical experiments and technological innovations, whereas those before are mainly given over to the pansophical scheme and the dissemination of knowledge and understanding through the medium of the written word, the ethos underlying them is the same.

Moreover, though there is next to nothing about the subject of natural philosophy in the earlier letters to Hartlib, it is evident from the handful of letters to Van Assche preserved in Amsterdam that Moriaen was a practising alchemist and iatrochemist at least as early as 1634, ie. during his second spell in Cologne. A letter of 8 March 1634 is largely given over to describing chemical preparations, mostly of a medicinal nature.[7] It is a salutary warning not to draw over-confident inferences from fragmentary documentation.

A possible reason for the change of emphasis in the Moriaen-Hartlib correspondence is that it was Hartlib, rather than Moriaen, who had turned more whole-heartedly to experimental philosophy during this period. Having declared his own disillusion with metaphysics, Moriaen went on to add, 'it is no wonder you [Hartlib] have fallen in love with experimental and mechanical philosophy'.[8] Though Hartlib too had certainly been interested in 'realia', and particularly in chemical and physical experiments, throughout his life, the *Ephemerides* distinctly chart a personal history in which over the years such subjects increasingly occupied his mind, at the expense of more abstruse metaphysical and theological speculations. Though the religious motivation underlying all his actions and studies remained the driving force, detailed experimental investigation of the 'creatures', the 'Book of God's Works', gradually ousted the exegetical and doctrinal interest in the 'Book of God's Word'. Such a development cannot be demonstrated by isolated examples out of context, and can be fully appreciated only if one reads through the whole of the *Ephemerides* in sequence. But two admittedly extreme cases from near the opposite chronological ends of the diaries may serve to illustrate the trend. There is nothing from the latter years remotely like this of 1639 under the heading 'MS Theo*logica*':

A *Question* Answered by Mr Gawdin to my Lady Barrington, whether the

> Essence or Being of all created *things* purely considered and only
> substantially as metaphisically abstract and separat from accidental
> qualityes and mutable formes (w*h*ich being is in everything real true and
> one and while it is in being most necessary to bee) whether I say this pure
> and precise being bee of the very essence or Being of G*o*d etc.[9]

Nor is there, conversely, anything in the early years to compare with the
report in 1656 of John Rushworth's 'optical undertakings in my dining roome
to know all what is done at Charing Crosse or in the Strand by meanes of the
Chimney with some extr*aordinary* cost'.[10]

The branch of experimental learning that came increasingly to dominate
Hartlib's interest from the late 1640s on was chemistry - or, rather, what
Allen G. Debus has dubbed 'the Chemical Philosophy'.[11] For chemistry, or
alchemy, rarely depicted itself at this period as a mere branch of knowledge: it
was, rather, a means of understanding and regaining dominion over the very
fabric of Creation. Debus aptly describes its goal as finding 'the key to a truly
Christian interpretation of nature.'[12] But, it will be argued, the alchemical
quest aimed at more than just understanding: the purpose of that
understanding was control and manipulation. Its aims were no less ambitious
than, and in many respects strikingly similar to, those of Pansophy, though its
means were very different.[13] Comenius, it seemed to many of his original
supporters, remained mired in didactics and declined into an increasingly
crotchety and belligerently eccentric old age. He fell out with one collaborator
after another, exasperating his patrons Louis and Laurens de Geer (the son of
Louis, who was at first more than happy to inherit his father's commitment to
support Comenius) and even his closest and most loyal supporters.[14] Figulus,
for instance, more in sorrow than in anger, wrote to Hartlib in 1658 that 'My
Fat*he*r in *Law* is likewise withering & decaying [...] I beginne to feare our
Pansophia, shall neuer come to perfection',[15] and that

> his vehement desire, of the wished for Change of all things, to see the
> Antichrist fall, & Christ in his Kingdome triumphing & reigning ouer the
> whole world, cannot permitt his Spirit to bee qviete: & likewise for his
> Pansophica & the like labours, which lye upon his [*sic*] dayly. I beleeue,
> in well considering his nature, & his age also, these things are
> irremediable, & there will bee no helpe for him, but hee thus must bring
> his bones into the graue.[16]

Hartlib was only one of many in the circle who turned increasingly to the
chemical philosophy to supply the universal reformation and enlightenment
that had so fervently been expected from Comenius's labours.

It is no longer possible for any serious historian of science to dismiss
alchemy and its elaborate symbolic jargon as charlatanism, superstition or
plain daftness, of no relevance to modern scholarship except as a reminder of
the quaint and exotic misconceptions of our forebears. This is, however, an
attitude that remains prevalent among those without a specialist interest in the
field. The latest edition of *Chambers Twentieth Century Dictionary* still
defines alchemy as 'the infant stage of chemistry' and describes its principal
goal as transmutation of metals, with no mention of the medical and
spiritualistic aspects of the discipline.

Glauber's biographer K.F. Gugel was, however, overreacting (with understandable defensiveness) to such preconceptions when he declared in 1955 that 'The convoluted symolic language [of alchemy] was just as comprehensible to the chemists of the day as modern formulae are to us now'.[17] Hermetic writing was certainly not incomprehensible to the initiated, but its elucidation depended on a combination of skills far more diverse than would be expected of a twentieth-century research specialist in any field. It demanded great practical experience, extensive familiarity with a vast range of rare literature, and in many cases access to a particular key obtainable only through personal contact with the author or his friends. It also demanded highly advanced reading skills of a type regarded nowadays as far more the province of the literary scholar. Symbol, metaphor and often very heavily veiled allusion, not to mention deliberate red herrings and self-proclaimed self-contradictions, were the stock-in-trade of these authors.

The impression of impenetrability and daunting erudition is as calculated and deliberate as in Pound or Joyce. Here, for instance, is George Starkey on transmutation, speaking 'not [...] one word doubtfully or mystically':

> In this our work, our Diana is our body when it is mixed with the water, for then all is called the Moon, for Laton is whitened, and the Woman beares rule, our Diana hath a wood, for in the first dayes of the Stone, our body after it is whitened grows vegitably. In this wood, are at the last found two Doves, for about the end of three weeks, the soul of the Mercury ascends, with the soul of the disolved Gold, these are infolded in the everlasting armes of Venus, for in this season the confection are all tincted with a pure green colour, these Doves are circulated seven times, for in seven is perfection, and then they are left dead, for they then rise and move no more, our Body is then black like to a Crowes bill.[18]

By the standards of the day this is in fact relatively clear. William Newman, in his recent study of Starkey,[19] brilliantly elucidates this and a number of similar passages by relating them to Starkey's other works, to the broader alchemical tradition, and to practical experimental detail that would have been attainable by an 'adept' of the day. Only a nodding acquaintance with alchemical symbolism is needed to identify 'Diana' (or 'the Moon') as silver, the 'water' as mercury and 'Venus' as copper. The 'souls' of the mercury and gold cannot be translated into modern chemical terminology since they are supposed extracts or 'essences' of what are now regarded as elementary substances. The more crucial details, however, are hidden very deep indeed, and it would be equally misguided to suppose that such writing was readily (if at all) accessible even to the best-qualified experts of the day. It is obviously with reference to this passage that the question in the *Ephemerides* is posed: 'Quid sint Columbæ Dianæ [*what may the doves of Diana be*]? which yet Mr Clod*ius* is to seek out for the p*er*fecting hims*elf* in the understanding of this mystery'.[20]

Great strides have been made by the likes of Newman in interpreting the real experimental details concealed behind such passages. Although there certainly were a good many frauds and hoaxters of the stamp of Subtle in Jonson's *The Alchemist*, the more serious writers often possessed immense practical expertise, and - especially in their private correspondence - were genuinely and successfully trying to communicate it. They were not, however, trying to communicate it to everyone. On the contrary, most alchemists were at considerable pains to make their work as difficult as possible to understand. The reasons for such obscurantism were various, and while self-interest may often have been at least part of the motivation, it was by no means always the whole of it.

It was a commonplace that arcana were to be revealed, if at all, only in veiled, symbolic terms, to ensure that the mysteries disclosed would be accessible only to those who had proved themselves worthy through years of diligent and unprofitable study. Even at the time, of course, this left every writer open to the countercharge that his (or, in rare cases, her) veiled symbolism in fact concealed not profound knowledge but vacuity or lies. The symbolism developed to express alchemical theory was extremely intricate, and furthermore, to make life especially difficult for the later student, there was very little attempt made to standardise it. A measure of agreement was established, and remains discernible today, on the symbolic nomenclature applied to some of the more basic substances. But when it came to finer detail, writers were prone to launch into a private or esoteric symbolism that was accessible only to those with access through personal contact or the still-thriving oral tradition to the intentions behind an often self-consciously literary façade.

In attempting to interpret alchemical recipes in terms of their reception at the time, we are faced with a dual task. On the one hand, there is the question of what the author intended to convey to those capable of understanding him. On the other, there is the question of what those who took him seriously but were not in fact fully capable of comprehending him did actually understand. It is not the purpose of this study to deduce the literal experimental details concealed by such allegories: that is a labour I am happy to leave to those better qualified to accomplish it. My concern here is rather with the ways in which such writing was understood and acted on by practising alchemists such as Moriaen and others of the Hartlib circle, who were less gifted and expert than Starkey, but by no means ignorant or uninformed, and whose lives were profoundly affected by their response to alchemical texts, however skewed and partial their understanding of them may often have been.

Charles Webster points out that 'to anyone immersed in decoding and unifying the symbolism of the Books of Daniel and Revelation, the hermetic literature would not offer insurmountable problems.'[21] This analogy with Scriptural exegesis is very apposite, but it should also be pointed out that while there was no shortage of people confident of their ability to decode Daniel and Revelation, the results of such decoding were spectacularly diverse. The same applies to the interpreters of hermetic writing. As Newman himself (whose remarkable work is by no means confined to literal elucidation) repeatedly stresses, the material products of the alchemist's laboratory were always considered less important than, and were interpreted within the context of, a broader religious and spiritual world-view. My subject here is the insight provided by the published writings and - far more - the private correspondence of such figures into the mental world they inhabited.

The notion of a distinctive scientific discourse, clearly differentiated from literary or religious writing and characterised by objectivity, clarity and accessibility (at least to those with the requisite training) was a new one, and was actively opposed by many thinkers, among them some of Hartlib's most cherished associates. Such opposition was not merely a case of old habits dying hard, or a bid to protect vested interests. It was in many cases both those things, but it was also and more fundamentally a defence of an entire religious and philosophical outlook, a whole way of making sense of life itself. The development of such a distinctive discourse was in itself symptomatic of the 'parcelling and tearing of learning into peeces' to which Comenius so vehemently objected.[22] The conflict between respect for the hermetic seal of the obscurantists and the promotion of a more open and literal discourse forms a recurrent theme in the remaining chapters of this study.

That said, it would be simplistic to suggest that there existed a clear demarcation between the two camps, or that such a distinction was consciously formulated either by writers or readers at the time. Of the figures associated with Hartlib, Starkey might perhaps be seen as the most committed and gifted representative of the obscurantist tendency, while Robert Boyle is still celebrated as a pioneer of a more objective, accessible and (in the modern sense) 'enlightened' scientific discourse, and openly championed the ideal of a 'free and generous communication of secrets'.[23] Yet Starkey and Boyle were, for a time at least, friends and collaborators, and undoubtedly respected one another's knowledge and insight. This is a question not of binary opposites, but of a broad spectrum with no clearly defined divisions. The observations of less exceptional students of alchemy, such as Moriaen, Heinrich Appelius, Benjamin Worsley and Cheney Culpeper, are of value precisely because they themselves had no clearly formulated notion of such a spectrum, let alone any definite idea of their own location within it.

Especially since Paracelsus, the notion of a medicinal and a spiritual aspect of alchemy was quite as important as the physical manipulation and transformation of created matter, the mere party trick of turning things into gold. Paracelsus himself had defined alchemy as nothing else but 'a preparer of medicine' ('eine bereiterin der arznei').[24] Johann Hiskius Cardilucius, in the introduction to his alchemical anthology *Magnalia Medico-Chymica* (1676) observed that 'alchemy is mocked and despised only by the ignorant, who do not know what it is, but think it no more than befooling oneself to make gold and silver': its true purpose, however, was to master the preparation of all created matter 'in most noble fashion, that you might be able most gently and lovingly to relieve any sick man of his ailments in a few hours'.[25] Alchemy could be seen in the broadest sense - analogically as well as literally - as a medical discipline. It was not limited to providing specific remedies for given illnesses, nor even to providing a panacea for all human ailments: it set out to cure matter itself and the human soul from the corruption that had entered them after the Fall.

Some of the claims made for the art seem staggeringly audacious. Death itself, some claimed, while remaining ultimately inevitable, could be dramatically postponed by the elixir of life.[26] The mythical Rosicrucian brotherhood supposedly spent most of their time curing the sick, without charge, through their alchemical prowess, and Christian Rosenkreuz himself was allegedly one hundred and six years old when when he died in 1484 or 1485.[27] They too despised transmutation for transmutation's sake, as though a man should be most dear to God merely because he can make great masses and lumps of gold [...] but we declare openly that this is false, and to true philosophers the matter stands thus: that making gold is to them a paltry matter and a parergon, than which they have many thousand greater works'.[28]

Though it may well be the case that the author(s) of the *Fama* and *Confessio* did not intend to be taken literally, there is absolutely no doubt that a great many people did take the works both literally and seriously.

Cardilucius stated entirely earnestly that Paracelsus had been an undoubted possessor of the elixir, and that his death at the unremarkable age of forty-seven was only due to the counter-effects of alcohol, to which the magus was notoriously given.[29] A strikingly similar account was given of the death of Starkey (another heavy drinker) in 1665. Whatever his ethical shortcomings, Starkey engaged that year in a genuinely heroic if totally misguided mission to preserve the populace of London from the plague by visiting victims and administering an infallible cure, the principal ingredient of which was powdered toad. Predictably enough, despite his powdered toad, he succumbed to the disease himself; but according to his friend and fellow iatrochemist George Thomson, Starkey's 'archeus', the inner principle that reacts to combat malign influences on the human organism, had been irredeemably weakened, partly by a depression induced by the slanders of Galenic physicians, but principally by the fact that on the day he contracted the disease Starkey had (by his own confession) consumed an 'unreasonable quantity of Small beer'.[30]

Starkey's death provides a good illustration of the tragi-comic divide between the aspirations and the achievements of medical alchemists. Seventeenth-century chemical medicine is often spoken of by modern scholars as 'progressive', at least in comparison to the practices of the more 'traditional' Galenists. However, while it was certainly more innovative, there is no evidence at all that it was any more effective. The hundreds of iatrochemical recipes preserved in the Hartlib archive are apt to leave a modern reader uncertain whether to laugh or to vomit. To be sure, there is no lack of unsolicited testimonials from satisfied patients of the efficacy of chemical medicines. However, without doubting the sincerity of such depositions, one may well question their objective truth. They often say more about the faith (or hope) of the patients than about the actual effect of the treatment. Improvements in health tend to be ascribed to the effects of the medicine, while downturns are interpreted as occuring in spite of it. It is also very likely that - in the short term at least - many of the less noxious preparations had a genuine but purely psychosomatic beneficial effect. That said, the naivety of seventeenth-century patients should not be exaggerated: they were as aware as their twentieth-century counterparts of dangerous side-effects. Hartlib's ascription of his final agony to a medicine sent through Moriaen has already been cited. The report in the 1635 *Ephemerides* of a 'most extra-ordinary-singular and approued Remedy ag*ainst* the stone' concludes, with possibly intentional irony, 'And one of the best property [*sic*] it hase [is] that if it does no good it will doe no harme'.[31]

But however misguided the attempts of medical alchemists to apply their learning for the relief and benefit of their neighbours may often have been in practical terms, the ethical and spiritual dimension must not be underrated in an account of their art. This emphasis on the medical aspect of alchemy is abundantly reflected in Hartlib's correspondence and publications. The *Chymical, Medicinal, and Chyrurgical Addresses* juxtapose a 'Conference concerning the Phylosopher's Stone' with an equally open-ended discussion as to whether there is such a thing as a panacea;[32] and Starkey's deliberately impenetrable 'exegesis' of George Ripley's account of transmutation with an advertisement for the 'Chyrurgical Balsams' of Moriaen's former assistant Remeus Franck. To Hartlib and his prospective readership there was evidently no incongruity. The vast majority of alchemical reports and recipes preserved in Hartlib's papers at least touch on, if they are not primarily concerned with, medicinal applications of the processes described.

The prospect of unlimited access to wealth doubtless had its attractions, and could be reassuringly rationalised - as in the case of any presumptively profitable enterprise - by the thought that such wealth would be devoted to pious ends. But the idea of profit for profit's sake incurred passionate opprobrium, in this discipline more than any other except perhaps doctrinal polemic: one is reminded of Protestant outrage at the venality of Papists who sought monetary gain through the marketing of masses, dispensations and absolutions. And in both cases, venality of purpose was seen as proof in itself of fraudulence. In German, the word 'Goldmacher' ('goldmaker') became a widely-used term of abuse directed by serious alchemists at those who envisaged nothing beyond personal material profit. One of Moriaen's sternest criticisms of Glauber was his mercenary streak: 'Another thing I dislike about Glauber is that he seeks to communicate such rare secrets to persons of rank, for they commonly abuse such precious things for their lust and greed'.[33] To sell genuine arcana to Epicure Mammon was an even greater sin than to sell him false ones.

The idea of an unprofitable transmutation, proving the adept's prowess and the possibility of the thing while remaining free of the taint of material greed, became something of an alchemical topos.[34] According to the 1649 *Ephemerides*, 'Mr Boyle hath a *Recipe* how to turne iron into gold but there is nothing to bee gotten by it. Yet it is worth the best consideration in reference to the Experiment of Iron and Antimony discovered in Mr Boyle's Letter'.[35] Gabriel Plattes' *Discovery of Subterraneall Treasure* (London, 1639) included a whole chapter (chapter nine) 'Wherein is shewed, how true and perfect gold may bee made by Art with losse to the workman'. 'If any one doubt the truth of *Alchimy*,' Plattes suggested, 'he may be satisfied by this triall; but instead of gaine he shall pay for his learning, by going away with losse'.[36] Glauber made the same claim in *Miraculi Mundi Continuatio* (1656), and again in *De Medicina Universali* (1657), a point Moriaen thought it worth drawing to Hartlib's attention:

> In this treatise [*De Medicina Universali*], he claims that his *aurum potabile* transmutes or develops not only mercury but all other metals into true gold, but without profit, and so of no value except to prove the truth and possibility of the thing, and to confirm this medicine as universal.[37]

Gold was significant not for its monetary worth, but as the most exalted and incorruptible substance on earth, the substance supplied abundantly by

God in Havilah, just outside Eden,[38] but which had since become so scarce. The human being who could raise another substance to this sublime state, even if the costs of the operation were so high as to entail a net loss to the transmuter in merely financial terms, appeared regenerate in the form God originally intended, having dominion over all the earth.

The faith invested by the alchemists in the lore of their subject was scarcely if at all less than their faith in Scripture. A striking illustration of this occurs in one of Poleman's numerous diatribes against Glauber. Informing Hartlib that he had no intention of visiting Glauber's laboratory and inspecting his 'conjuring tricks' ('gauckelspiel'), he explicitly compared the latter's wilful perversions of alchemical wisdom with heretical misinterpretations of Holy Scripture:

> I have ever and always greatly disliked his books, to the point of feeling utterly nauseated by them, and I can scarcely read a paragraph therein without conceiving a just wrath against the perverted man, so stubbornly and speciously does he twist and trammel the writings of the wise, far more than the most vicious and pernicious heretics distort Holy Scripture: and this wicked man misleads the innocent and ignorant onto such hideously false paths that they shall never find their way to the truth on them. How could I in conscience visit so wilful a cheat?[39]

As with Scripture, there was scope for endless dispute as to how to interpret the canonical texts and indeed as to what constituted the canon, but the conviction was equally profound in both cases that what the true canon said, once properly established and interpreted, was incontrovertible truth.

Enlightenment was to be sought by the twofold route of practical experiment and personal divine revelation. This parallels the twin emphasis of such inspirational Protestant theologians as Böhme on the practical expression of faith through works (which is not to be confused with justification by works) and a personal relationship with God. The classic emblem of this is the plate at the end of Heinrich Khunrath's *Amphitheatrum Sapientiæ æternæ* (Hanover, 1609), showing an adept kneeling at prayer before an altar in his laboratory, surrounded at once by the apparatus of religion and that of practical experiment. 'Laboratorium' and 'oratorium', laboratory and house of prayer, were one. There was no question, for the 'chemical philosophers', of choosing between divine and experimental revelation: they amounted to the same thing.

Chemistry versus Alchemy?

The alchemical fraudster is a stock figure of medieval and early modern European literature, but it is often unclear whether the works in question represent a rejection of the very notion of alchemy or merely a warning to distinguish the true adept from the false. Chaucer parodied such charlatans in the *Canon's Yeoman's Tale*, a cautionary fable reproduced in Elias Ashmole's alchemical verse anthology *Theatrum Chemicum Britannicum* (1652),[40] not because Ashmole mistook it for a genuine alchemical tract, but as a warning against false adepts. The classic example in English is Jonson's *The*

Alchemist. Sebastian Franck's *Ship of Fools* (*Narrenschiff*) has a place of honour for 'the great dunghill of alchemy' ('das große Bschiß der Alchimey'), and Donne in *Ignatius his Conclave* gives a hilarious account of Paracelsus arguing his higher claim over Copernicus and Machiavelli to a seat at the right hand of Satan for services to the detriment of mankind (all three are beaten hands down by Ignatius Loyola, the founder of the Jesuits). Donne has a great deal of fun with the Paracelsian doctrine that like cures like, i.e. that the remedy of a disease is to be sought in the source of that disease, and that noxious substances, suitably treated by the alchemist's art, thus become medicines. He has Paracelsus boast that

> whereas almost all poysons are so disposed and conditioned by nature, that they offend some of the senses, and so are easily discerned and avoided, I brought it to passe, that that treacherous quality of theirs might bee removed, and so they might safely bee given without suspicion, and yet performe their office as strongly.[41]

Hartlib's death at the hands of Moriaen's well-meaning friend Kreußner shows just how pertinent Donne's satire was.

Chemical practitioners of the seventeenth century were keenly aware of such charges and repeatedly defended themselves against them. The denunciation of dupes and charlatans is a major theme in the works of almost every serious writer on the subject. For one thing, there was the fear of being tarred with the same brush; for another, there was a strong incentive for the alchemist in search of patronage to cast aspersions on the probity of other aspirants to the same funding.[42]

Plattes 'Caveat for Alchemists' in the *Chymical, Medicinal, and Chyrurgical Addresses* is a catalogue of alchemical confidence tricks, aimed not at discrediting alchemy itself but at sparing serious would-be adepts the time and expense of learning to recognise cheats the hard way. In it, Plattes approvingly, if rather vaguely, cites the *Canon's Yeoman's Tale*. 'This Cheat is described in old *Chawcer*, in his *Canterbury Tale*,' observes Plattes, and having summarised the story concludes by saying that the dupe 'was earnest with the cheater to teach him his Art, but what bargain they made I have forgotten, for it is twenty years since I read *Chawcers* book'.[43] Far from rejecting the philosophy itself, however, Plattes announced at the end of the tract that he had petitioned Parliament 'that I may demonstrate my ability to do the Common-wealth of *England* some service' by reforming husbandry and medicine

> and lastly, to shew the Art of the transmutation of Mettals, if I may have a Laboratory, like to that in the City of *Venice*, where they are sure of secrecy, by reason that no man is suffered to enter in, unless he can be contented to remain there, being surely provided for, till he be brought forth to go to the Church to be buried.[44]

He had presumably concluded that, with further refinement, the loss-making method of transmutation described in his *Discovery of Subterraneall Treasure* could be rendered profitable. He also asserted this possibility, emphasising the potential benefits to the State as a whole, in his Utopian tract *Macaria*

(1641). In this, the 'Traveller' who describes the ideal kingdom lends his interlocutor, the 'Scholar', a 'booke of Husbandry' designed to show how Macarian perfection might be attainable in England. The 'Scholar' is particularly impressed by the fact that in this book,

> you shew the transmutation of sublunary bodies, in such manner, that any man may be rich that will be industrious; you shew also, how great cities, which formerly devoured the fatnesse of the Kingdome, may yearely make a considerable retribution without any mans prejudice, and your demonstrations are infallible: this booke will certainly be highly accepted by the high Court of Parliament [...] with all my seven Liberall Arts I cannot discover, how any businesse can bee of more weight than this, wherein the publike good is so greatly furthered.[45]

There is no record of Plattes' having in fact made an alchemical petition to Parliament, and Hartlib later told Winthrop that 'Platts never made any demonstration befor *the* Parliament of *the* possibility of *the* Lapis for ought I know'.[46] But this probably reflects lack of opportunity rather than lack of will.

Moriaen offered a simpler and more general rule of thumb for detecting alchemical fraudsters: anyone selling his secrets for money was manifestly a charlatan, since if his methods were genuine, his ability to produce precious metal would make money a matter of complete indifference. There was, however, a handy get-out clause: 'But if he seeks a collaborator and cannot set the work on foot alone, that man gives him enough who lets him work at his expense'.[47] Alchemical expense accounts were seldom modest.

Contracts relating to alchemical funding fall into at least two distinct categories. In the one case the 'adept' simply sold his secret to a wealthier but less enlightened patron. More often, however, potential patrons were themselves practising alchemists, and in such instances the proposals tended to be cast rather in terms of research agreements than plain trafficking in information, and the question of finance, while remaining crucial, became rather less blatant. One such document is a letter from the chemist Friedrich Kretschmar[48] to Hartlib, Clodius, Dury and a fourth whose name has been carefully obliterated from the manuscript. I agree with Turnbull's reading of Brereton.[49]

The gist of the proposed deal was as follows. Having been shamelessly betrayed and abandoned by his previous associate, Hartprecht (who, however, did not have the wisdom to use his ill-gotten knowledge correctly), Kretschmar had been left stranded and destitute, barely able to support his laboratory and his large family. However, his desperate entreaties to God had been rewarded with the discovery of a method of extracting a grain of gold from an (unspecified) quantity of silver which, repeated often enough, would eventually transmute all the metal. After a couple of pages of pious outbursts about this, he abruptly came to the point by proposing a very businesslike contract in five numbered clauses. In return for a full revelation both of the materials involved in the process and the method of effecting it, Hartlib and his friends would undertake 1) to provide £600, either from themselves or from a sponsor 'whom they deem worthy of this truth' ('den sie dieser warheit wehrt achten'); 2) never to impart the knowledge to unworthy people;

3) never to set it down clearly and precisely ('klar und deutlich') on paper; 4) to inform Kretschmar (or his heirs should he be dead) of any refinement or development of the process they might subsequently discover; and 5) to sell on his behalf, for a small commission, a large quantity of a cure for the plague he had just prepared.

The document is a treasure-trove of alchemical clichés. Such agreements to pool knowledge were forever ending with one side or both claiming to have been swindled by the other, as Kretschmar said he had been by Hartprecht. And it was rarely that anyone claimed to have found the Stone itself: what was normally offered, as here, was a first step in the right direction, not yet profitable enough to cover its own costs but pointing towards great future achievements.[50] Still more typical is the aura of intense piety and secrecy and the insistence on keeping the mystery hidden from those who might use it for improper purposes. Kretschmar was most insistent Hartlib should show the letter to no-one but the other three addressees, a stipulation Hartlib characteristically broke. Clause 3 (never to set down the details) is the standard undertaking that so bedevils modern attempts at reconstructing the real chemical processes involved in such undertakings. This was a sales pitch which at once enhanced the value of the goods on offer and flattered the proposed recipients, who had been specially selected as fit trustees of the arcanum - which is not necessarily to say that the effect was mere calculation. Kretschmar's most successful piece of audience-targetting was an extra promise to reveal a new medicine based on the same materials which he was certain would cure bladder stones. Hartlib was already taking one of Kretschmar's remedies for the stone, and told Boyle it 'is certainly most excellent, and absolutely the best that ever I have used'.[51] The passage relating to this new cure has been underlined in a different ink, probably by Hartlib himself.

The business sense tempering the mysticism in this proposal is at least matched in the witheringly sarcastic reply to it composed by Clodius.[52] He demanded statistics: exactly how much gold was yielded by a given quantity of silver; was it 'common' or 'expensively prepared' silver (note how readily the term was accepted as having a number of distinct meanings); how much did it cost to reconstitute the left-over silver after the gold had been extracted? And who would bear the costs should any of the plague medicine fail to sell? Perhaps the most striking feature of the letter is that for all his wariness and scepticism, Clodius did not for a moment seem to doubt that Kretschmar really had produced gold. Indeed, he affected not to be particularly impressed by the fact. 'For, Sir, we are not so ignorant here that we could not produce a little gold from an ounce [of silver], but either the process does not cover its own costs or it does not work in bulk'.[53] He could himself by such a method offer a fair return on a £100 investment, but '[I] assure you we are convinced that your way must be very profitable since you ask six hundred pounds for it'.[54]

More damning still was the judgment of Joachim Poleman. Despite all Kretschmar's strict injunctions to secrecy, Hartlib had obviously sent a copy of the proposal to Poleman, who in several letters over the following few months spoke contemptuously of Kretschmar as the archetypal false alchemist, accusing him of having bought his goldmaking conjury ('goltmacherische taschenspielereÿ') from the arch-deceiver ('Haubtbetruger') Glauber[55] and warning Hartlib against 'the sweet hissing of such a cunning serpent'.[56] Not that Poleman, any more than Plattes, disbelieved in alchemy itself, of which he too was an ardent practitioner. His contempt - which he expressed frequently and vitriolically - was for charlatans such as Kretschmar and Glauber, whose conjuring tricks redounded 'to the great discredit of that more than kingly art, true Chymia'.[57]

The standard strategy of the defenders of 'true Chymia' was to distinguish not between chemistry and alchemy, but between the true philosopher and the false, both of whom might go under the name of either chemist or alchemist. There is a need for a detailed philological study of the usage of the words 'alchemy' and 'chemistry' (or 'chymia') and their derivatives with a view to establishing what difference there was between their usages, and how those usages developed and altered.[58] Etymologically, the two words amount to the same thing. The precise origin of the term is disputed, but the derivation in both cases is from the Greek *chymia* and/or *chemeia*: the 'al' in 'alchemy' is merely the Arabic definite article, reflecting the fact that the art reached Western Europe from Greece by way of North Africa, where the Arabs were its principal practitioners in the Middle Ages. In most European languages, 'alchemy' is the older form: the 'al' began to be dropped in the sixteenth century by humanist scholars who recognised and were repelled by such linguistic bastardy.[59] Initially, the choice of term seems not to have implied any semantic distinction, but merely the level of the given writer's awareness of and concern for etymological purity. But between the middle of the sixteenth and the end of the seventeenth centuries, separate associations began to accrue to the originally synonymous words. These changing semantic associations in turn reflect increasingly divergent understandings of the art of studying and manipulating created matter. (The word 'chemistry' derives from 'chemist', a chemist being a practitioner of 'chemia'. The *OED* suggests that at its first appearance around the beginning of the seventeenth century it had pejorative connotations, as in 'sophistry', but in Hartlib's papers it seems to be merely a variant form of 'chemia'. Neither German nor French found any need for such an extra term, and they still use 'Chemie' and 'chémie' respectively for 'chemistry' in the modern sense.) An exhaustive account of this development would fill a book in itself. All I shall offer here are some pointers and suggestions, based principally on the extensive chemical/alchemical material in the Hartlib Papers, and thus representing the crucial transitional stage of the third, fourth and fifth decades of the seventeenth century.

There can be little doubt that by the end of the seventeenth century, it had become possible to distinguish between the two terms in the manner made standard by eighteenth-century rationalists and still widely accepted today, seeing chemistry as a 'true' and 'rational' science, alchemy as a 'false' and 'superstitious' myth or magic if not outright charlatanism. (That is not to say such a distinction was by then universally accepted. On the contrary, the vehemence with which alchemy was derided by rationalists such as J.C. Adelung in the eighteenth century is evidence of how seriously it continued to be taken in many quarters during the 'Age of Reason'. One does not waste ammunition on an opponent who is already dead.[60]) But no such distinction could have been made at the beginning of the century, and it was barely beginning to be made by the time of Hartlib's death in 1662.

In the following examples, the two words appear to be used without distinction. (In this and the following paragraphs, emphasis has been added to citations by the use of bold type. In my translations here, I have used *chemist, chemistry*, etc. to render all derivatives of *chymia*; and *alchemy, alchemist,* etc. for all derivatives of *alchymia*. The reader is requested to shelve for present purposes all semantic preconceptions about either word.)

The author of one anonymous and undated tract among Hartlib's papers inveighed in the same breath against the '**common herd of alchemists**' and '**pseudo-philosophical chemists**'.[61] Sophronius Kozack in his *Liber Spagyricæ* mocked at 'ignorant apothecaries, **lying alchemists** and presumptuous surgeons',[62] having just said that a true physician must be, among other things, a **master of alchemy**.[63] George Starkey[64] contrasted the '**half-learned knowledge of alchemy**'[65] of 'deceivers and sophists'[66] with the true and faithful student who 'at once acquires the name of chemist, and soon afterward earns the title of Philosopher',[67] learning operations that are beyond the reach of the '**common chemists**'.[68] Starkey himself had identified mercury as the '**true key to the art of alchemy**'.[69] Glauber recalled having had to suffer the jibes of the ignorant rabble jeering '**Alchimist, Alchimist!**', who failed to distinguish '**true alchemy** from vagabond rogues or **false alchemists**'.[70] In none of this does the choice of the term 'alchemy' carry a greater suggestion of mysticism, esotericism or magic, either approvingly or pejoratively. Much of the time the two terms were still being used interchangeably, almost synonymously. If there is a distinction to be drawn between them in the writings of this period, it is not the distinction that is drawn today. Herwig Buntz speaks of a 'separation of alchemy from chemistry' ('Trennung von Alchimie und Chemie') in the seventeenth century, but the work he cites as a ground-breaking example of the *latter* is a book by Andreas Libavius entitled 'Alchemia' (1597).[71]

There are, however, many instances where a distinction does seem to be made, though it is often difficult to deduce quite what that distinction is intended to be. One self-promoting list of experiments proclaimed that the author had 'many things in **chemistry, alchemy,** medicine, the mechanical arts and natural magic'.[72] Heinrich Appelius, informing Hartlib about Glauber's furnaces, remarked 'they will be very useful for a **chemist or an alchemist**'.[73] He later added, 'I think those that have skill in **chymicall et alchymisticall** matters [...] will be best able to judge of his [Glauber's] inventions'.[74] Hartlib heard in 1652 that one Dr Fogarty had acquired 'all the MS. of Hugens [probably Constantijn Hujgens] [...] They are all in Latin several Volums Medicinal **Chymical and Alchymical**'.[75] Dury spoke of ploys to inveigle information out of people, 'as **Chimists** sometimes or **Alchimists** use to doe when they would dive into the secrets of nature which others pretend [i.e. claim] to have'.[76]

Some of this may be mere tautology, a common enough feature of seventeenth-century writing in general (and of Dury's in particular). But tautology was a rhetorical or stylistic device designed either to clarify unfamiliar terms (as in 'your Tubus or Telescopium') or to add weight to a discourse and to enhance the writer's perceived authority by showing off his or her command of language: it characteristically juxtaposes synonyms or near-synonyms that are etymologically distinct and do not look or sound unduly similar. The effect becomes transparent if obvious cognates are used.

Tautology is not an adequate explanation of this repeated placing side by side of these two terms as though in opposition.

There is one document in particular which suggests a distinction compatible with all the types of usage described above: it is again a letter from Appelius to Hartlib, and is a personal assessment of what advantages a friend of Hartlib's (unnamed but almost certainly Benjamin Worsley[77]) might reasonably expect from a visit to Glauber. Though inclined to favour the idea, Appelius prefaced his remarks with this caveat:

> I doubt not but *the* Gentleman knowes how fickel, difficult, dangerous et chargable matter is **Chymia especially Alchimia** [...] **Chymia** egregia promittit, et præstat, sed non sunt omnium temporum nec personarum, Condimenta dat non Alimenta, Coronam non Vestem. [*Chemistry promises and delivers great things, but they are not for all times and all people; it gives the spices but not the substance, the crown but not the clothes.*] [...] **Alchimia** adhuc est difficilior [*alchemy has so far been more difficult*]: yet intend I not to make *the* friend afraid: naturalis impetus hic Coryphæus est, si uspiam est [*a natural impulse is the leader here if anywhere*].[78]

Appelius's terms here are hardly crystal clear, but the general implication is surely that alchemy is a distinct field not *from* chemistry but *within* it. It is the most 'difficult, dangerous et chargable [ie. expensive]' part of it, but it is also the core, the yolk of it, providing sustenance rather than mere flavouring through an understanding of essences as opposed to outward forms. Just as Bacon's 'Natural Histories' were a preparative to the 'experiments of fruit' that would once again make Nature Man's servant; just as Comenius's didactics were a preparative to the opening of the 'Janua Rerum', the gateway to real things; just as Pell's *Idea of Mathematics* posited all preliminary mathematical study as a preparative for grasping the method that would solve all mathematical problems whatsoever; so the theoretical aspects of chemistry were a preparative to penetrating its core, alchemy, the spiritual understanding of created matter and mastery of the 'soul of the world'. All alchemists were chemists, but not all chemists were alchemists. The distinction is between the mere student and the practitioner or 'adept', between passive understanding of Nature's forms and active dominion over her spirit. The chemist was as it were the cartographer of a newly discovered country; the alchemist colonised it.

The Key to Creation

The seventeenth century was alchemy's Indian summer. Its practitioners had no sense of nurturing a science in its infancy, a 'prelude to chemistry';[79] on the contrary, they looked to the imminent culmination of all knowledge. Like Pansophy, alchemical theory presupposed a universe comprehensible to humankind by dint of the fact that everything in it was interconnected, producing a harmony that in turn revealed the will of God to the enlightened listener. The simultaneous birth of Pansophy and resurgence of alchemy represent two dying convulsions of the microcosm-macrocosm theory.

The 'Chymicall Gentleman' Cheney Culpeper[80] wished to learn more about the effect of 'cold' (understood at the time as a potentially definable and measurable quality opposite to heat rather than simply a lack of the latter) on 'putrefaction' and 'multiplying of the spirit of nature', a 'multiplying' which would manifest itself in increased fertility. Given the terminology of the time and the known interests of Culpeper and his correspondent, Worsley, this evidently refers to the transmutation and multiplication of metals rather than to an agricultural process in the literal sense. Culpeper was explicit about having hit on the idea through a reflection on macrocosm-microcosm analogies:

> not but that I acknowledge alsoe a spring and an autumn as well in our lithe [sic: presumably a scribal error for 'litle'] world as in the great but my desire is that if wee desire to see a fruitful summer, wee must pass through the winter quarters, for if wee looke into nature wee shall find winter to be a naturall cause of the fruitfullnes in summer.[81]

Underlying this animistic view was the conviction that all Creation was imbued with a materially identifiable life-force, variously designated 'world spirit' ('spiritus mundi'), 'world soul' ('anima mundi'), 'universal spirit' ('spiritus universalis') and the like. Paracelsus called it an 'aerial nitre'.[82] As ever, it is very difficult if not impossible to determine just what was understood by these terms, if, indeed, there was any consensus as to their definition, but the chemical literature of the period is full of practical experiments aiming to isolate and analyse this spirit, illustrating the way in which the new experimental philosophy was seen by the alchemists not as a challenge but an ally. 'Salt' in particular - a term of even greater ambiguity as used at the time - came to assume an importance it would be virtually impossible to overstate. Robert Fludd thought he had isolated the material spirit of life from wheat as 'a pure and divine volatile salt of wondrous properties'[83] and J.B. Van Helmont was 'convinced that the vital spirit must be saltlike and aerial in nature'.[84] Perhaps the most spectacular claims for salt were made by the colourful figure of J.R. Glauber, who will provide the focus for the following chapter.

'Salt' is the dominant theme in much of Glauber's writing. Like most authors who accepted the microcosm-macrocosm theory - and Glauber embraced it wholeheartedly -, he saw nothing odd in setting down side by side recipes for a salt preparation to kill maggots in cheese and another to turn base metals into gold, for preparing 'aurum potabile' and 'philosophic dung' ('philosophischer Mist').[85] He was typical too in combining, almost in the same breath, conclusions drawn from laboratory experiment and from Scriptural exegesis and seeing the two as complementary. He pointed out that Christ referred to his disciples as 'the salt of the earth' (Mark 9:49-50), proving that salt is divinely privileged above all other substances just as the disciples were divinely chosen above all other men,[86] and went so far as to speak of Christ himself as 'a pure divine salt' ('ein lauter Gottlicher Saltz').[87] Its value as a fertiliser and preservative proved that it contained the miraculous spark of life itself, associating it in Glauber's mind with the sun, likewise a great fructifier, and with the first divine act of Creation, making it superior and anterior to the four Aristotelian elements: 'Salt is a symbol of eternity, for it is not altered or reduced in fire, air, water or earth, but long preserves all things from decay. Salt was the first fiat at God's Creation, and from this fiat arose the elements'.[88] Hard as it may be to imagine God's first words having been 'let there be salt', Glauber went on to explain how salt emanating from the sun's fire passes down through air into the sea water (which, he claimed, is far saltier in sunny climes[89]) and thence into the interstices of the earth, animating and fecundating as it goes. In short, 'All fruitfulness and nutrition, then, comes from salt, salt from the sun, and the sun from God the creator of all things'.[90]

This identification of sunlight with 'salt' finds a clear echo in Moriaen's descriptions of his optical experiments:

> Concerning burning glasses, I have noted this too: if finely ground antimony is ignited through them by the sun, it burns away strongly and yet loses none of its weight, but becomes heavier by this means, which is proof indeed that the sun's rays impart natural salt and impregnate [the antimony] with it'.[91]

The conclusion is not as wild as it may at first sound. The nature of light was one of the great mysteries of seventeenth-century science, and many leading thinkers tending towards atomism, including Gassendi and Newton, inclined to the view that it was composed of extremely small atoms, i.e. was a material substance, albeit of an exceptionally rarefied nature. Ally this with a belief that salt is a primordial building-block of Creation, and it becomes entirely logical to expect that sunshine should consist at least partially of salt.

Metals and minerals were generally seen not as inanimate, but as organic substances growing in the earth like vegetables (though far more slowly). Bruce T. Moran gives a fascinating account of how in 1618 the alchemist Johann Popp 'proved' this theory to the delight of his patron Moritz of Hessen by growing crystal flowers from lead.[92] A contemporary (and open-ended) discussion of the idea can be found in 'A Discourse about the Essence or Existence of Mettals' by Gerard Malyne, the (unpaginated) Appendix to the *Chymical, Medicinal, and Chyrurgical Addresses*. Comenius took it entirely for granted:

> if one wishes to distinguish Man's end and the means to his end by comparing him with other creatures, one will not concentrate upon his points of likeness to metals or stones or animals (inasmuch as he is born and grows and feeds and moves and uses his senses) but upon his points of excellence.[93]

Boyle too (or at least his fictional self-personification, the 'Sceptical Chymist' Carneades) thought the most plausible account of the origin of mineral matter, including metals, to be that it grew in the earth: he cited the formation of stalactites as an example.[94] He also thought it probable that minerals altered in nature in the course of their development, though he characteristically warned that 'the growth or increment of Minerals being usually a work of excessively long time, and for the most part perform'd in the bowels of the Earth, where we cannot see it, I must instead of Experiments make use, on this occasion, of Observations'.[95] Many less cautious spirits took such natural growth and transmutation of metals as axiomatic, and assumed that since Nature, being the creation of God, aspired always toward perfection, they reached the highest stage of their development in gold. Alchemists saw themselves not as perverters or mutators of nature but as catalysts in a natural process. Their art was the husbandry of matter, and especially of metals. Thus, for instance, Glauber gives a method of 'planting' a gold 'seed' in the 'earth' of copper and regulus of antimony and 'watering' it with saltpetre to stimulate its growth:

> and here the gold takes the place of a seed, and the copper and regulus of antimony the place of the earth in which the seed feeds and multiplies itself, and the saltpetre the place of the rainwater that moistens the earth and makes it fruitful. The longer the gold lies growing in this earth, the greater will be its increase[96]

Though the sexually-cum-astrologically-based tradition that saw each metal as being born of the astral 'seeds' with which each 'planet' impregnated the earth was by no means universally accepted even among the Spagyrists, its implications were deep-rooted and continued to influence scientific thought into the eighteenth century if only at a subconscious level. It is essential to bear in mind that only seven metals were distinguished at this period, corresponding to the seven 'planets': from Saturn came lead; from Jupiter, tin; from Venus, copper; from Mars, iron; from Mercury, mercury (the one hangover in modern English of chemistry's astrological pedigree); from the Moon, silver, and from the Sun, gold. There was no reason for the Copernican reorganisation of the model of the planetary system to dent this astrological and microcosmical interpretation of the nature of metals: on the contrary, the centrality it acccorded the sun served rather to confirm that gold occupied a privileged position in the hierarchy of created matter, and that other metals drew their life from it and aspired to develop into it. As Glauber put it, 'Nature strives continually to bring her children to perfection, but base metals are not perfect. Why should we not be able to come to Nature's aid and improve them?'[97] The Latin names and astrological symbols for the 'planets' were used as synonyms and shorthand respectively for the corresponding metals until well into the eighteenth century, even by thinkers who had nothing but derision for the theory underlying such nomenclature. This ingrained habit, together with the deeply-rooted belief that seven was a magic or mystic number, probably did much to retard the realisation that there are in fact rather more than seven metals. Though other metals were known and named, such as bismuth, antimony and zinc, these were taken to be 'imperfect', 'immature' or 'half' metals, which had not yet grown into true ones.[98]

The mystical-alchemical theosophy of Jacob Böhme, which was highly influential on many of these thinkers, set out to define God himself as, effectively, a chemical reaction (though obviously of a highly exalted, spiritual nature). God consisted, he claimed, of seven 'source spirits' ('Quell-Geister'), each with a different 'quality': the sour, the sweet, the bitter, heat, love, sound and the 'corpus' which comprehended the first six. All seven constantly gave birth to each other and affected or 'qualified' one another in, as it were, an eternal and infinite chain reaction.[99] Böhme, it should be pointed out, was not himself a practising alchemist, though the influence of alchemical literature (especially Paracelsus) on his idiosyncratic account of

God, Creation and the Universe is unmistakeable. Nor was he so presumptuous as to purport to have analysed God in this fashion by experiment. He claimed a single and irrefutable source for all his knowledge of such matters: God had told him personally. But his association of alchemical theories and language with insight into the deepest mysteries of God and Nature is highly symptomatic of the aspirations of the chemical philosophers.

Creation itself was seen by many as an alchemical process, the separating out into discrete elements of the initial Chaos. The early chapters of Genesis were frequently invoked as images of and sanction for the alchemist's labour. Culpeper, for instance, sought to produce 'such an excitation of the Spirit of nature as that it may (as in the beginning) moove in and upon the waters'.[100] It followed that to practise alchemy was to emulate God - an idea strikingly exemplified in a tract sent to Hartlib from Hamburg,[101] which he passed on to Moriaen, J.F. Schlezer and others for comment. The author of this work, a now otherwise unknown septuagenarian going by the name of Stapula,[102] not only wished to replicate the action of the Holy Spirit in Creation, he maintained that he had isolated that Spirit by experiment. The piece advertises a miraculous 'spirit of mercury' or 'philosophical water' ('spiritus mercurii', 'philosophisches wasser') which would preserve seeds from frost, increase the yield of a crop three thousandfold and cure all diseases, 'and this is the quintessence of the Universal Spirit that moved upon the face of the waters (Genesis 1)'.[103] To be sure, this remarkable claim of in vitro revelation was too much for Hartlib's correspondents. Moriaen characteristically criticised it as undemonstrated speculation: 'I see indeed that the author's philosophy goes beyond his experience'.[104] But, equally typically, he suggested the discovery was probably not without value, albeit the claims made for it were preposterously exaggerated. Schlezer suspected the 'philosophical water' of being merely ammonia ('Spiritus Vrinæ').[105] Another commentator, who remains anonymous, objected more sternly to the virtually blasphemous implication of the claims: 'it is expressly stated in the text [of Genesis] that this spirit was the Spirit of God, but it is absurd for a chemist to try to make a quintessence into the Spirit of God'.[106] Yet the fact remains that the claim was made and that Hartlib seriously canvassed opinions on it. This philosophy not only saw but set out to analyse the world in a grain of sand and heaven in a wild flower.

An exchange such as this helps to suggest the tightrope alchemists found themselves obliged to walk. Just as Comenius had been criticised for a presumptuous mingling of divine and human knowledge, for attempting through his merely human Pansophy to gain access to an omniscience that was only accessible to his Creator, so - perhaps even more so - were alchemists vulnerable to the charge of playing God. Hence the defensive iteration of pious rhetoric that is a feature of almost all writing of the genre. Over and again, these thinkers and experimenters insisted that their knowledge had been vouchsafed them by God himself, that they were acting under his tutelage and on his instructions. Their dilemma is implicit throughout the myth of Genesis itself. On the one hand, people were created in the image of God, and specifically instructed to take charge of the rest of Creation: clearly it behoved them to emulate their Maker.[107] On the other hand, the first two great curses brought down on them were precisely for overstepping the bounds of their delegated responsibility and aspiring to divine status themselves. 'And the Lord God said, Behold, the man is become as one of us, to know good and evil: and now, lest he put forth his hand, and take also of the tree of life, and eat, and live for ever: Therefore the Lord God sent him forth from the garden of Eden'.[108] The same thing happened at Babel: it was to be a tower 'whose top may reach unto heaven', but God again seems to have been palpably alarmed at such presumption: 'this they begin to do: and now nothing will be restrained from them, which they have imagined to do. Go to, let us go down, and there confound their language, that they may not understand one another's speech'.[109] Naturally, alchemists were at pains to stress that when they replicated the Creation act in miniature in their laboratories, they were acting as faithful stewards, not as usurping masters. The question on which no consensus could be reached was where to draw the line between the two, and it would be rash to take at face value the alchemists' rationalisations of their schemes. As with the writings of missionary colonialists and pansophic educationalists, the fundamental impulse behind these works can be seen, I would suggest, as a desire for reassurance that humanity has both the right and the ability to comprehend and control the world about it.

The influence of such concerns and convictions on the laboratory practice of the alchemists is illustrated in two strikingly similar experiments aiming to isolate the life-spirit, one described by Moriaen in somewhat fragmentary fashion (and at second hand, as he frankly admitted) in the course of three letters between April and July 1658,[110] the other, apparently independently, by Glauber in Part IV of *Des Teutschlands Wohlfahrt*,[111] published the following year. Both versions involved 'magnetising' a raw material by impregnating it with sunlight and subsequently using the 'magnet' to attract from the night air something described by Moriaen as 'salt of nature' ('sal naturæ') and by Glauber as 'a water, in which water is concealed the general nutriment of the air'.[112] This substance was then purified by distillation (Moriaen) or evaporation of the superfluous fluid (Glauber), and what remained exposed again by night, purified again, and so forth, over a period of some thirty days in Moriaen's version, or a hundred in Glauber's. What remained at the end was, according to Moriaen, a 'liquor' containing the sperm of both the sun and the moon, or in Glauber's account a 'salt' in which 'the astral life-giving rays of the sun' had been made 'visible, tangible, corporeal and solid'.[113]

Moriaen called his liquor the 'Universal menstruum' but gave no clearer indication of what he thought it was or what was to be done with it; however, the mention of solar and lunar seeds clearly points to an alchemical purpose, the sun and moon being the ruling 'planets' of gold and silver respectively. Glauber was marginally more forthcoming on this point: his preparation was a medicine (though he neglected to say what for) and it could transmute metals (but he forgot to mention how). What comes down to us is a great cry of Eureka but no very clear definition of what was supposed to have been found. That it struck a chord in contemporary minds, however, is evidenced not only by the fact that Moriaen returned to the subject four times within three months, obviously at Hartlib's urging, but by Hartlib's underlining relevant passages in the manuscripts or having scribal copies and translations made of them. He also discussed with Boyle a later version of Moriaen's experiment, of which there is no trace in the surviving papers. In 1659, Hartlib advised his young friend that 'Concerning the instrument of catching and condensing the sunbeams, I have a promise of a large account from Mr *Morian*'.[114] And he elicited a lively reaction from Poleman, who urged Hartlib to send him full details:

> I thank you most warmly for the extracts you sent of Herr Moriaen's manuscript on concentrating the spirit of the world. But among other things, Herr Moriaen says in his account that he has revealed to you a method of catching the water of the air by means of calcined pebbles: I pray you seek this out and send it to me as soon as possible.[115]

Close comparison of the two experiments leaves Glauber's account looking suspiciously like a rewrite of Moriaen's with certain crucial details left out. The point cannot be proved one way or the other without further documentary evidence, but I do not think it out of the question that Glauber based his version, without acknowledgment, on information given him by Moriaen. Since Moriaen made no claim to have devised or even conducted the experiment himself, there is no reason to suppose that if Moriaen had had it from Glauber he would have concealed the fact from Hartlib. He said he had learned it 'from the mouth of my cousin' ('aus meines Vettern mund), the 'cousin' in question having taken part himself in the experiment. The German word 'Vetter', like the English 'cousin', was at this date used very loosely to designate any relative beyond the immediate family (though Moriaen's German grammar makes it clear this relative was male): since he gave no indication of how long ago he had learned the process, it is conceivable that the reference is to his alchemically-inclined brother-in-law Peter von Zeuel, but this is pure conjecture.

Whether or not Glauber and Moriaen were aware of how similar their experiments were, the two accounts exemplify the contrasting presentation of public and private alchemical exchange. Glauber totally omitted to define the nature of his raw material; Moriaen somewhat more helpfully described his as a coarse powder obtained by grinding a type of flint or pebble[116] to be found by the Rhine. Moriaen was quite explicit in stating that what his 'magnet' initially attracted from the air was 'salt'; Glauber said no such thing, but did suddenly and bafflingly start referring to the residue after evaporation as 'salt'. Similarly, Glauber abruptly remarked that the evaporation drew off superfluous liquid without affecting the 'seeds' the magnet had attracted, but gave no hint as to what these seeds were or where they had come from; Moriaen was far more specific with his solar and lunar spermata.

Glauber's omissions are deliberate, for like most alchemists who actually went to press, his aim was not to communicate the whole mystery (whether or not he believed himself to know it). It was rather to attract the interest of a particular audience. Whether in Glauber's case that intended audience consisted solely of well-heeled potential patrons or included anyone whose piety, wisdom and application rendered them worthy of alchemical enlightenment is a moot point. In all probability he had both categories in mind: and should his work fall under the eyes of someone who belonged to both categories at once, so much the better. It is in any case certain that he was in the habit of sending presentation copies of his new publications to figures of high social standing who had shown signs of interest in the chemical philosophy.[117] Moriaen, on the other hand, knew very well who his audience was: it was Hartlib and Clodius in the first instance, and anyone to whom they saw fit to pass on the information. He was clearly not seeking any personal gain through the communication, and in contrast to most such private reports there is no injunction to secrecy. Moreover, far from hinting at further information that he might be induced to impart, he repeatedly apologised for having no more to offer. It is a genuine example of 'free and generous communication of secrets'.

Both accounts, though, Moriaen's no less than Glauber's, seem frustratingly incomplete. In particular, they are very vague as to the nature and use of the experiment's end product. In Glauber's case, this is hardly surprising, for all the reasons just stated. In Moriaen's the matter is less clear-cut. It may be that he saw no reason to expand on the definition of 'universal menstruum' because he thought Hartlib would regard it as self-evident. On the whole, however, this seems unlikely. Neither Moriaen nor Hartlib ever claimed to be an adept. Hartlib was an interested observer and sponsor of other men's labours in the field, but clearly no more than that. Moriaen certainly was a practising alchemist, but he never pretended to be a very successful one. It is likely that the lacunae in the account simply represent the limitations of Moriaen's own knowledge and understanding of the business.

Nonetheless, however vague he may have been as to what the 'universal menstruum' actually was, he seems to have been quite sure that whatever it was, this was it. The same applies to the 'ludus Paracelsi' he sent Hartlib through Albert Otto Faber in 1661, and to the method of turning antimony into gold he believed he had discovered in the early 1650s. (This will be discussed in Chapter Seven.) Glauber and Moriaen found what they were looking for because they defined their results in terms of what they were expecting to find. By the same token, many alchemists must have concluded that what they had produced was a form of gold, or the elixir, or the universal spirit, because they were assured by respected authority and/or what they took to be divine inspiration that that was what their method would produce. It was one thing to dismiss the theories of pagans such as Galen and Aristotle as ignorant or misguided and to refute them by experiment, but the study of true Scripture and the insights achieved through pious Christian meditation could only serve to illuminate and explain experimental data. This is not to accuse these thinkers of intellectual laziness or dishonesty, merely to attempt to understand their habits of thought by placing them in historical context.

The letters and documents of the natural philosophers directly or indirectly associated with Hartlib in the mid-seventeenth century, far from showing any gathering doubts about the claims of alchemy, manifest a mounting and at times near-hysterical enthusiasm. Confronted with unprecedented social upheavals - the Thirty Years War in Germany and surrounding lands, the civil wars in England - and with the explosion of information and new philosophies posited in the previous chapter as the challenge that inspired Comenian Pansophy, they found in alchemy a system of thought that reconciled the evidence of their senses with the demands and promised rewards of the Christian faith to which they clung with almost desperate tenacity. There was, in their minds, no antithesis between the pragmatic inductivism of Bacon and the mystic Paracelsianism of Böhme, and they actively encouraged the development of new technology and experimental science, which they thought could only contribute to their work. The papers abundantly demonstrate that, as is now widely recognised, the revival of alchemy and the growth of the 'new' science were not merely parallel but inextricably intertwined. Though empiricism was in time to sound the death-knell of alchemy, it is wholly anachronistic to speak in terms of a conflict between the two at this date. Francis Bacon, dismissing alchemy as outmoded superstition, thought he was speaking of the past, but might equally be seen as having predicted the future, when in 1605 he acknowledged that

> surely to alchemy this right is due: that [...] the search and stir to make gold hath brought to light a great number of good and fruitful inventions and experiments, as well for the disclosing of nature as for the use of man's life'.[118]

Bacon meant to suggest that such useful discoveries were an unintentional by-product of the vain labours of would-be gold-makers. In fact, the disclosure of nature and use of man's life were very much part of the alchemical agenda, but they were by no means the whole of it. The underlying impulse, like that of Bacon's own projected Great Instauration, was dominion. I suggested at the end of the last sub-chapter that alchemists, as opposed to mere chemists, might be seen not as mappers but as colonists of the created world. Such an account is of course anachronistic, representing a twentieth-century analysis that would have been quite incomprehensible to a seventeenth-century practitioner of alchemy. Alchemical rhetoric speaks not of dominating or colonising Nature, but of helping it, husbanding it, curing it. Nor, for that matter, did 'philo-Judaists' such as Moriaen, or the missionaries who set out for the supposedly New World, regard or project themselves as conquerors: they genuinely believed, or many of them did, that they were doing the benighted Jews and native Americans a favour by guiding (or driving) them towards the light, accelerating their progress along a path that was divinely pre-ordained. Like the inhabitants of nations overcome by Thomas More's Utopians, one could only expect them, in the long run, to be grateful for the experience.

All metals aspired to become, indeed were destined to become, gold. Jews (and, by some accounts, heathens) were likewise destined to mature into Christians. Colonists, Pansophists and alchemists were only acting as catalysts, helping the rest of Creation on its providentially pre-ordained way, raising it to the standard of physical and spiritual health it had been vouchsafed them to recognise. Or so they convinced themselves.

The impulse underlying both Pansophy and alchemy is that underlying the Judaic Creation myth itself. The Book of Genesis is essentially an affirmation of the divine sanction accorded to mankind to assert control over the rest of Creation, and to a given race and creed to assert control over the rest of humanity. Put another way, it is a rationalisation of the impulse to exercise such control. Judaism's equally anthropocentric daughter religions, Christianity and Islam, accepted wholesale the notion of humanity's privileged position within the sublunary sphere, and adroitly transferred the status of chosen race and creed, with all the responsibility and licence that status implied, to a variety of European and Arab civilisations. While alchemy in early modern Europe tended on the whole to downplay the importance of national identity (the figure of the 'Cosmopolite' was a stock-in-trade of the alchemical tradition, and one which Starkey in particular made an integral part of his self-projection), the notion of a supremely privileged, divinely sanctioned elect resurfaces as strongly as ever in the topos of the magus or adept inspired directly by God and manipulating the very fabric of the planet.

It was suggested earlier that Christian proselytisers regarded Jews (or whatever other group they were seeking to 'enlighten') as raw material to be remoulded in their own image. James Holstun, in his extremely perceptive and thought-provoking study of Protestant Utopianism, depicts Comenius's educational ideology in very similar terms, and relates it to the endeavours of early colonists to set up new model societies on the 'virgin' soil of the Americas - and to the economic and ideological colonialism of our own time.[119] He draws attention to Comenius's notion of 'didachography', his oft-repeated metaphor of the infant mind as a blank page on which virtue and truth may be inscribed by the enlightened educator:

> Nowhere does Comenius refer to the student as an autonomous subject or even as a being with any trace of prior individuality. He (or she - Comenius proposes the education of both sexes) is only the blank paper on which didachography prints. But the sheer repetitiveness of the printing becomes millennial: 'For the moment, it is enough to have shown that our discovery of didachography or the panmethodia can multiply learned men in precisely the same way that the discovery of printing has multiplied books [...] And since we struggle to implant piety itself after planting learning and morality in the souls of all who are consecrated to Christ, we can hope for the fulfillment of those divine prophecies that we are commanded to hope for: "The earth shall be full of the knowledge of God, as the waters cover the sea" (Isa. 11:9)'.[120]

Once again, the aim of alchemy can be seen as analogous to, or even an extension of, that of Pansophy. Alchemy sought to demonstrate the possibility of returning Creation itself to its original status as blank page, when the earth was without form, and void.[121] That page had been written on by the word that was in the beginning, that was with God and was God,[122] but the text had subsequently been corrupted by sin. Just as Comenian education would mould the uncorrupted minds of infants in godly fashion, as missionaries would build a new Jerusalem on the undefiled soil of the New World, so the alchemists would rewrite Creation in better accord with the original divine intention. Of course they did not think they were usurping God. They believed that God intended them to do so, and it is certainly not my intention to question the sincerity of that belief. My suggestion is rather that the God on whose authority they were acting was himself a projection of their own deep-seated impulse to mastery.

Notes

1   It is certain that there were substantial losses from the archive. See Hartlib to Worthington, 2 Nov. 1661, *Worthington Diary* II, 67, on the 'distraction or embezzlement' of many books and manuscripts he had entrusted to an unnamed friend for safekeeping, and 6 Feb. 1662, ibid., 107, on the loss of more through a fire in his house. While he was living with his son in Axe Yard, his friend Samuel Wartensky

was alarmed to find that his possessions were 'a prey to plunder by all' ('omnium exposita rapinæ' - Wartensky to Hartlib, 23 July 1661, HP 32/3/40A). Other papers were almost certainly abstracted from the collection after his death.

2   There is one mention of him in a letter from Comenius to Hartlib, 25 May 1646, HP 7/73/3A, stating that Moriaen would send Hartlib Comenius's new publications from Amsterdam. Apart from this, he is mentioned only in the letters of Dury's brother-in-law Heinrich Appelius.

3   'bin woll eher ein großer liebhaber und verfechter meta*phy*sicarum et meta*phy*sicorum gewest, wie Ich aber darnach ad scientias reales et usuales kom*m*en, sind mir die speculationes inutiles stinkend word*en*' - Moriaen to Hartlib, 10 Feb. 1648, HP 37/129A.

4   *The Advancement of Learning, Works*, III, 287.

5   *Comenius' Självbiografi*, 148 (cf. Young, *Comenius in England*, 31).

6   Boyle to Isaac Marcombes, 22 Oct. 1646, *Works*, ed. Birch (1744 edition) I, 20. The identity of this 'new philosophical college', referred to elsewhere by Boyle as the 'Invisible College', has been much debated: for a summary of opinions, see Webster, *Great Instauration*, 57-67, and 'Benjamin Worsley: Engineering for universal reform from the Invisible College to the Navigation Act', *SHUR* 213-35. Webster's own suggestion that it was an informal association of younger scientists centred on Boyle, Worsley and Katherine Ranelagh, and possibly including the Boate brothers, John Sadler, Robert Child and John Winthrop, seems to me the most plausible, though as Webster points out there is no more than circumstantial evidence for anyone's membership but Boyle's.

7   UBA N65a, 8 March 1634 (not 10 March as the UBA catalogue and Van Der Wall (*Serrarius*, 661) state, misreading the Gothic 8 which is written at 90° to the modern one). Chemistry is also discussed in letters from Cologne of 6 Sept. 1636 and 17 Jan. 1637 (UBA N65c and N65d).

8   'das mein herr in *Philosophia* experimentali & mechanica sich verliebet ist nicht zue wundern' - Moriaen to Hartlib, 10 Feb. 1648, HP 37/129A. It is unclear whether 'verliebet' is here a past participle or a present indicative: the phrase could equally be translated 'that you are falling in love with experimental and mechanical philosophy'; there can be little doubt, however, that Hartlib's infatuation with those subjects began well before 1648.

9   HP 30/4/27A. Gauden's reply to the question, dated 16 June 1637, is preserved in full in the papers, HP 26/14/1A-15B. This is the same Gauden whose *Love of Truth and Peace* recommended Dury and Comenius to Parliament (see above, pp. 128-9).

10   HP 29/5/77B.

11   Allen G. Debus, *The Chemical Philosophy: Paracelsian Science and Medicine in the Sixteenth and Seventeenth Centuries* (2 vols.), New York 1977.

12   *The Chemical Philosophy* I, xi.

13   Cf. Webster, *From Paracelsus to Newton*, 10.

14   Cf. *HDC*, 382-413 on Comenius and his assistants, especially Kinner; and Rood, *Comenius and the Low Countries*, 77-87, on strained relations with the de Geers.

15   Figulus to Hartlib, 19 July 1658, HP 9/17/11A; Blekastad, *Peter Figulus. Letters to Samuel Hartlib*, 216.

16   Figulus to Hartlib, 2 Aug. 1658, HP 9/17/15B; Blekastad, *Figulus Letters*, 219.

17   'Die geschraubte Symbolsprache war den Chemikern seiner Zeit genau so verständlich, wie es die moderne Formel uns heute ist' - K.F. Gugel, *Johann Rudolph Glauber 1604-70: Leben und Werk* (Würzburg, 1955), 39.

18   Starkey, 'Sir George Riplye's Epistle to King Edward Unfolded', in *Chymical,*

Medicinal, and Chyrurgical Addresses, 19-47, esp.20 and 42.

19 William Newman, *Gehennical Fire: The Lives of George Starkey, an Alchemist of Harvard in the Scientific Revolution* (Harvard, 1994).

20 *Eph 51*, HP 28/2/24B.

21 Webster, *From Paracelsus to Newton*, 10.

22 *A Reformation of Schooles*, 6.

23 The phrase is from the description on the title page of Boyle's contribution to the *Chymical, Medicinal, and Chyrurgical Addresses*, 'An Epistolical Discourse of Philaretus to Empyricus', which can virtually be read as the group's manifesto. It is 'An Invitation to a free and generous Communication of Secrets and Receits in Physick'.

24 Paracelsus, *Werke*, ed. Karl Sudhoff (Berlin, 1922-33), VIII, 38, cit. Heinrich Schipperges, 'Strukturen und Prozesse Alchimistischer Überlieferungen', in Emil Ploss et. al., *Alchimia: Ideologie und Technologie* (Munich, 1970), 67-118, esp.108.

25 *Magnalia Medico-Chymica*, 12: 'Alchimey wird nur von den Unkündigen (so nicht wissen was sey/ sondern nur dafür halten/ es sey nichts anders darinn/ denn daß man sich narret mit Gold- und Silbermachen) verlachet und verachtet: Aber durch dieselbige Kunst magst du aus allen greifflichen Dingen Saltz/ Kelch/ Staub/ Wasser/ Safft/ Oel/ auf das alleredleste zurichten/ dadurch du einen krancken Menschen in wenig Stunden gantz sanfft und lieblich von seinen Gebrechen erledigne magst.'

26 See Webster, *Great Instauration*, section 4 (246-323).

27 *Confessio Fraternitatis*, 67 (37 in the Van Dülmen edition).

28 *Fama Fraternitatis*, 125 (29 in the Van Dülmen edition): 'als ob die mutatio metallorum der höchste apex und fastigium in der philosophia were, und derselbe Gott besonders lieb sein müsse, so nuhr grosse Goldmassen und klumpen machen köndte [...] So bezeugen wir hiermit öffentlich, daß solches falsch und es mit den wahren Philosophis also beschaffen, daß ihnen Gold zu machen ein geringes und nur ein parergon ist, derengleichen sie noch wol andere etlich tausend bessere stücklein haben.'

29 *Magnalia Medico-Chymica*, 14.

30 Newman, *Gehennical Fire*, 205, citing George Thomson, *Loimotomia; or the Pest Anatomized* (London, 1666), 100.

31 HP 29/3/48B.

32 'Whether or no, each Several Disease hath a Particular Remedy?', *Chymical, Medicinal, and Chyrurgical Addresses*, 89-99 (translated from the proceedings of Théophraste Renaudot's 'Bureau d'Addresse').

33 'Es gefelt mir auch nicht aller dings an Glaubern das er eben hohen Persohnen solche rare Wissenschaft mitheilen will, den die pflegen dergleichen köstliche sachen doch nur gemeiniglich zu ihrer wollust und geitz zu misbrauchen' - Moriaen to ?, 31 Jan. 1651, HP 63/14/4A.

34 See the epigraph to this chapter.

35 *Eph 49*, 28/1/35A: the informants are Boyle himself and Worsley. There are no letters from Boyle among Hartlib's surviving papers, and his 'Experiment of Iron and Antimony' has not been identified. It seems likely that Boyle's letters (of which there were undoubtedly a considerable number) were among those plundered from the archive in Hartlib's last years or after his death, either by figures who recognised the potential value of Boyliana or by friends or agents of Boyle himself concerned to erase evidence of his association with Hartlib, whose close association with Oliver Cromwell and the Parliamentary cause meant that many were concerned to distance themselves from him after the Restoration.

36   *A Discovery of Subterraneall Treasure*, 42.

37   'Er bekent in diesem tractat das diß sein aur*um* pot*abile* nicht allein den [*mercurium*]
     sondern auch alle andere metallen in gutt goltt transmutire od*er* gradire ab*er* ohne nuz
     und also unnötig darzue zue gebrauch*en* als allein die mügligkeit und warheit zue
     beweisen, wie auch diße medicinam als Universalem zue bewehren' - Moriaen to
     Hartlib, 5 Oct. 1657, HP 42/2/22A.

38   Genesis 2:11-12.

39   'seine bücher in v*nd* allezeit [haben mir] sehr missgefallen, dass ich gar ein grossen
     äckel dafür bekommen, vnd [...] kaum ein paragraphum darin lesen kan, dass ich über
     den verkehrten man nicht ein gerechten zorn concipire, weil er so trotziglich vnd
     speciosè der weisen schrifften viel gräwlicher drähet vnd zwacket, als die
     allergreiligsten vnd ärgesten kätzer die H*eilige* Schrifft verkehren; vnd verleitet dieser
     böse man die einfaltigen vnd vnwissenden auf solche grewliche irr wege, auf welchen
     sie nimmermehr zur warheit kommen können. Mit was für gewissen solte ich wohl
     solchen muthwilligen verführer besuchen?' - Poleman to Hartlib, 12 Sept. 1659, HP
     60/10/2A. The analogy with Scripture comes over even more strongly in German
     since the same word, 'Schriften', covers both human writings and holy writ.

40   Facsimile reproduction with an introduction by A.G. Debus, London, 1967: the
     Canons Yeomans Tale is at pp. 227-56.

41   Donne, *Ignatius his Conclave*, ed. T.S. Healy (Oxford, 1969), 21 (Donne's own
     translation of his Latin original).

42   Cf. Bruce T. Moran, *The Alchemical World of the German Court: Occult Philosophy
     and Chemical Medicine in the Circle of Moritz of Hessen (1572-1632)*, Sudhoffs
     Archiv Beiheft 29 (Stuttgart 1991), *passim*.

43   *Chymical, Medicinal, and Chyrurgical Addresses*, 81-3.

44   Ibid., 87.

45   Plattes, *A Description of the Famous Kingdome of Macaria* (London, 1641), 11-12.
     As Webster suggests, the book in question was probably Plattes' own *Arts Mistress*,
     which is now lost if indeed it was ever completed (*Utopian Planning and the Puritan
     Revolution*, 86).

46   Hartlib to Winthrop, 16 March 1660, HP 7/7/2B, replying to Winthrop's query at
     HP 32/1/4A (16 Dec. 1659).

47   'Sucht Er aber Laboris socium vnd kan seine wißenschafft allein nicht ins w*er*kh
     stellen, d*er* gibt Ihm genug wan Er ihn das werckh auff seine kost*en* machen läst' -
     Moriaen to Hartlib, 24 March 1639, HP 37/14A.

48   Kretschmar was a diplomat in the service of Elector Friedrich ('the Great') of
     Brandenburg, and was in England in 1657-58, petitioning Cromwell to release the
     funds raised by an official charitable collection for the Bohemian and Polish exiles
     (copy of the petition at HP 54/35A), and approaching the Austin Friars Consistory
     for further assistance for them (Hessels III, nos. 3441, 3445). While in London he
     made the acquaintance of Hartlib and his friends, and seems to have been involved
     with Clodius's 'Chemical College' (Webster, *Great Instauration*, 302).

49   22 July/1 August 1659, HP 26/64/1A-4B; cf. Turnbull, 'Johann Valentin Andreæs
     Societas Christiana', *Zeitschrift für deutsche Philologie* 73 (1954), 407-31, esp.414
     n.53. William Brereton (1631-79) was a founder member of the Royal Society and
     from 1664 third Lord Brereton. He had studied at Breda under Pell and was close to
     the Hartlib circle; it was he who purchased Hartlib's papers after their owner's death.
     See James Crossley (ed.) *The Diary and Correspondence of John Worthington* I
     (Manchester, 1847), 212-13, and the 'Introduction' to *SHUR*, 4-7.

50   Bruce T. Moran cites many similar examples in *The Alchemical World of the*

German Court (Stuttgart, 1991).

51 Hartlib to Boyle, 7 Jan. 1658, Boyle, *Works*, VI, 99.

52 A draft of this letter in Clodius's hand and a fair scribal copy, both undated, are appended to the original Kretschmar letter, HP 26/64/5A-7B. Turnbull states rather bewilderingly that 'eine Abschrift befindet sich bei den Briefen Johann Morians in Hartlibs Papieren, und jener konnte es verfaßt haben' ('there is a copy among the letters of Johann Moriaen in Hartlib's papers, and he may have been the author') ('J.V. Andreæs *Societas Christiana*', 414 n.53). This (most uncharacteristically for Turnbull) is completely erroneous. The document is not located among Moriaen's letters, and the hand of the draft is unmistakeably Clodius's.

53 'Den mein H wir sindt alhie nicht so vnwissend, dz wir nicht könten [...] auß einer Vntze ein wenig goldes bringen, aber hier entweder es zahlet nicht die vnkosten oder es gehet nicht an im großen.'

54 'versichere M*einen Herrn* dz man davor gewißlich helt dz sein weg sehr profitable muste sein weil er 600lb davor begehret.'

55 Poleman to Hartlib, 12 Sept. 1659, HP 60/4/56B-57A.

56 'dz liebliche zischen einer solchen listigen schlangen' - Poleman to Hartlib, 15 Aug. 1659, HP 60/10/1A.

57 'zur großen schmach der mehr als königlichen kunst, der wahren Chymia' - Poleman to Hartlib, 19 Sept. 1659, HP 60/4/58A-B. Poleman is referring here to yet another German alchemist in Amsterdam, Liebhart.

58 On this subject, see A.J. Rocke, 'Agricola, Paracelsus and "Chymia"', *Ambix* 32 (1985), 38-45. The article is useful for defining the (al)chemical genres: 'esoteric' (religio-philosophical), 'exoteric' (transmutational) and 'empirical' (technological and pharmaceutical), but as I hope to show, the demarcations between these three were far from rigid, and the semantic distinction that applies 'alchemy' to the first two and 'chymia' to the third was far from being generally accepted by the mid-seventeenth century

59 Rocke, op. cit., 38-9 and *passim*.

60 Adelung, *Geschichte der menschlichen Narrheit* (Leibzig, 1785), *passim*. Cf. Debus, 'The Paracelsians in Eighteenth-Century France: A Renaissance Tradition in the Age of Enlightenment', *Ambix* 28 (1981), 36-54; reproduced as chapter 14 of *Chemistry, Alchemy and the New Philosophy: studies in the history of science and medicine* (Variorum Reprints, London, 1987).

61 '... alchemistarum vulgo', 'Chemici Philosophastri' (HP 18/12/11B).

62 'Ignari pharmacopæi, mendaces alchimistæ, temerarij chyrurgi' (HP 25/20/7A).

63 'Famulantur autem Medicinæ, Physica, Botanica, Anatomica, Chyrurgica, Alchimistica Pharmaceutica; omnes has artes cognoscere tenetur qvisqvis ambit titulum Medici' (HP 25/20/6B).

64 The untitled and unascribed Latin tract at HP 18/7/1A-20B is a complete copy of Starkey's *Metallorum Metamorphosis*, which was later published under his pseudonym 'Philalethes' in the collection *Musæum Hermeticum Reformatum et Amplificatum* (Frankfurt, 1678), 743-74. See William Newman, 'Prophecy and Alchemy: The Origin of Eiranæus Philalethes', *Ambix* 37 part 3 (Nov. 1990), 97-115, for identification of Philalethes as Starkey.

65 'Nihil enim præter dispendium (et nummorum et temporis) à semidocta Alchymiæ scientia' (HP 18/7/1B; *Musæum Hermeticum*, 743).

66 'Non etenim (qvia plurimi repriuntur, Alcymiam tractantes, deceptores sophistæ) hæc perinde) aut falsitates aut ineptiæ arguitur' (HP 18/7/2A-B; *Musæum*, 745).

67 'Chymistæ actutùm nomen induit; mox [...] protinus Philosophi titulam vendicat'

(HP 18/7/1B; *Musæum*, 744).

68 'Chymici vulgares' (HP 18/7/4A; *Musæum*, 748).

69 '... veram (Artis Alchymiæ) clavem' (HP 18/7/17B; *Musæum*, 770).

70 'die wahre Alchimia von den Landtläuferischen Buben oder falschen Alchymisten' - Glauber, De tribus *lapidibus ignium secretorum* (Amsterdam 1667), 6-7.

71 Herwig Buntz, 'Die europäische Alchimie vom 13. bis zum 18. Jahrhundert', in Ploss et al., *Alchimia: Ideologie und Technologie*, 119-210, 194.

72 'In Chymicis, Alchymicis, Medicinâ, Mechanicis artibus, Magiâ Naturali, plurima habeo' (HP 1/33/106A-B). The undated tract is entitled 'N. Reneri, Professoris Ultrajectini, Experimenta'. This is perhaps Cyprien Regneri ab Oosterga, who became professor at Utrecht in 1641 (cf. *Correspondance de Mersenne* X, 203), though it is not clear where the initial N comes from. It could simply be a mistake.

73 'einem Chymico oder Alchymiste [...] dienen sie sehr wol' - Appelius to Hartlib, 5 Sept. 1644, HP 45/1/13A.

74 Appelius to Hartlib, 26 Aug. 1647, HP 45/1/33B.

75 *Eph 52*, HP 28/2/27B.

76 Dury to [Worsley?], 25 Aug. 1655, HP 4/3/121A.

77 On Worsley and his visit to the Netherlands, see below, pp. 217-26.

78 Appelius to Hartlib, 6 Nov. 1647 (dated 27 Oct. O.S.), HP 45/1/27A.

79 John Read, *Prelude to Chemistry: An Outline of Alchemy, Its Literature and Relationships* (London, 1936).

80 See M.J. Braddick and M. Greengrass, 'Introduction' to *The Letters of Sir Cheney Culpeper (1641-1657)*, Camden Miscellany XXXIII (Cambridge, 1996), 115-50, and Stephen Clucas, 'The Correspondence of a XVII-Century "Chymicall Gentleman": Sir Cheney Culpeper and the Chemical interests of the Hartlib Circle', *Ambix* 40 (1993), 147-70; also Chapter Seven below.

81 Culpeper to Worsley, n.d. but probably late 1647, HP 13/223A.

82 On the 'aerial nitre', see Allen G. Debus, *Chemistry, Alchemy and the New Philosophy, 1550-1700* (Variorum Reprints, London 1987), ch. 9, 'The Paracelsian Aerial Nitre'.

83 Debus, op. cit., ch. 10, 253; Robert Fludd, *Philosophical Key*, ed. Debus (New York, 1979).

84 Debus, ibid., 256.

85 *Miraculi Mundi Continuatio* (Amsterdam, 1657), 85.

86 *De Natura Salium* (Amsterdam, 1658), 14.

87 Ibid., 115.

88 'Das Saltz ist [...] ein Symbolum Æternitatis, weiln weder im Fewer/ Lufft/ Wasser/ noch Erden alteriret oder geringert wirdt/ sondern alles vor verderben eine lange Zeit bewaret. [...] Das Saltz ist bey der Schöpfung GOttes das erste Fiat gewesen, vnd auß dem Fiat sind hernach die Elementa entstanden' - ibid., 43-44.

89 Ibid., 10-11.

90 'Komt also alle fruchtbarkeit/ vnd Nahrung vom Saltze/ das Saltz von der Sonnen/ die Sonne von GOtt dem Schöpffer aller dingen' - ibid., 117.

91 'Von den brenn gläßern hab ich gleichwoll auch diß gesehen, wan man ein klein gestoßenen antimonium an der Sonne damit anstecket so rauchet Er stark hinweg und verliert gleichwoll nichts an seinem gewicht sondern wird schwerer dardurch, das dan freylich ein beweiß ist das der Sonnen stralen das sal naturæ hinein bringen und damit imprægniren' - Moriaen to Hartlib, 14 June 1658, HP 31/18/30A.

92   *The Alchemical World of the German Court*, 130-31.

93   *Panegersia* (1657), trans. A.M.O. Dobbie (Shipton on Stour, 1990), 10.

94   Boyle, *The Sceptical Chymist*, 356-67.

95   *Sceptical Chymist*, 356.

96   'vnd ist daß Goldt alhier anstatt eines Samens/ das [*Kupfer*]/ vnd Regul. Antim. aber an statt des Erden/ darauß das [*Gold*] sich nehret vnnd vermehret/ vnd der Salpeter anstat des Regen-wassers/ dadurch daß Erdtreich befeüchtet/ vnd fruchtbahr gemacht wirdt. Ie länger nun daß [*Gold*] in diesem Erdtreich liegt/ vnd wächset/ je mehr es zuwachses darauß stehet' - *Miraculi Mundi Continuatio* (Amsterdam, 1657), 67.

97   'Die Natur sucht allzeit jhre Kinder zur perfection zubringen/ vnd die geringe Metallen seynd nicht perfect. Warumb solte man der Natur nit zu hülff kommen/ vnd dieselbe verbessern können?' - *Furni Novi Philosophici* IV (Amsterdam, 1650), 37.

98   Cf. Link, *Glauber*, 77.

99   *Aurora, oder Morgenröthe im Auffgang, Sämtliche Schriften* I, ed. Ernst Peuckert, (Stuttgart, 1955), 85-132. I have drastically edited Böhme's account of these seven 'Quell-Geister', which I make no pretence of understanding in any detail.

100   Culpeper to [Worsley?], 9 May 1648, HP 13/218B.

101   HP 63/14/23A-24A, undated. The tract was sent by Joachim Lange on 14 October 1653.

102   So Schlezer told Hartlib in his account of the figure (16 Dec. 1653, HP 63/14/26A); Schlezer's terms imply that this was a pseudonym. According to Schlezer he was 72 years old and lived in Hamburg, but no further evidence about him has been discovered.

103   'vnd ist dieses die Quinta Essentia des Universal Geistes, welcher Genesi primo Auff dem Wasser geschwebet' - HP 63/14/23A.

104   'sehe wol dz des Authoris Philosophia höher gehet als seine Erfahrung' - Moriaen to ?, 28 Nov. 1653, HP 63/14/24B and 30A.

105   HP 63/14/26A.

106   'expresse im text stehet, dz derselbe geist sey der geist Gottes gewesen, ein absurdum aber ist zu sagen, dz ein chymicus wolle eine quintam essentiam, den Spiritum DEI machen' - HP 63/14/33A, n.d.

107   Genesis 1:26-30. I use the plural advisedly: 'male and female created he them', though the creation of Eve is not mentioned until the next chapter.

108   Genesis 3:22-3.

109   Genesis 11:6-7.

110   The fullest accounts are at HP 31/18/29B-30A and 31/18/40B-41A.

111   Reproduced in *Glauberus Concentratus oder Kern der Glauberischen Schrifften* (Leipzig and Breslau, 1715), 465-66.

112   'ein [Wasser] [...] in welchem [Wasser] die allgemeine Lebens-Speise der [Luft] verborgen' - *Glauberus Concentratus*, 465.

113   'die astralisch lebendig-machende Sonnen-Strahlen [...] sichtlich/ greifflich/ corporalisch und fix' - Ibid.

114   Hartlib to Boyle, 5 April 1659 (*Works* VI, 117).

115   'Fur die communicata ex MS Morianis de Concentrandu S*piritu* Mundi bedancke Ich mich gar herzlich [...] es saget aber H Mor*ian* in dieser Description vnter And*er*n Er habe dem H. vor diesem eine weisse entdecket, durch Calcinirte Kiesel-steine [...] dz wasser d*er* luft zu fangen [...] als bitte Ich solch*en* aufzusuch*en* v*nd* ehestes zu vbersenden' - Poleman to Hartlib, 5 Dec. 1659, HP 60/4/159A.

116 In Latin passages, the term consistently used is 'silices', in German, 'Kießlinge'.
117 Link, *Glauber*, 103-4.
118 Francis Bacon, *The Advancement of Learning*, I; in *Works* III, 289.
119 James Holstun, *A Rational Millennium* (New York and Oxford, 1987) 308-315.
120 Ibid., 309-10, citing Comenius, *The Great Didactic* (trans. M.W. Keatinge from *Didactica Magna* (Amsterdam, 1657)) (New York, 1967), 293-4
121 Genesis 1:2.
122 John 1:1.

CHAPTER SIX

Universal Medicines: Johann Rudolph Glauber and his Reception in England

'[Glauber] ist ein Mensch voller verstand und wißenschafften in re medico-chimica Ia so [*sehr?*] daß Er gleichsam darinnen sich veriret und nicht weiß welches er am ersten furnehmen oder ins werkh richten soll' ('[Glauber] is a man of great understanding and knowledge in medical and chemical matters; so much so, indeed, that he loses himself in them, as it were, not knowing what to undertake or set on foot first') - Moriaen to Hartlib, 27 August 1647, HP 37/121A.

'Paracelsus of the Seventeenth Century' or 'German Robert Boyle'?

Of all the many 'Chemical Philosophers' with whom Moriaen became associated in the course of his long involvement with alchemy, the one personally closest to him and on whom he sent the longest and most detailed reports was his highly controversial countryman Johann Rudolph Glauber (1604-1670).[1] It is now generally accepted that Glauber was among the most historically significant practical chemists of his day, though assessments of the scientific value of his work still vary considerably. Because of Moriaen's personal friendship and practical collaboration with the man, his comments on Glauber are of particular value. They supply some hint of what is most irrevocably lost to later scholars, the essential oral component of alchemical communication, in the context of which published and even manuscript material was intended to be understood.

Though numerous monographs on him have been written, many details of Glauber's personal history remain obscure. The principal primary source of information hitherto available on his life has been his own autobiographical writings - a notoriously unreliable form of evidence. These autobiographical fragments, which are scattered in typically disorganised fashion throughout his work, were mostly written in response to accusations published by Christoph Fahrner, an assistant and protegé with whom Glauber fell out in 1654.[2] They are thus highly polemical and defensive, and particularly in the cases where Fahrner's charges appear to have had at least an element of truth in them, Glauber did not scruple to doctor the facts in order to refute them. The other main source has been contemporary publications about him, almost all of which were written by personal enemies such as Fahrner and are hence equally partisan and unreliable.

Hartlib's papers, especially the letters from Moriaen, supply a number of lacunae in the biographical data so far available on Glauber, particularly for the 1640s and 1650s. They are also a rich source of informal contemporary comment on the man and his work, covering the whole gamut from enthusiastic approval through interested comment, scepticism and frank bafflement to outraged condemnation. This chapter will present a considerable body of new biographical evidence to supplement the extant accounts, and draw on the Hartlib archive to provide a more sophisticated analysis of the reception of his work in his own age than can be gleaned from printed sources. Though the letters preserved by Hartlib are by no means free of partisanship and personal agendas, neither are they public denunciations or defences, and a measure of balance is supplied by the sheer variety of sources and opinions. The case of Glauber also provides a very interesting and well-documented example of the workings of Hartlib's information network as applied to a given subject or individual.

Glauber's life and work were both consciously modelled on those of Paracelsus: he has been described as the 'Paracelsus of the seventeenth century'.[3] He wandered as restlessly through Europe as his forebear before finally settling for good in the Netherlands in his fifties. Like Paracelsus, he wrote in the vernacular, though in Glauber's case this was as much a consequence of linguistic limitation as of principle. He despised received academic wisdom, though as Boyle was to complain of the Spagyrists in general, he was not always so cautious of doctrines of the non- 'academic' variety. He laid great emphasis on exact observation and physical experiment, and displayed exceptional practical expertise, particularly in technological and agricultural matters.

Like Paracelsus, he was a spectacularly controversial figure during his lifetime, and has continued to be the object of both uncritical praise and excessive vilification in the centuries since his death. What both camps have generally agreed on, however, is that an evaluative judgment of Glauber depends on the question of whether he is to be seen as an alchemist or a chemist - a question which, as was argued in the previous chapter, is wholly anachronistic.[4] Adelung thought him a complete charlatan, but he is seen far more sympathetically by most of his more recent biographers. Pietsch calls him 'a founder of chemical technology' ('einen Ergründer der chemischen Technologie'); for Gugel 'he became one of the founding fathers of German chemistry' ('wurde er zu einem der Väter der deutschen Chemie überhaupt').[5] Jan V. Golinski agrees with Pietsch in seeing Glauber as a pioneer of precise and lucid scientific terminology,[6] but J.R. Partington, while acknowledging him to have been 'a very skilled practical chemist', criticises him as 'an extremely untidy, verbose and often obscure author', 'too fond of praising himself and posing as a benefactor of mankind in general and Germany in particular'.[7]

Paul Walden, on the other hand, goes so far as to call him 'the German Robert Boyle'.[8] This is about as illuminating as calling Shakespeare the English Racine. Both can be seen as the leading exponents in their respective countries and generations (Glauber was already about 23 when Boyle was born) of the same discipline, but in almost every other respect they were diametrical opposites. Boyle was an aristocrat with a thorough classical education, a man of independent means which enabled him to devote his time and energy to his beloved science without being distracted by the problem of funding. Glauber's origins were in the artisan class and he was largely self-taught, facts he stressed in his autobiographical writings with truculent pride if not outright inverted snobbery:

> I am glad to admit that I never went to prestigious schools and never wanted to: had I done so, I might never have gained such understanding of Nature as, without wishing to boast, I now possess; I do not in the least regret that from my youth I had my hands among the coals and by this means learned the hidden secrets of Nature. I seek to take no man's place, I have never aspired to eat fine gentlemen's bread, but preferred honestly to earn my own, with regard to this motto, ALTERIUS NON SIT QUI SUUS ESSE POTEST.[9]

The motto ('let him belong to no one else who can belong to himself') is taken directly from Paracelsus,[10] a reference Glauber would have expected a reader with any knowledge of the chemical tradition to recognise. Chemistry was the trade by which Glauber earned his living, partly by teaching, both publicly and privately, partly by seeking employment and (for all his declared distaste for eating fine gentlemen's bread) patronage from men of rank, and partly by marketing a whole range of products, principally distillation ovens and other equipment, mead and wine made from various fruits, and chemical medicines.

Boyle's thought was exceptionally systematic and sequential: he was among the first clearly to formulate and practise a method of consistent scepticism and experimental verification, rejecting all prior authority and tradition, of what is now called empiricism (though the word had other connotations at the time, implying random guesswork if not outright quackery). The insistence on trusting only the evidence of the senses, the 'light of nature', was nothing new, having been commonplace already in medieval alchemical writing and become even more strident in Paracelsus and his followers, especially (in his earlier work) Glauber. What is revolutionary about Boyle is that he followed the idea through and made it the central tenet of his scientific method rather than a mere rhetorical tag. His style is incomparably more organised and sophisticated (though at times hardly less verbose) than Glauber's: indeed, Glauber's frequent coarseness is singled out for criticism in Boyle's *Sceptical Chymist*.[11]

Glauber's thought and writing, by contrast, were spectacularly unorganised, and he had the practical auto-didact's defensive contempt of theory and method. As Gugel points out, although he described his profession (on his second marriage certificate) as 'apothecarius', he never attempted to gain a qualification from the Amsterdam Collegium Medicum, as practising apothecaries were theoretically required to do.[12] Gugel considers this surprising, but it probably reflects the same disapproval of monopolies and mistrust of academic establishments that characterised the attitude of so many English iatrochemists to the College of Physicians.[13] There is no documentary evidence about his education. His father was a barber,[14] and it is not clear what first attracted him to natural philosophy, though the combination of a quick brain, lively imagination, practical dexterity and strong ambition are in themselves perhaps explanation enough. Thanks to the keen interest taken in chemistry, and the substantial sums laid out on it, by many German princes and indeed the Emperor himself,[15] few professions offered such potential rewards for a gifted man without formal training or private means as that of investigator of nature.

Boyle's thorough scepticism led him to be chary of all tradition and received wisdom from whatever source, to take nothing on trust until he had himself seen it experimentally verified. Glauber, like the majority of iatrochemists, ostensibly held the same opinion, but in fact reserved his mistrust for the authorities sanctioned by the Schools, investing in the Hermetic writers, particularly Van Helmont, 'the most learned and experienced philosopher of his day',[16] and above all his hero Paracelsus, a faith every bit as blind as that of the Schoolmen in their sacred cows. He portrayed it as part of his mission on earth to unravel and state in plain terms the mysteries embedded in Paracelsus's often well-nigh impenetrable pronouncements, into which he had gained unique insight by the parallel routes of meditation and practical experiment. His methodology, in later years at least, ran to such procedures as solving what he took to be anagrams in his forebear's work, in a manner distinctly akin to the approach of the chiliasts who applied numerology to the prophetic books of the Bible in order to date history in advance, and his belief in the transcendent truth of these texts was almost as fervent as theirs in Scripture.

Finally, while Boyle's thought developed towards a scientific methodology recognisable and indeed still practised today, Glauber in his old age turned away from the practical chemistry for which he is now best known - his observations on acids, alkalis and salts, his production of fertilisers and fruit wines, his studies of the therapeutic effect of spa waters - and turned instead to a wholly contemplative and mystical approach, depicting his earlier labours as a superficial and mechanical preliminary to the true transcendent insights into the secret fires of the earth, the transmutation of metals and the universal animating spirit which he gained only after abandoning practical experiment. The development of Glauber's scientific thought from the merely practical to the transcendent could serve as a paradigm of the progression through 'chemistry' to 'alchemy' suggested in the previous chapter, though the utter rejection in his last years of practical experimentation makes his a rather extreme and idiosyncratic case.

Heyday in the Netherlands

Between the still almost totally obscure *Wanderjahre* of his youth and his move to the Netherlands in c.1640, Glauber was for a time Court Apothecary to Landgrave Georg II of Hessen-Darmstadt, in Giessen and Marburg. He occupied this position by 1635 at the latest.[17] Why he left the post remains entirely unknown, but it is certain he was in Amsterdam by 1640, for it was there that he married Helena Cornelisdottir on 20 January 1641.[18] This was his second marriage, the first having come to an untimely end, according to Glauber, some two years earlier when he surprised his wife in bed with his servant.[19] If Glauber's account of the business is true, he then separated from his first wife, leaving her to wander into France with her paramour. He is rather vague about the details, saying of his second wife, 'two years passed before I married this wife after the first',[20] but whether this means two years after the first marriage or two years after its annulment (if indeed it was officially annulled) is not clear. Fahrner accused him of adultery and bigamy, which he of course denied, but with a suspicious lack of verifiable evidence.

Glauber had not, he claimed, intended to settle in Amsterdam, but had merely been making a business visit. He cited two compelling grounds for taking on another wife in spite of the previous unfortunate and cautionary experience: he had fallen ill, and he disliked Dutch food: 'I went to Holland on business, but because of the change of air I fell ill, and being unable to stomach Dutch food, I was obliged to remarry, that I might be better looked after'.[21] An additional and more convincing incentive is suggested by the fact that the couple's first child, Anna, was born almost exactly seven months after the date of the wedding, on 29 September.[22]

It may well have been at this time that Glauber made friends with Moriaen. It is the first time both men were demonstrably in the same place, and as two German emigrés with a pronounced interest in chemistry, it would hardly be surprising if they became known to one another. They were certainly acquainted by 1642, for on returning to Amsterdam in September that year after two months' absence, Moriaen mentioned to Van Assche that on account of this he had not seen Glauber for some time.[23] This is his first surviving mention of the man, but makes it obvious he already knew him well. According to Moriaen, Glauber at some unspecified point spent 'a long time' as a guest or lodger in his house,[24] and it seems very likely that this refers to some at least of the period between Glauber's arrival in Amsterdam and his marriage.

On 9 May 1643, Moriaen told Van Assche that Glauber had moved into a new house in Amsterdam.[25] This was on the Elandsgracht,[26] and is doubtless the house described in Glauber's *De Tribus Lapidibus*, which the chemist had bought from a 'lover of the art' ('Liebhaber der Kunst', ie. an alchemist), who had had it built expressly to house a laboratory. Glauber gave a grand account of the establishment he set up here with the intention of performing 'something proper on a large scale in Alchemy'.[27] It featured, he claimed, six large stone outbuildings with mighty chimneys, 'all sorts of ovens, large and small, various small and large bellows'[28] and a staff (number unspecified) of labourers and apprentices.[29] Among the visitors to this impressive-sounding public laboratory were Moriaen, who received instruction in metallurgy from Glauber,[30] and Dury's future brother-in-law Heinrich Appelius.

In a letter to Hartlib of 7 June 1644, Appelius assumed his friend in London would already have heard all about Glauber from Moriaen: 'I would have sent you Glauber's *Uses of the New Philosophical Oven*, but I suppose you will have heard all about such matters from Herr Moriaen, and if not, he is the best person to ask, for he surely knows more about such things than I'.[31] Apparently, however, Appelius was wrong, for some two or three weeks later, he sent a copy of 'Glauber's oven' ('Glauberi ofen'), presumably at Hartlib's request, mentioning again that 'Herr Moriaen and other physicians who have some of his things are well satisfied with him'.[32] But either Hartlib did not follow up the suggestion of directing his enquiries to Moriaen for another two-and-a-half to three years, or Moriaen did not bother replying until then.[33] This lends considerable weight to the conjecture that there was a lapse in Moriaen's relations with Hartlib between these dates. From this point on, however, Glauber became far and away the most discussed figure in the correspondence, and Moriaen took over from Appelius as Hartlib's principal source of information on the German chemist.

The tract sent by Appelius was an advertisement for Glauber's new laboratory. A copy, in Appelius's hand, is preserved among Hartlib's papers, entitled 'Furni Noui *P*hiloso*p*hici Utilitates od*er* Beschreibung d*er* eig*en*schafft*en* eines sond*er*baren new erfundenen *P*hiloso*p*hisch*en* distillir ofens [...] Zu Amsterdam gedruckt beÿ Broer Ianß. Ao 1643' ('Uses of the New Philosophical Oven, or a description of the particulars of a singular new philosophical digesting oven, printed at Amsterdam by Brother Jans, 1643).[34] No copies of the printed version of this pamphlet seem to have survived, and it is not mentioned in any bibliography of Glauber. Pre-dating his first previously recorded publication by three years, it is the earliest known piece of writing by him (see Appendix One).

In contrast to the later but very similarly entitled *Furni novi Philosophici* (1646-49), the work that was to make Glauber's name throughout Europe, the advertisement gives no indication whatsoever of how the furnace was constructed or how it worked. Instead, it describes, in deliberately vague terms, the processes it could perform and the products it could yield. The fact that only one oven is mentioned suggests that Glauber's later description of his laboratory in *De Tribus Lapidibus*, equipped 'with all manner of small and large furnaces', had benefited from a certain amount of retrospective embellishment. It may be, however, that Glauber was using one oven for public displays and others for his private research: it is clear from Appelius's report that there was at least one other oven in the house. The advertisement concludes with an invitation to 'the lover of truth and the spagyric art' to visit Glauber and have the furnace's operations revealed to them: Glauber would not withold his mysteries from the curious visitor. Not, at least, if the visitor came armed with a suitable fee. Appelius was charged 30 Imperials to see both furnaces and their more basic operations: he thought this a reasonable sum.[35] The more specialised processes, however, had to be paid for separately. The sums involved are revealed in detail by Appelius in a later letter,[36] and make it clear that the charge of 30 Imperials was very much a budget-class deal. Between them, these documents supply quite a detailed price list of the marvels on display in a mid-seventeenth century public chemical laboratory.

A particularly striking feature of the list is that Glauber was already speaking of the 'secret philosophic fire', probably some highly corrosive acid, which was to become one of his deepest obsessions in later years. The prices quoted by Appelius were what he and his friend[37] had themselves paid - a fact of some significance, since Appelius gave every impression of being thoroughly satisfied with the deal. This tends to verify that Glauber's claims were genuine, or at least appeared so to two experienced chemists of the day who had investigated them in person. Deliberately vague though much of Glauber's terminology is, it is not mere attention-grabbing publicity.

The total fee mentioned by Appelius is 420 Imperials, or about £100. Had Glauber had many such eager customers, his business would have been a very profitable one indeed: £100, it may be remembered, is what Comenius a few years earlier had considered an adequate annual income. Glauber was doubtless also selling the products of his laboratory, such as medicines, pesticides, preparations for purifying or preserving food and drink, and the like. But it seems there were few both able and willing to run to expenditure on this scale for the satisfaction of their curiosity, and the overheads must have been considerable. The chemist himself later described the enterprise as 'nothing but much expense and little return for it'.[38] Moreover, Glauber, whose health was precarious throughout his life (which is hardly surprising given that the senses of taste and smell ranked first among the analytical apparatus of mid-17th-century chemistry), repeatedly complained that the damp and noxious Amsterdam air disagreed with him. On 22 July 1644, Appelius, writing from Amsterdam, reported that Glauber planned to leave the city in three weeks time and seek a more comfortable place of residence further up the Rhine.[39]

All that has previously been known of Glauber's movements in the Netherlands is that besides Amsterdam he dwelt at some point in Utrecht and Arnhem. This information is drawn from the truculently incoherent *Glauberus Ridivivus*:

> It is true that I could not stand the damp air of Amsterdam and sought healthier air in Utrecht and Arnhem; then for the sake of earning my keep I had to settle again in Amsterdam, but I never lived in Leiden as you [Fahrner] pretend, and if I had lived there, what would it have mattered if Leiden had suited me better than another place, who could object to my living there?[40]

Information in Hartlib's papers make it possible to establish the chronology of these movements with much greater accuracy, thanks to the regular news about Glauber sent by Moriaen and Appelius. Though the very vehemence with which Glauber denied a stay in Leiden inevitably arouses the suspicion that he had been there and had reason to conceal the fact, the absence from their reports of any mention of such a stay tends to suggest on this occasion he was in fact telling the truth.[41] He moved to Utrecht in August 1644,[42] and was back in Amsterdam briefly from March to at least the end of August 1647 before decamping to Arnhem.[43] He returned to Amsterdam probably between May and August 1648.[44] Unfortunately, nothing in the papers sheds any new light on the reasons for all these moves.

Both Pietsch and Gugel conclude that after leaving Amsterdam the first time, Glauber returned to the service of the court of Hessen-Darmstadt. This is because Glauber appears to cite the siege of Marburg by invading troops from Hesse-Kassel, which occurred on 2 November 1645, as his reason for leaving this employment. But as Link points out,[45] this does not add up. Glauber's account of the episode is jumbled together with the lurid tale of his first wife's adultery. Writing in 1656, he declared that

> twenty-odd years ago I took a wife in Giessen, then I was summoned to supervise the prince's court apothecary, but when Hesse-Cassel made war with Hessen-Darmstadt and sought to take Marburg by force of arms, everything changed, and whoever could fled to safety; I moved then down the Rhine to my gracious Lord [= Georg II of Hessen-Darmstadt?] in Frankfurt and then Bonn, and during this time surprised the said wife from Giessen one day committing adultery with my then manservant in my bedroom; I then moved to Holland *for the first time* over a year later [emphasis added].[46]

The passage thus seems to place the siege of Marburg (1645) a year *before*

Glauber's first move to the Netherlands (1640). Link suggests three possible explanations. Hessen-Darmstadt and Hesse-Kassel had been at war since 1618, and it is conceivable that the military threat to Marburg mentioned by Glauber was indeed merely a threat, not the actual siege of 1645. Or Glauber's memory may have been at fault. Thirdly and by far the most likely, it may be that the deliberately vague and confusing details are a smokescreen for the real reason (whatever that may have been) why he left the landgrave's service.[47] As will be shown below, this would not make it the only piece of deliberate misinformation in his autobiography.

Gugel and Pietsch also both assume Glauber was back in Amsterdam by 1646, on the grounds that his first major published works, *Furni novi philosophici* I and *De auri tinctura* (often referred to as *De auro potabili*), appeared there that year.[48] It was not, however, necessary to be in Amsterdam to have works printed there. He could have sent or brought them over from Utrecht, either direct to the printer - Moriaen's old associate Hans Fabel - or to friends in Amsterdam, Moriaen being an obvious candidate. Book I was out by September 1646, shortly to be followed by *De Auri tinctura*.[49] Writing from Amsterdam towards the end of 1646, Appelius told Dury that 'the Author protesteth by his friends, that hee intendeth to write nothing but what hee hath, and yet daily can doe without fallacie, not what he hath observed or lighted upon by chance',[50] a turn of phrase strongly suggesting that Glauber was not yet in Amsterdam to do the protesting in person. According to Moriaen, he was on his way to settle there again in early February 1647,[51] and Appelius reported his arrival in March.[52]

It was at just this juncture, it seems, that Moriaen's regular correspondence with Hartlib was resumed, and it is obvious that his relations with Glauber were now very close. Though only part One of *Furni Novi Philosophici* had appeared in print, he was able to give detailed and accurate accounts of the ovens that were to be described in parts Two to Four (1647-8).[53] Indeed, he planned to set up the 'second oven' (ie. the one described in Part Two) in his own house and to use it for the production of chemical medicines,[54] though there is no firm evidence as to whether he actually put this proposal into effect.

Moreover, it emerges that not only had Moriaen given the chemist lodgings at his house in Amsterdam, he and Odilia were the godparents of two of Glauber's children.[55] This bears witness to the remarkable latitudinarianism of both men, since Glauber was, nominally at least, a Roman Catholic. It is barely conceivable Moriaen was unaware of this. One of the more irrelevant charges later laid against Glauber by Fahrner was that he was a hypocrite in matters of religion, altering his allegiances to suit whatever set of circumstances he found himself in at the time and to ingratiate himself with people of influence. This elicited one of Glauber's most convincing and coherent refutations, indeed a fine and really quite bold defence of non-sectarian religion. He made no bones about having attended Catholic, Lutheran and Calvinist churches, nor about having had some of his children baptised Catholic and others Evangelical: he had, he said, simply done whichever was more convenient, seeing either as equally valid. He considered himself a Catholic, but pointed out that the Lord

expressly says in several places, Come unto me all ye who labour and are

heavy laden and I shall refresh you etc. And it was for everyone, not only
for Catholics, Lutherans or Arminians etc. but also for all Jews, Turks
and heathens that Christ in his perfection died and gained Heaven[56]

If Glauber really had been playing the Vicar of Bray, he would hardly have
published a declaration so calculated to offend all the established Christian
orthodoxies, one which makes him sound more like a Behmenist or a
Collegiant, or at any rate an 'impartial' spirit very much of Moriaen's own
stamp, than a kow-tower to any denominational authority.

The evident closeness of their relationship did not, however, make
Moriaen an uncritical admirer of his friend. Already at this stage he was
commenting on Glauber's inability to concentrate on a given subject or follow
his experiments through to a definite conclusion. Later, this inconstancy of
purpose would be a source of continual annoyance to Moriaen, though he
always stressed that Glauber was genuinely talented and that 'he has been
granted a considerable light into Nature'.[57] One feature of that inconstancy, as
Moriaen saw it, was his habit of constantly uprooting himself and setting off
for Germany, but then returning to Amsterdam instead. It was not until 1650,
a full decade after his first arrival in the Netherlands, that Glauber finally took
his leave and departed for his native country.

Flight into Germany

At least as early as 1644, Glauber had been hankering to return to his
homeland. Reporting his move to Utrecht that year, Appelius stated that he
had intended to go to Germany but was prevented by the continuing state of
war.[58] Again when he moved to Arnhem in 1647, it was intended as the first
leg of a journey home: 'he would faine goe higher, in[to] Germany, & set up
their such workes whereby he might maintaine his family most liberally [...]
so that hee expects onely [ie. is only waiting for] peace in Germany for this
Country agrees not with his nature'.[59] This is one of the reasons Glauber
himself later gave for his eventual return to Germany in 1650: that he wished
to see his homeland again after peace had been established.[60] Even his most
sympathetic biographers have assumed that this was merely an excuse and that
the real reason for his departure was a financial collapse and a bid to escape
his creditors. However, Moriaen's and Appelius's evidence suggests it was
in fact the truth, albeit financial problems were almost certainly the immediate
impulse. Glauber also claimed he was cheated in the selling of his house in
Amsterdam, his laboratory equipment being wrongfully sold as part of the
furnishings, and that it took him a two year legal campaign to reclaim his
lawful possessions.[61] This perhaps accounts for his return to Amsterdam
from Arnhem in 1648 and the fact that instead of proceeding to Germany as he
initially intended he did not, in the event, leave the Netherlands until two years
after the signing of the Peace of Westphalia (1648).

It has not previously been possible to establish whether Glauber made his
move in the spring of 1650 or that of 1651. The latter has, reasonably
enough, been favoured, on the grounds that Glauber's son Alexander was
baptised in Amsterdam in 1651.[62] But Moriaen's letters place the move
squarely in March or April 1650. He told Worsley on 4 March that Glauber

'hath now finished all hee thinks to doe heere' and was preparing to leave. He planned initially to go only as far as the Rhineland (or so he told Moriaen), to Duisburg or Wesel.[63] Brun had reported the previous year that he was planning to go to Cologne.[64] However, he soon changed his plans and plunged on north-east to Bremen, in the heart of Lower Saxony, where Moriaen thought him settled by the end of April.[65] He was still there in July,[66] but for unexplained reasons he set off again some time in the next two months, heading south this time, by way of Frankfurt to Wertheim, where he was living by 7 October 1650,[67] though still considering a move back to Frankfurt or on to Nürnberg. Glauber's account of this implies that the whole journey was of a piece,[68] which would be barely credible even without the evidence of Moriaen's letters to prove it was a matter of fits and starts, of constantly revised plans. He may well genuinely have wanted to see his homeland again, but to plan such a circuit would be taking a preference for scenic routes to extremes. A likelier motivation for the bizarre route is an attempt to shake off creditors on the one hand and repeatedly frustrated hopes of employment or business opportunities on the other.

Glauber also claimed that, far from sneaking out of Amsterdam in secret to escape his creditors and a pending court case for debt, as Fahrner (very plausibly) charged, he had merely gone on ahead alone to check that the route was safe for his family, and that having found it was, he summoned them to follow him by boat to Bremen, from where they completed the rest of the journey together.[69] Even the cautious Link sees no reason to doubt Glauber's word in this matter.[70] But Moriaen's letters reveal that Glauber left Bremen in September 1650 at the latest,[71] whereas Helena Glauber was still in Amsterdam for the baptism of her son the following year. When and how she and the children eventually did join him is not clear, but Glauber's version of the story is pure fiction.

There are two possible reasons why Glauber should have bothered with this invention. The first is to gloss over the fact that he left a pregnant wife and nursing mother to fend for herself, and fend off the creditors, for at least the better part of a year. If, that is, Helena *was* pregnant when he left: and herein lies the second likely reason. Having admitted to one cuckolding already in this book, Glauber doubtless did not wish to draw attention to the fact that he had not seen his wife for a good nine months at least before the birth of 'his' son. The available evidence unfortunately does not reveal when in 1651 Alexander Glauber's baptism took place. If it was in early January, and if Glauber did not in fact leave Amsterdam until early April 1650, it is possible he was indeed the child's father, but the odds are not favourable. This would also help explain Glauber's apparently gratuitous remark, in the story of his first marriage, that in spite of her treachery he would not have cast his first wife off if they had had any children living.[72] The comment was perhaps more relevant to the second wife than the first. This piece of disinformation has led Gugel to be consistently a year out in his datings of Glauber's movements from this point until his final return to Amsterdam in 1656, since he assumes he cannot have left Bremen until after Alexander's birth.

In Wertheim, Glauber rented a large house and set up a new public laboratory in which to teach transmutation of metals, and set about exploiting a mine, the nature of which is not clear.[73] It was also (according to Moriaen) at this juncture that he started claiming to have discovered the fabled universal solvent, alcahest.

The initial funding for these projects, which must have represented a considerable outlay, was presumably supplied by Glauber's new patron, Johann Philipp von Schönborn, Elector and Archbishop of the Imperial City of Mainz (some hundred kilometres to the west of Wertheim), though it has not previously been known that Glauber was associated with him this early. On 13 June 1651, Glauber specifically mentioned Johann Philipp as his patron, from whom he expected an unspecified advantage in exchange for the revelation of an unspecified secret.[74] Moriaen took Glauber to mean a privilege for his books, but it may be that what he was after was a patent for his process of extracting tartar from wine lees. He later described this in his *Gründliche und Wahrhafftige Beschreibung wie man auß den Weinhefen einen guten Weinstein [...] extrahiren soll* (1654), which he dedicated to the Elector. According to this dedication, he received a privilege for the process from Johann Philipp in 1652.

Faced with this large and diverse work-load, Glauber took on two students as apprentices-cum-assistants.[75] One of these was sent to Holstein on business, apparently to display some of Glauber's products or processes to the court there. He was supposed to deliver some alcahest to a correspondent of Hartlib's in Amsterdam (probably Moriaen) on his way back, but failed to do so. Glauber immediately concluded there was some sort of treachery involved.[76] He was, probably with some justification, of a highly suspicious nature, which in later years developed into something approaching full-blown neurosis. Glauber started imagining his enemies to be bribing his children to reveal his secrets, or lurking in gangs at street corners in the hope of killing him.[77] Even allowing for the wild overstatements habitual in seventeenth-century polemic, some of Glauber's outbursts, evidently written or dictated at great speed and quite extemporaneously, sound genuinely and alarmingly unhinged.

Despite the quarrels with his apprentices, Glauber seemed comfortably placed in Wertheim, in favour with the Elector, his mine and public laboratory flourishing. This situation too, however, was soon to be disrupted, as the owner of the house he was renting sold it and the buyer promptly evicted him. Glauber moved this time to the relatively nearby Kitzingen - still within the Elector's sphere of influence - and devoted himself more exclusively to his enterprises of manufacturing and improving wine and extracting tartar from wine lees.[78] Here he also had a medical practice, for which (or so he later claimed) he made no charge, accepting only voluntary donations which he distributed among the local poor.[79] He remained in Kitzingen for some three years, producing another daughter, Johanna, in June 1653, and publishing parts 2 and 3 of *Operis Mineralis* (1652),[80] part 1 of *Miraculum Mundi* (1653), part 1 of *Pharmacopoea Spagyrica* (1654) and the *Gründliche und wahrhafftige Beschreibung* of 1654 mentioned above.

Gugel describes this last work as Glauber's parting gift to the Elector and the district that had treated him well for some years. This may be true as far as it goes, but if so it is the first of many examples of Glauber's offering as a gift what had ceased to be of any use to him. The explicit motivation behind this and the ensuing torrent of publications was to forestall the attempts of his estranged assistant Christoph Fahrner to pass off what he had learned from

Glauber as his own work.

Glauber had met Fahrner soon after his arrival in Kitzingen in mid-1651, and took him on as a trainee and assistant, under a vow of secrecy.[81] Fahrner later claimed that Glauber had duped him by promising to reveal the Philosophers' Stone and then refusing to do so. Glauber maintained he had taken Fahrner on only to work on his schnaps production, tartar extraction, vinegar making and wine improvement, and promised him no other secrets than these, 'by which means, if you had kept faith with me, we might both in a short while have richly provided for all our children': he had never offered 'to reveal any metallic art, which I neither could nor wished to perform'.[82]

This does not chime very well with Moriaen's earlier report that Glauber not only claimed to understand transmutation but had taught it publicly in Wertheim. It must, however, be doubted whether Moriaen's report is an entirely accurate representation of what Glauber had told him - or indeed whether what Glauber had told him was an entirely faithful representation of what Glauber was doing. If Glauber really was, as Moriaen stated, offering instruction to the general public in the transmutation of metals, he was breaking the most sacred alchemical taboo. The 'great work' was not to be made available to all and sundry, or not at least until the world itself had been transmuted into a terrestrial paradise by direct divine intervention. It seems likelier that what Glauber was doing, as in his earlier public laboratory in Amsterdam, was demonstrating the results of his methods to the public rather than explaining the methods themselves, and that these supposed results now included transmutation (to which he had not laid claim in *Furni Novi Utilitates*).

Gugel asserts somewhat defensively that though he believed in the possibility of transmutation, Glauber repeatedly stated that he himself had never achieved a successful transmutation.[83] However, while Glauber did indeed deny his own transmutational prowess when it suited him - as here, to make Fahrner's charge appear absurd -, he also repeatedly claimed precisely the opposite. Not only in the account of the Wertheim laboratory, but in other reports from 1657 and 1659, Moriaen passed on unequivocal claims by Glauber that he could turn base metals into gold: in the latter case, indeed, Moriaen himself believed he had seen him do so. [84]

According to Fahrner, not only did Glauber withold his alchemical secrets, even his wine treatments were valueless. Glauber countered that any failures they had met with were the result of Fahrner's incompetence. What truth there is in either account it is now largely impossible to determine. The polemics on both sides are almost exclusively ad hominem and obviously wildly exaggerated. Fahrner accused Glauber of being a time-server in religious matters, an adulterer and a bigamist; Glauber accused Fahrner of everything from inadequate facial hair to uxoricide.[85]

Whatever the full facts behind the dispute, it is clear that Fahrner did indeed set about selling some of the secrets he had learned from Glauber. Whether he also, as Glauber claimed, incited other former employees to do likewise is not verifiable, but since Fahrner himself did not deny the main charge, claiming only that he had offered his knowledge to far fewer people than Glauber made out, it seems certain the accusation was substantially true.[86] This treachery, Glauber claimed, moved him to go to press with all his knowledge. The account is the more convincing for the fact that, far from painting an over-sanctified picture of Glauber himself, it frankly contradicts the purely philanthropic motivation he laid claim to elsewhere. If he was not to enjoy all the profit of his art for himself, he said, he could at least ensure, by making it public, that Fahrner would not do so either:

> by which revelation the whole human race, its aged and sick, will gain great delight and salve, which I might perhaps not have done had the godless Fahrner not wrung it from me through his treachery, lies and calumnies, but Fahrner will earn a reward like Judas Iscariot's.[87]

Starting with the *Gründliche und wahrhafftige Beschreibung*, exposing in some detail the process even Glauber stated he had originally contractually agreed to confide to Fahrner, works flooded from his pen in the following years, all purporting to make a gift to mankind of what Fahrner had tried to steal for himself.[88] Moriaen at least found this self-projection entirely credible, and though he thought the quarrel reflected badly on both parties, he believed it would benefit the world in general by encouraging Glauber to publish.[89]

When Glauber left Kitzingen is uncertain, but it was probably soon after publishing *Gründliche und wahrhafftige Beschreibung* in 1654. He later gave as his grounds for leaving that the local distillers, envious of his success and under the influence of their own produce, had resolved to use violence against him: 'seeing that I was likely to come to blows with a gang of drunken thugs, I sought to take my family to a place of safety'.[90] It was perhaps during this move that he suffered another setback to his health, reported in a lost letter from Moriaen to Hartlib and mentioned by the latter to Boyle:

> Mr. *Morian* writes again of *Glauber*, that he hath had a very dangerous fall from a waggon, spitting much blood, and if the fever prevail upon him he fears for his life; which I pray God may be yet continued for giving many good hints, at least[,] to the studiers of nature and arts.[91]

He then spent some time in Frankfurt am Main, which he was forced to leave, he claimed, for fear of being murdered by Fahrner's cronies.[92] Next, he worked for 'persons of high princely rank' ('hohen fürstl*ichen* Personen') as an assayer in mines near Cologne. In this instance, Moriaen's letters provide confirmation of Glauber's own published statements, which have previously been the only evidence for his stay in Cologne, and suggest that by 'princely persons' Glauber meant the Elector himself.[93] Link concludes, by correlating Fahrner's and Glauber's accounts, that Glauber spent about a year in Frankfurt, from mid-1654 to mid-1655. Moriaen, however, said he was on the brink of moving to Cologne in October 1654,[94] though whether that intention was followed through is not revealed. This remains another very obscure period of Glauber's life, on which Hartlib's papers otherwise shed no new light. He comes back into focus with his return to Amsterdam in 1656, this time for good.

Last Years in Amsterdam

In *Glauberus Ridivivus*, published in 1656, Glauber declared - somewhat paradoxically in view of his statement elsewhere in the same book that one reason he kept moving was to escape Fahrner's murderous intentions - that 'now here I am in Amsterdam and I live on the Kaisersgracht, in a well-known place, not in a corner; if you [Fahrner] or anyone else have anything to say to me, come here and say it; you shall have a straight answer'.[95] Here he continued working on his celebrated and much discussed *aurum potabile*, with which according to Moriaen he now claimed he could transmute all metals, albeit unprofitably. It was also, more importantly, a universal medicine.[96] He also experimented, apparently successfully, with a salt-based fertiliser.[97] Potentially even more profitable were a method he claimed to have invented to convert common salt into saltpetre,[98] and his proudest achievement, 'sal mirabile'. This is sodium sulphate, known to this day as 'Glauber's salt' and still used in medicine. It is possibly the basis of the alcahest he had already claimed to have discovered in 1650, for he affirmed that 'my *sal mirabile* fundamentally dissolves not only all metals but all stones and bones, yea, coal itself, which no other corrosive can dissolve; I could write a great book about this miraculous solution'.[99] The excitement engendered by such ideas is well illustrated by Moriaen's pouncing on this passage after a hurried inspection of the work and copying it out at once to send to Hartlib.[100]

Plans for Moriaen to visit Glauber, or vice versa, were constantly being renewed after the latter's return to the Netherlands in 1656, but were repeatedly frustrated by one or the other's ill health, or by bad weather. Indeed, in July 1658, Moriaen reported that Glauber had 'a violent desire to leave Amsterdam',[101] and planned to join Moriaen in Arnhem, though there is no indication of the reason. However, nothing came of the proposal, and Glauber remained based in Amsterdam until his death.

He was evidently soon thriving once more, for at least by 1659 he had set up yet another new laboratory, part public and part private. Moriaen finally managed two visits to Amsterdam in the summer and autumn of 1659 in order to inspect this. Another visitor that summer was Kretschmar, who told Hartlib:

> Herr Glauber's public and private laboratory has now been set on foot, and he has many friends visiting him, especially good old Joh Moriaen of Arnhem, with whom I have met several times. He is staying in Herr Glauber's own house, and will perhaps be able to tell you more than I can of Herr Glauber's affairs.[102]

Both Glauber himself and his new laboratory were described by the travelling French scholar Samuel de Sorbière in 1660.[103] Sorbière, who was no novice in scientific matters, was greatly impressed both by the chemist and his equipment. After a long passage expressing haughty contempt for Paracelsian mumbo-jumbo, for 'the Panaceas, the Alcahest, the Zenda and Parenda, the Archeus, the Enspagoycum, the Nostoch, the Ylech, the Trarame, the Turban, the Ens Tagastricum and the other visions Van Helmont and his fraternity serve up to us',[104] he was careful to absolve Glauber: 'By none of this speech, Sir, do I intend to insult Glauber, nor any of those who, like him, set their hand to the work, and whom I should rather encourage. He is undoubtedly the most excellent or the noblest of them all'.[105] Indeed, so well-appointed was Glauber's laboratory that Sorbière, for all his sarcasm about alchemical jargon, was inclined to think he must have mastered the secret of transmutation in order to maintain it and his large family (eight children by this time) in such fine style.

But there is a telling detail in Sorbière's account: he and his companions guessed Glauber's age to be sixty-six. In fact, he was at least ten years younger than that.[106] The years of handling assorted poisonous and corrosive materials were taking their toll, and Glauber's health was soon to give way completely. Serrarius visited him in February 1662 and 'found him yet very sick, though in a recovering way for life thoug not for perfect health.'[107] For much of the rest of his life he was bedridden. According to another travelling French scholar, Balthasar de Monconys, who visited him in 1663, he 'no longer works, and has no ovens'.[108] In 1668 he offered what remained of his library and laboratory for sale, producing a catalogue of his books and equipment.[109] It appears from this that Monconys overstated the extent of Glauber's decline, since the catalogue includes sixteen ovens and stills. It does seem fairly certain, however, that Glauber's ill health prevented him almost entirely from conducting any further practical laboratory work.

Nonetheless, he managed in his last eight years, before being finally released from what must have become a very trying and dispiriting existence in March 1670, to produce a further eleven works besides the catalogue of his effects. In terms of numbers of titles this represents forty percent of his total output, though it should be said these are all short single-volume works, and in terms of bulk of content account for only half that proportion.[110] But they still represent a significant section of his work, and though they have received less attention than his earlier productions on the grounds that they are less 'scientific', they are of considerable interest in assessing the development of his thought, as he turned perforce from practical experiment and consoled himself instead with mystical speculation.

He took to denouncing practical experiment as a superficial, mechanical operation, and to lauding instead the 'secret fire' he claimed to have discovered, probably an acid of some form, which could do more in a hazelnut shell than could be done by ordinary fire in the greatest furnace.[111] He indulged too in various pieces of fanciful etymology and mystical anagrammisation to demonstrate his long-standing conviction, originally arrived at by experimental practice, that salt constituted the essence of life. The Latin words for salt and sun, 'Sal' and 'Sol', he decided, both derived from the same word in the original, divinely-inspired pre-Babelian language in which words perfectly and directly signified their objects. Furthermore, the only difference between them was A and O, Alpha and Omega.[112]

There can be little doubt that Glauber's rejection of laboratory work was to some extent at least a case of sour grapes. One of the advantages of his 'secret fire' was that the adept did not even need to get out of bed to work with it:[113] it is surely pertinent that when Glauber wrote this, he had been physically incapable of getting out of bed for the best part of seven or eight years. Nonetheless, these musings of his old age were not a wholly new departure following his physical collapse, and should not be too lightly dismissed. Such ideas had had a place in his thought from the very first, from the promise in *Furni Novi Utilitates* to reveal the 'secret fire of the philosophers', and had gained rather than lost weight with him as his technical expertise increased. Long before he was forced to give up practical experiments, he was busying himself with isolating and analysing the 'soul of the world', interpreting the microcosmic 'signatures' of salts, and offering chemical accounts of Creation itself. This 'mystical' aspect of his thought was not separate from, let alone opposed to, his practical work, and only became divorced from it when the latter became impossible for him. Like so many of the figures associated with or promoted by Hartlib and his circle, Glauber has been widely praised as a precursor, or even a 'father', of modern science, but was in fact intent on guiding human enquiry onto paths utterly divergent from those that the most enduringly influential scientific thinkers (such as Boyle) opted for in the latter half of the century.

Glauber's Reception in the Hartlib Circle

The most valuable supplement the Hartlib Papers can add to the individual history of Glauber is a broader and more contextualised view of contemporary reaction to the man and his work. They also reveal much about the international dissemination of his writings and equipment, which Hartlib did a great deal to promote. Glauber's first public laboratory in Amsterdam began to acquire a reputation in 1643, with the publication of *Furni Novi Utilitates*. This was precisely the time when Hartlib, after the failure of his plan to launch a pansophic reformation of learning by establishing a College of Light in England under the directorship of Comenius, began to turn more wholeheartedly to the study of nature as a means of achieving universal illumination, and he immediately latched onto Glauber's work as a possible means of promoting this. The earliest surviving mention of Glauber in his papers is in a letter from Appelius of 7 June 1644 mentioning the *Furni Novi Utilitates*,[114] but it is obvious Appelius was returning to a subject that had been broached earlier.

Several extracts of Glauber's works are to be found among Hartlib's papers, but Hartlib must have possessed all, or almost all, the Glauberian works that appeared during his lifetime. Appelius sent him Part I of *Furni Novi Philosophici* and probably *De Auri Tinctura*.[115] Moriaen sent the subsequent four parts of *Furni Novi*, as well as *Operis Mineralis, De Medicina Universali, De Natura Salium*, the *Apologia* against Fahrner, and other unspecified books. He also promised to send *Trost der Seefahrenten*, until he discovered that copies had already been sent directly to England by the publisher. This work was published simultaneously in Amsterdam by Jansson and in Arnhem by Jacob von Biesen: it appears from Moriaen's letter that it was Biesen who was sending copies to England to pre-empt Jansson - proof in itself of how ready a market there was in this country for Glaubers productions.[116] From 1658 onward Moriaen was trying to assemble a complete collection of Glauber's publications, to send them bound together to Hartlib,[117] though whether he in fact did so is unrecorded.

Hartlib in turn distributed the works he received, or copies of them, to other chemical enthusiasts. He had *Furni Novi Utilitates* translated from German into Latin and recopied for circulation. He aroused the interest of

William Petty, John Sadler and Cheney Culpeper.[118] In 1648 he sent a 'Glauberianus Tractatus' (probably *Furni Novi Philosophici*, or part of it, possibly *De Auri Tinctura*), to Comenius's estranged assistant Cyprian Kinner in Poland.[119] Robert Child acknowledged receipt from Hartlib of the first two books of *Operis Mineralis* (1651) early in 1652,[120] about a year after Moriaen had sent them, and further unspecified works in August.[121] Henry Jenney sought to obtain further information about Glauber through Hartlib, as did John Winthrop Junior in America.[122] While he did not pursue the promotion and distribution of Glauber's work with quite the same wholeheartedness and zeal as he had done that of Comenius, Hartlib was probably the most important channel through which Glauber became known in England, and also encouraged his dissemination abroad.

Not only Glauber's writing but also his equipment was brought to England, or replicated there, by various of Hartlib's associates. However varied the judgments on his theoretical writings and chemical products, there has never been any doubt that his technological innovations were genuine and valuable: not even his fiercest detractors denied this, though some questioned their originality.[123] The *Ephemerides* of 1654, citing Boyle as a source, record that 'Dr Rigely an Auncient Physitian of the College [...] bought vp all Glauberian furnaces especially the 2d with a new Head, which also Mr Boyle hath'.[124] Clodius also sampled this '2d oven' and 'performed that by it in the space of 6. houres, which could not bee done by other meanes in 24. or 12.' - though Clodius, typically enough, added that it was 'not so vniversal as he brag's' and that Clodius could improve on it.[125] Moriaen sent a retort for Glauber's second oven to one Mr. Sotheby, with a wooden model showing how to instal it.[126] Culpeper was frequently on tenterhooks awaiting receipt of new models or specifications.

Hartlib was also instrumental in commissioning early translations of Glauber. His papers include a complete English version of the *Gründliche und Wahrhafftige Beschreibung*, the work on tartar extraction Glauber had written for the Elector of Mainz, [127] and an account by Glauber of 'the Vertues of Mr Glaubers Alkahest', also in English translation.[128] It is not certain that these translations, which were never published, were written by or for Hartlib, but he is an obvious candidate. The first published English version of any of Glauber's work was a compilation of *Furni Novi* and *De Auri Tinctura*, which appeared in 1651 or 1552[129] from the pen of one 'J.F.M.D.' This was John French (Medicinæ Doctor), a chemist associated with the circle at this period, and it is virtually certain that the impetus for his efforts came from Hartlib. French himself declared in the preface to his *Description of New Philosophical Furnaces* that he had found 'the greatest part of the treatise in private hands already translated into English by a learned German',[130] and had consequently been moved to complete the work. Given that Hartlib is known to have been collecting Glauber's works and was personally associated with French at the time, it is very likely that these 'private hands' were his. Whether he himself was also the 'learned German' who had already made a start on the translation is more doubtful: he is not otherwise known as a translator on this scale and it is difficult to see how he could have spared the time for such an undertaking. He cannot, however, be ruled out. Another possibility is that the 'learned German' was Haak, who was a prolific translator.[131] Moriaen had earlier suggested he translate Gabriel Plattes into

German,[132] indicating that he was seen as suitable for such work, though there is no evidence that he in fact ever did so.

What is certain, however, is that Hartlib subsequently urged French to undertake further translation of Glauber, a fact which lends considerable weight to the hypothesis that it was he who suggested and supplied the original texts for French's version of the *Furni Novi*. Hartlib recorded that 'The 30. of Nov. 1652 I lent to Dr French the 2. et 3. Part of Glaub. to be translated into English'.[133] This cannot mean parts 2 and 3 of *Furni Novi*, for French had already translated these and almost certainly published them.[134] The reference is surely to *Operis Mineralis*, which Hartlib had received from Moriaen earlier that year, though if French did undertake this work it was never published.

Whoever French's predecessor as translator of *Furni Novi* was, he must already have finished Part One some time before March 1647, as Cheney Culpeper had by then started, given up on and decided to restart a translation of the English, presumably into Latin. He specifically remarked that he was not working from the original: 'truly', he complained, 'I finde it a greater busines to translate it out of Englishe then it wowlde haue beene out of Dutche [ie. German] if I had vnderstoode that langwage'.[135] It had been handed over to William Petty for completion, but he had changed his mind or refused, moving Culpeper to take it up again himself.[136] Hartlib, rather untypically, seems to have worried about whether Glauber might object to this, since one of a battery of questions fired at Appelius must have concerned Glauber's attitude to translation of his work. Appelius answered reassuringly that Glauber had told another would-be translator that 'there was no necessity to aske leave of him, seeing *the* book were no more his, but all mens'.[137] Self-publicity being a major purpose of Glauber's going to press in the first place, he had little reason to object.

In this case, the correspondence leaves no doubt whatsoever that Hartlib was the instigator of the project. The translation cost Culpeper much pains, and he apologised repeatedly to Hartlib for the fact that it was taking him far longer than he had expected.[138] He was perhaps feeling a little put-upon, for he added pointedly that he was doing it 'upon your desires'.[139] He would appear to have given up on the project in the end; at all events no Latin translation of the *Furni Novi* ever appeared in England.

Hartlib even nursed hopes of persuading Glauber to move to England to teach at Gresham College. In 1647, Appelius advised:

> But to gett Gl. in Hunns.[*expanded by Hartlib to* Hunniades] place, that shall not bee, because hee is this summer gone from Amsterd. to Arnheim, to bee *the* nigher Germany, whither hee intends to goe up *the* next yeere, to settle him et so to live by his art.[140]

Johannes Banfi Hunniades (1576-1646), also known as Hans Hungar, was a Hungarian alchemist and mathematician who had moved to England by 1633 and at some point taught alchemy and mathematics at Gresham College. He was described on engravings by Wenceslaus Hollar, dated 1644, as a former practitioner of the hermetic and mathematical disciplines at Gresham ('Olim Anglo-Londini in Illustri Collegio Greshamensi Hermeticæ Disciplini Sectatoris et Philo-Mathematici').[141] The astrologer William Lilly in 1644 spoke of his achievements as having been equalled 'by few else, if any at all, Professors in Chimistry',[142] adding that Hunniades was planning to return to Hungary. This move must have been in the air by April 1643, when Appelius asked Hartlib whether Hunniades was still in London or had gone back to Hungary.[143] Since he left Gresham in or before 1644 (the date of Hollar's engraving), the suggestion of replacing him with Glauber in 1647 presumably means the post had been vacant since then.

It has been suggested that Hunniades' post at Gresham was Professor of Mathematics,[144] but Lilly's remarks and the evidence of the Hartlib papers suggest a stronger emphasis on chemistry. The legend on Hollar's engravings mentions his 'Hermetic' before his mathematical work at Gresham. Hartlib noted in 1640 that 'A Laboratory is erecting in Gresham-Colledge by Sir K. Digby and others [...] Hunneades is the erecter or builder of it'.[145] Most convincing of all is this suggestion of 'getting Glauber in Hunniades' place', for Hartlib was certainly better-informed about Glauber than to suppose him either qualified or likely to be inclined to teach mathematics. Glauber was no scholar and had no pretensions to be one: his expertise lay entirely in the field of chemistry. In a draft version of one of Hartlib's numerous proposals for the Office of Address, probably dating from this period, a number of concrete schemes are mooted including 'The Erecting and maintaining of Glauberus New Laboratorie'.[146] However, this item has been struck through, probably on account of the disheartening news sent by Appelius, and does not appear on what is obviously a later draft of the same document.[147]

Hartlib's idea was in any case hardly realistic, if only on linguistic grounds. He had obviously considered this problem, as Appelius in the same letter reported that Glauber 'understands latyn well, et can also make his minde knowne therein, if I remember well',[148] which suggests something a good deal less than fluency. Moriaen mentioned that Glauber was uncomfortable expressing himself in Latin,[149] and Sorbière later noted, though not unkindly, that on the occasion of his visit Glauber 'made us no excuses for his poor Latin'.[150] It is certain he did not know English.[151] But the suggestion is a striking testimony of the extent of Glauber's reputation among the chemical fraternity in England only a year after the publication of his first two book-length works, as well as further confirmation of Hartlib's tireless activity in recruiting manpower for English education, and manoeuvring the educational ethos towards a concern with 'realia', with 'useful' knowledge and applied sciences.

Further evidence of this general early enthusiasm for Glauber is provided by the commendatory remarks by Appelius and Moriaen already noted. Glauber also inspired considerable interest in Boyle. Early in 1648, noting Boyle himself as the source, Hartlib recorded that

> Helmont's stone wherby hee cured the stone in bladder kidney called Ludus Paracelsi is a stone which is found neere Antwerp prepared by Helmont. This stone one of Helmont's friends hath gotten and shewn or promised it to Morian, which hee hath promised for Mr Boyles sake to give to Glauberus that hee may prepare it and make the Ludus Paracelsi of it.[152]

Boyle had only just turned twenty when this was written, and it is a striking indication of how deeply imbued his early thought was with the convictions of the Spagyrists. Eight years later, he was still taking an approving interest in Glauber's work, maintaining that

> In Tr*actatus* Glaub*eri* de Prosperitate Germaniæ [ie. *Teutschlands Wolfahrt* I, which came out that year], the annexed dis*course* of salpeeter De Nitro is the most substantial rational et real piece, wherin many secrets are discovered w*hich* hims*elf* [Boyle] had before.[153]

Perhaps the most assiduous collector of Glauberian writings and equipment was Cheney Culpeper, whose complex and ambivalent assessment will be considered at more length in Chapter Seven.

However, in a striking re-run of the history of the Hartlib circle's responses to Comenius, initial high enthusiasm was increasingly displaced by scepticism and disillusion. Just as with Comenius, the more Glauber wrote, the less Hartlib's friends saw their initial expectations fulfilled. When Robert Child in 1652 received the first two books of *Operis Mineralis* from Hartlib, he could make little sense of them, though he nonetheless asked in April, 'pray let me se all Glaubers workes if possibly [*sic*]'.[154] Henry Jenney failed to obtain the promised results from a Glauberian experiment relating to husbandry, but had the grace to admit it was perhaps a mistake on his part rather than dishonesty on Glauber's that had led to the failure.[155] He was one of very few with the humility to adopt the stance later recommended by Moriaen, that people should not automatically blame Glauber for their inability to replicate his experiments.[156]

Doubts about Glauber's honesty recur throughout the papers. The naturalist and historian Georg Horn complained that Glauber was more assiduous in making promises than in keeping them.[157] At one point in 1648, even Culpeper's enthusiasm seems to have been briefly quenched by adverse reports: 'Mr Petty his late carriage, & that Monsieur Glauberus is like to turne a Wheeler, hathe bred in me a resolution, not to trouble my thowghts any farther with these kinde of people'.[158] The following August, however, he was again excitedly looking forward to news about Glauber's 'ouens, & wayes of distillation; w*hich* I wonderfully approue'.[159]

A recurrent charge, and perhaps one of the weightier ones, was that Glauber was given to selling processes he had not in fact tested. Erasmus Rasch, for instance, declared: 'Glauber, in my opinion, commits a great sin by undertaking to teach others things he does not know himself'.[160] Earlier, however, he had been keen to learn Glauber's method of making aqua fortis and spiritus salis, and complained to Hartlib that Clodius, who was obviously very well up on Glauberian chemistry, or at least gave himself out to be so, had not sent him the promised recipes for these.[161]

Moriaen himself, during the 1650s, became increasingly dubious about Glauber's claims and motives. After reporting his friend's discovery of 'sal mirabile', he went on to remark that if what Glauber said was true, he had indeed discovered the alcahest or something very like it, in which case it would certainly cure Hartlib's bladder stone, an ailment Moriaen feared he was developing as well. But hard on the heels of this optimistic report came a sombre caveat:[162]

> He has been putting me off in this fashion for a long time now, and
> leading me to the summit of Mount Pisga; whether anything will come of
> it this time and what good things he will bring me, only time will tell; I
> can no longer depend on him, having been disappointed so often and for so
> long.[163]

And indeed, when Moriaen asked Glauber for some sal mirabile, so that he
might try to prepare the alcahest and treat his stone, the usual story unfolded:
Glauber claimed to have no sal mirabile to hand, and sent instead some
'tinctura nitri', together with the unhelpful remark that Moriaen's bladder
stone was probably hereditary.[164] It was just the same with Glauber's much-
vaunted fertilising salt ('fruchtbarmachendes saltz'): he promised to send
Moriaen some, but by April 1658 'I have still heard nothing, and now sowing
time is almost over',[165] and by July he was still waiting.[166] By June 1658 he
was thoroughly exasperated: 'it will be a wonder if anything further comes
from him, for I have never known his like for inconstancy of purpose'.[167]

Nonetheless, the two men appear to have remained on friendly terms. In
July 1657, the time when Moriaen was recovering from the violent fever he
had fully expected would kill him, and was reflecting anxiously on what
would befall Odilia if he died, Glauber reassured him that should the worst
happen, he would take it upon himself to guarantee her welfare. Moriaen
thought this reflected very well on the chemist.[168] After his visit to
Amsterdam in 1659, when he had an opportunity to view all Glauber's
processes for himself, Moriaen wrote excitedly that all his doubts had been
resolved, and that having personally witnessed Glauber's transmutation of
metals into gold and production of medicines, he could no longer doubt the
validity of any of his claims.[169] Poleman, however, subsequently maintained
that a friend of his had relieved Moriaen of some his delusions about Glauber,
presumably during this visit:

> You should know that Herr Moriaen no longer thinks so highly of
> Glauber as he did, for he has been convinced that the yellow metal of
> which his so-called aurum potabile is made is no true gold and will not
> stand thorough testing, as I have been told by a trusted friend who has
> proved this to Herr Moriaen on a sound basis, and whom Herr Moriaen
> had to admit was right.[170]

Unfortunately, the lack of material from Moriaen himself after this date makes
it impossible to judge whether there was any truth in this claim of a chemical
conversion.

In 1660, an anonymous correspondent who I believe is Kretschmar[171]
evidently thought he was doing Hartlib and his friends (Clodius, Dury and
Brereton) a great favour by sending - without Glauber's knowledge or
consent - a very detailed description of the equipment in the last Amsterdam
laboratory and the processes carried out there. If Glauber's laboratories can
be seen as an early example of chemical industry, then this is an early example
of industrial espionage, a world away from the ideal of 'free and generous
communication':

> I hope by God's grace I have it largely right; it was a wonder I managed to
> see the ovens despite the fact that he keeps the laboratory close shut now

they are built, and lets no one in. It has cost me all my slender means and there is nothing further I can do but faithfully reveal it all to you, begging once again for God's sake keep it utterly secret from everyone, especially Herr Moriaen, that I have told you, and let Glauber not learn of it. Once again for God's sake keep it utterly secret from everyone, especially Herr Moriaen, that I have told you, and let Glauber not learn of it.[172]

If this is indeed from Kretschmar (who, like Moriaen, frequently incurred Poleman's scorn for believing Glauber's fairy tales), it may well be that he was offering these details as an added incentive to the addressees to participate in his own transmutation project. The response to this decidedly underhand piece of intelligencing is not preserved, but it is highly unlikely that Hartlib, at least, would have been impressed by such methods of gaining wisdom.

In 1660 and 1661, Fahrner's published attacks on Glauber were supplemented by three polemical works from other pens. These were the *Glauberus Refutatus* of the self-styled 'filius Sendivogii', Johannes Fortitudino Hartprecht,[173] the *Sudum Philosophicum* of one 'Antiglauberus', whom an anagram in his title reveals as Johannes Joachim Becher,[174] and the *Gründliche Widerlegung* of 'C.D.M.A.S.'.[175] There is little comment on these works in Hartlib's archive, but two pieces of evidence about them are of some interest. Though Poleman was elsewhere less than complimentary about the 'filius Sendivogii', he was always ready to approve an attack on Glauber, and in telling Hartlib about Hartprecht's *Sudum Philosophicum* he supplied the bibliographical detail that this work, which was published without indication of place, in fact came out in Amsterdam: 'the Son of Sendivogius has thoroughly demonstrated that he [Glauber] is a complete ignoramus in true philosophy in his *Ludum* [sic] *Philosophicum*, which is now under the press here [Amsterdam]'.[176]

'C.D.M.A.S.' accused Glauber of being semi-literate, of employing an assistant to render his books readable, of not understanding Paracelsus properly, of atheism, and of having killed a number of people with his 'aurum horribile'. The author has so far remained unidentifiable, though as Link remarks it is not unlikely, given that his work was published there, that he lived at the time in Leipzig.[177] An anonymous letter in the Hartlib Papers includes a quotation from one 'Charls de Montendon from Leipzigk concerning his Purpose and Booke against Glauber'. In the extract, which is dated 4 March 1661, Montendon speaks of being at the 'Altenburg-Court' (near Leipzig), where Glauber had 'fallen vpon' him. The reference appears to be to a legal accusation rather than a physical attack, and presumably he means that Glauber fell on him by proxy, since there is no other indication at all of Glauber's having gone to Leipzig at this period, and indeed it is very doubtful whether his health would have permitted him to do so. Montendon went on to declare (not very lucidly, at least to anyone unfamiliar with the details of the affair) that Glauber had cheated him and that he (Montendon) was publishing 'a Treatise on purpose entituled - A needful Refutation of Glaubers hitherto divulged Vn-Truths' - an unequivocal reference to the *Nothwendige Refutation auff etliche Johann-Rudolph Glaubers zu Amsterdam unwahre bißhero außgelaßene Bücher*.

We have, then, a name to put to 'C.D.M.A.S.', Charles De Montendon - perhaps Altenburgensis Studiosus? Unfortunately that is about all we have.

Montendon mentioned himself in this extract that his mother tongue was French, and that he knew German well enough to write in it. The only other mention of Montendon in the papers is in the anonymous alchemical copy letter of 1660, quoted above, which I attribute to Friedrich Kretschmar. The author mentioned that he was enclosing a copy of a letter in French from one Peter Mariceus in Amsterdam to 'Monsr. Charle de Montendon of Yserton from Saphaÿen, who is now staying with me here'.[178] But there is no indication where the letter is from, the enclosure has not survived, and I cannot confidently identify either 'Yserton' or 'Saphaÿen', though Yverdon in Savoy is a possiblilty.[179] That is as much as it has been possible to ascertain. However, it seems worth exposing this loose thread in the hope that someone will find something to attach it to. The extract from Montendon is given in full as Appendix 2.

All four men who published against Glauber in his lifetime (Fahrner, Hartprecht, Becher and Montendon) were themselves chemically inclined. So were the harshest critics whose comments survive in Hartlib's papers. Foremost among these was Poleman, whose diatribes are composed in a very similar spirit to those of Fahrner and the others, except that Poleman does not appear to have had any personal grudge against Glauber beyond the conviction that he brought discredit on the noble art of alchemy. Some of his comments have already been cited: there are a great many more. He reported with evident satisfaction that one Schöfler 'is slopping about in Glauber's stinking so-called alcahest and has made such serious mistakes with it that it well nigh cost him his life'.[180] Despite his claim that 'it nauseates me to think any further on Glauber's trickery',[181] he devoted a great deal of time and ink to vilifying his enemy.[182] 'As for Glauber's pranks' he maintained, 'it is truly not worth giving up so much as quarter of an hour to contemplate them, for they are nothing but trickery and empty boasts'.[183]

The range of opinions represented in the papers is spectacularly wide. The accusations of dishonesty and fraudulence somewhat outweigh the commendations, and the widespread enthusiastic interest of the 1640s tends to be replaced by disillusion and rejection in the 1650s. There is, however, no clear consensus at any point, and it should be added that even among Glauber's professed detractors a good many, like Rasch, were keen to obtain his works and, especially, his equipment. One of the more balanced judgments, which neatly sums up the tone of much of the polemic, is that of Appelius: 'for my own part, I have no reason to think him a cheat, but he despises others, and others despise him, as is the way with almost all artists, for none cries up any but his own wares'.[184]

Hartlib himself apparently remained perplexed as to which of the widely differing reports he should believe. Though he was still collecting Glauber's works assiduously at least as late as 1659, the stream of accusations from the likes of Rasch and Poleman, and news of the work of Becher, Hartprecht and Montendon, led him to become increasingly suspicious. In 1660, he told Winthrop:

> our german adepti with whom I shall be better acquainted ere long, count no better of Glauber then a mountebank, one *that* continues to cheat all sorts of people by his specious artifices and one *that* knows nothing in *the* true Philos*ophical* work Alkahest Elixir, &c &c There are some who are

> resolved to take him into task, to discover *the* error and falshood of his
> philosophy and experimentall knowledges & his willfull cheates and
> cousenages.[185]

This, however, is followed by the quintessentially Hartlibian rider, 'I have
suggested *that* some would also note whatever was true and good in all his
writings'.[186]

It is obviously impossible to reduce such a broad spectrum of opinion to
any simple formulation of the contemporary response to Glauber. It is quite
clear, though, that the most savage attacks came from what one might call the
'old school' of Hermetic chemists: men such as Rasch, Hartprecht and
Poleman, who were deeply committed to the notion of alchemy as essentially
a mystic experience and a matter of personal revelation, from which it was
important to exclude the common herd, even when publishing - indeed,
especially when publishing. This peculiar ambivalence to the notion of
publication finds striking expression in Poleman's comments on the
manuscripts of Starkey, which were sent to him by Hartlib in 1659. Poleman
was hugely impressed by these cryptic productions and wished to see them
brought to press at once - indeed, he expressed an interest in arranging this
himself.[187] There could be no harm in doing so, he declared in so many
words, since they were so thoroughly obscure that there was no danger of
anyone's understanding them: there were 'no arcana clearly enough expressed
in them for any man to be able to make them out. And that is the very truth,
for which reason they may safely be published'.[188]

Clearly, however, Poleman did not regard himself as 'anyone': these
mysteries were not impenetrable to him. The purpose of publication,
presumably, was to reach out to that tiny, elect body of similarly enlightened
adepts whose learning and insight qualified them to share in this virtually
sacred knowledge. The very fact that they were capable of understanding it
guaranteed that they were worthy to do so. To the proponents of such an
outlook, Glauber's direct, popular style and (comparatively) explicit
terminology was anathema. This is not, to be sure, what they ostensibly
attacked him for: the endlessly repeated charges were that he was at best
mercenary and at worst a charlatan and confidence trickster whose fake
medicines were lethal, whose writings led would-be adepts onto false paths
and who brought the noble art of alchemy into disrepute by his association
with it. However, the very vehemence of their onslaughts suggests they felt
threatened by him in some way, and this concern for a gullible public whom
they were themselves at such pains to keep in the dark is not overly
convincing. What really upset them, I would suggest, is that Glauber was
trying to make chemistry accessible to the commoner.

Others such as Boyle, Hartlib and Moriaen, who took a rather less elitist
view of the chemical art, were inclined to give Glauber more credit, and to
acknowledge at least his practical achievements. Boyle, as has been
mentioned, was keen to apply his furnace-making technology and thought
highly of his work on saltpetre; Moriaen was particularly impressed by his
contributions to agriculture and longed more than anything to learn the secrets
of his fertilisers and artificial wines. Poleman, by contrast, sneered at such
mundane achievements, remarking (not unreasonably) that if Glauber's aurum
potabile and alcahest were half so miraculous as he claimed, he would not

waste his time on gardening, or on merely technical processes such as smelting copper ore, and would have no need to offer such products or processes for money.[189]

But among those who did not simply dismiss everything connected with the man as manifest charlatanism, his practical and technical achievements were generally esteemed, even when his more grandiose claims were mistrusted. What many increasingly came to find wanting in his work, however, was the spiritual element, the transcendent insights into God and the harmony of the universe that were the ultimate goal of the 'Chemical Philosophy'. Attempts to apply Glauber's more mundane achievements to these mystical ends provide the subject of the final chapter of this study.

Notes

1   On Glauber, see J.C. Adelung, *Geschichte der Menschlichen Narrheit* (Leipzig, 1785) II, 161-92; H. Kopp, *Beiträge zur Geschichte der Chemie* (Braunschweig, 1869), 160-63; Kurt F. Gugel, *Johann Rudolph Glauber: Leben und Werk 1604-1670* (Würzburg, 1955); Erich Pietsch, 'Johann Rudolph Glauber: Der Mensch, sein Werk und seine Zeit', *Deutsches Museum Abhandlungen und Berichte* 24 (1956), Heft 1, Munich 1956, 1-64; J.R. Partington, *A History of Chemistry* II (London, 1961), 341-61; *NDB* VI, 437-8, and the excellent summary by Katherine Ahonen in *DSB* V, 419-23. Far and away the fullest and most objective account to date of Glauber's life and work, distinguishing carefully between pure myth, plausible speculation and verifiable fact, is Arnulf Link, *Johann Rudolph Glauber 1604-1670: Leben und Werk* (doctoral dissertation, Heidelberg, 1993); this also gives an excellent bibliography. I am deeply indebted to Dr. Link for supplying me with a copy of his thesis, which is not obtainable in England.

2   See section 3 of this chapter. Glauber's principal autobiographical works are *J.R. Glauberi Apologia Oder Verthädigung Gegen Christoff Farners Lügen vnd Ehrabschneidung* (Mainz, 1655); *Johann Rud: Glaubers Zweyte Apologia, Oder Ehren-Rettung Gegen Christoff Farnern [...] unmenschliche Lügen vnd Ehrabschneidung* (Frankfurt am Main, 1656), *Glauberus Ridivivus [sic]* (Amsterdam, 1656), and *Joh. Rudlophi Glauberi Testimonium Veritatis* (Amsterdam, 1657). There are, however, biographical asides in a great many other works, especially *De tribus Lapidibus Ignium secretorum* (Amsterdam, 1667).

3   'Paracelsus des 17. Jahrhundert' - Wolfgang Schneider, *Geschichte der Pharmazeutischen Chemie* (Weinheim, 1972), 130, cit. Link, *Glauber*, 8.

4   For an extensive summary of assessments of Glauber from his own time to ours, see Link, *Johann Rudolph Glauber* (doctoral dissertation, Heidelberg, 1993), 8-13. Link's own work is an honourable exception in this respect, presenting a much more integrated view of Glauber's natural philosophy and relating it more fully to contemporary currents of thought. Katherine Ahonen's *DSB* entry should also be exempted.

5   Pietsch, *Glauber* 51; Gugel, *Glauber* 69.

6   'Chemistry in the Scientific Revolution: Problems of language and communication', *Reappraisals of the Scientific Revolution*, ed. David C. Lindberg and Robert S. Westman (Cambridge, 1990), 367-96.

7   *A History of Chemistry* II, 343, 349.

8   'den deutschen Robert Boyle' - entry on Glauber in Günther Bugge (ed.), *Das Buch der großen Chemiker* I (Weinheim, 1974; first pub. 1929), 153.

9   'Ich gestehe das gern/ daß ich niemahlen auff Hohen Schulen gewesen/ auch niemahlen drauff begehrt/ wann solches geschehen/ ich vieleicht zu solcher Erkäntnus der Natur/ so ich ietzunder (ohne Rum zu melden) besitze/ nimmermehr kommen were: Reuhet mich also gantz nicht/ daß ich von Jugend auff die Hand in die Kohlen gestecket/ vnd dardurch die verborgene Heimligkeiten der Natur erfahren habe. Ich suche niemand zu vertreiben/ habe auch niemahlen darnach getrachtet grosser Herren Brodt zu essen/ sondern viel lieber solches durch mein eigen Hand/ neben Betrachtung dieses Spruchs (ALTERIUS NON SIT QUI SUUS ESSE POTEST) Ehrlich zu erwerben' - Glauber, *Deß Teutschlands Wolfahrt* I (Amsterdam, 1656), 80.

10   It appears above the most famous portrait of him, by Augustin Hirschvogel (1538), reproduction in Pagel, *Paracelsus* (Basel and New York, 1958) 28.

11   Complaining in the 'Preface Introductory' of those who 'rail instead of arguing, as hath been done of Late in Print by divers Chymists', Boyle adds the marginal note 'G. and F. and H. and others, in their books against one another' (*Sceptical Chymist*, A5v), a thinly disguised allusion to Glauber, Fahrner, and J.F. Hartprecht, who also wrote against Glauber (see below, p. 204).

12   Gugel, *Glauber*, 13.

13   Cf. Webster 'English Medical Reformers of the Puritan Revolution: A background to the "Society of Chymical Physitians"', *Ambix* 14 (1967), 16-41; also *The Great Instauration*, 250-56.

14   *Glauberus Ridivivus*, 65.

15   This was especially true of Rudolf II, but rather less so of his successor Ferdinand II. It has been alleged that Glauber himself was associated with Ferdinand's court in 1625-26 (Gugel, *Glauber* 13-14) but Link exposes this as unsubstantiated conjecture (Link, *Glauber* 18). On the patronage of German princes, see William B. Ashworth Jr., 'The Habsburg Circle', and Bruce T. Moran, 'Patronage and Institutions: Courts, Universities, and Academies in Germany; an Overview: 1550-1750', in Bruce T. Moran (ed.), *Patronage and Institutions: Science, Technology and Medicine at the European Court 1500-1750* (Boydell, 1991), 137-67 and 169-83.

16   'der aller gelährteste vnd erfahrneste Philosophus bey seinen lebezeiten' - *De Tribus Lapidibus*, 4.

17   Link, *Glauber*, 27.

18   Link, *Glauber*, 29-31; Gugel, *Glauber*, 16.

19   *Glauberus Ridivivus*, 50 and 65.

20   'sind 2 Iahr verlauffen gewest/ ehe ich diese nach der ersten Geheurat' - ibid., 65.

21   'bin [...] nach Hollandt wegen einiger geschäfften verreist/ da selbsten aber wegen verenderung der Lufft Kranck worden/ vnd weilen ich die Hollandische Kost nicht aller Dings vertragen können/ ich nothwendig mich wieder in Eehestant (desto besser wartung zu haben) begeben mussen' - *Glauberus Ridivivus*, 65.

22   Though both these dates have been available to Glauber's biographers since 1949 (Dirk Wittop Koning, 'J.R. Glauber in Amsterdam', *Jaarboek van het Genootschap Amstelodamum* 43 (1949), 1-6), none of them has drawn the obvious inference.

23   UBA N65f, 23 Sept. 1642.

24   Moriaen to ?, 7 Feb. 1647, HP 37/118A: 'hab Ihn lang beÿ mir im hauß gehabt'.

25   UBA N65g.

26   Link, *Glauber*, 31.

27   'etwaß Rechtes ins grosse in Alchimia' - Glauber, *De Tribus Lapidibus*, 9.

28   'allerhandt klein vnd große Oefens [...], vnterschiedliche klein vnd grosse Blaßbälge'.

29   Ibid., and see Link, *Glauber*, 32-3.

30 Moriaen to Van Assche, Nov. 1644, UBA N65h.

31 'Utilitates furni noui Philosophici Glauberi wolte ich jetzt geschickt haben, halte aber, der H wird von H Morian selbiger sachen schon gnugsam berichtet sein, wo nicht kan er sich am gewissesten bey ihm erkundigen [...] dann ihm ohne zweifel mehr davon bewust als mir' - Appelius to Hartlib, 28 May/7 June 1644, HP 45/1/6A.

32 'H Morian, vnd andere Medici/ die was von ihm haben, seind mit ihm wohl zufrieden' - 22 June 1644 (or possibly 2 July if Appelius is using Old Style), HP 45/1/8A.

33 Moriaen's first mention of Glauber in the Hartlib archive is in a letter dated 7 Feb. 1647, obviously written in reply to specific questions, but not necessarily to Hartlib (HP 118A-119A). The next, which is definitely to Hartlib and sets out at some length to supply 'was mein H sonsten wegen H Glauberi zu wißen begehret' ('whatever else you wish to know about Herr Glauber') is dated 27 Aug. 1647 (HP 37/121A-122B).

34 HP 63/14/48A-49B. Hartlib had a Latin translation made for circulation, of which there are two manuscript copies (HP 16/8/1A-4B and 25/22/1A-4B).

35 Appelius to Hartlib, 7 June 1644, HP 45/1/6A: 'man kriegt sie [seine Sachen] wol vmb ein leidlich gelt von ihm'; 13 Aug. 1644, HP 45/1/12A: 'Glauberus hath his furnaces communicated to my Docteur, et to me'. The charge of 30 Imperials is specified in Appelius's footnote to his copy of Glauber's advertisement (HP 63/14/49B).

36 Appelius to Hartlib, 6 Nov. 47, HP 45/1/37A-B. Hartlib was interested enough to add notes of these figures to his copy of the original advertisement: see Appendix 1.

37 Appelius says no more about this friend than that he was a doctor. It may well have been the influential natural philosopher François de le Boë ('Sylvius') (1614-1672), with whom Appelius was friendly at the time. On Sylvius, see Partington, *History of Chemistry* II, 281-9.

38 'nichts als viel geldt außgebens/ vnd weinig dargegen einkommens' - *De Tribus Lapidibus*, 10.

39 Appelius to Hartlib, HP 45/1/9A: 'Glauberus der Chymicus will erst vber 3 wochen von hinnen den Rein hinauff reisen, vnd sich an einen bequemen ort zu wohnen niedersetzen'. The phrase is rather odd, since the Rhine does not run through Amsterdam.

40 'daß ich aber die Feuchte Lufft zu Amsterdam/ nicht wohl vertragen können/ vnd eine gesundere Lufft zu Vtrecht vnd Arnheim gesucht/ ist wahr [...] habe mich wieder vmb besserer Nahrung willen nach Amsterdam setzen mussen/ aber niemahlen zu Leyden gewohnet wie du [Fahrner] auffschneitest/ vnd hette ich daselbsten gewohnt/ waß wehre es dan gewesen/ wan Leyden besser vor mich gewesen wehr alß ein anderer Orth/ wer wurde mich verdacht haben daselbsten zu wohnen?' - *Glauberus Ridivivus*, 65-6.

41 Even Gugel, who generally takes Glauber at his word, states as a matter of fact that Glauber at some point lived in Leiden (*Glauber*, 17).

42 Appelius to Hartlib, 22 July 1644, HP 45/1/9A, stating he planned to depart in three weeks, and 5 Sept. 1644, HP 45/1/13A, saying he had arrived there.

43 Moriaen wrote on 27 Aug. that Glauber planned to set off the following day (HP 37/121B). Appelius also mentioned his imminent departure on 26 Aug. (HP 45/1/33A).

44 When Benjamin Worsley arrived in Amsterdam in late Feb. 1648, Glauber was obviously not there as he was communicating with Worsley by post (Moriaen to Hartlib, 27 Feb. 1648, HP 37/131A), but Appelius's letter of 2 August (HP

45/1/39B) indicates that they were in personal contact and mentions Glauber's 'verhäusung' (move of house), probably meaning the move from Arnhem to Amsterdam. Since there is no mention of him in Moriaen's letter of 28 May 1648 (HP 37/133A-134B), though he knew Hartlib to be deeply interested in the progress of Worsley's contacts with Glauber, it seems likely the move had not yet happened. For details of Worsley's visit and contacts with Glauber, see below, pp. 217-26.

45 *Glauber*, 29-30.

46 'vor etlichen vnd Zwanzig Iahren [ie. before 1636] zu Giesen ein Weib genohmen [...] bin in die Fürstliche Hoff-Reichß Apotecken selbe zu versehen erfordert worden [...] nachdem aber Hessen Cassel/ mit Hessen Darmbstadt einen Krieg anfangen/ vnd Marpurg mit Kriegs Macht nehmen wollen/ ist alles verendert vnd wer gekonnt sich in sicherung salvirt hatt/ wie ich dan also von dannen mich nach Franckfurt den Rein herunter nach Bon zu meinem Gnädigen Hern begeben/ vnd in wehrender zeit obgedachtes Weib von Giesen/ einmal in meiner Kammer/ bey meinem damaligen Diener in Ehebruch erdappt [...] bin nach solchem fall vbers Iahr darnach erst nach Hollandt [...] verreist' - *Glauberus Ridivivus*, 65.

47 Link, *Glauber*, 30.

48 *De Auri Tinctura sive Auro Potabili Vero* (Amsterdam, 1646): the short title form *De Auri Tinctura* avoids confusion with the later *Tractatus de Medicina Universali, sive Auro Potabili Vero* (Amsterdam, 1657).

49 Appelius to ?, 13 Sept. 1646, HP 45/1/25A. *De Auri Tinctura* was not, therefore, as Partington states (*History of Chemistry*, II, 344), Glauber's first published work, having been narrowly preceded by *Furni novi* I.

50 Appelius to Dury, 16 Oct. 1646, HP 45/1/28A.

51 Moriaen to ?, 7 Feb. 1647, HP 37/118A.

52 Appelius to Hartlib, 23 March/2 April 1647, HP 45/1/38A. However, Moriaen some months later mentioned that Glauber had arrived in Amsterdam in May (to Hartlib, 27 Aug. 1647, HP 37/121B). This probably represents one of Moriaen's frequent memory lapses.

53 Moriaen to Hartlib, 27 Aug. 1647, HP 37/121B-122A.

54 Moriaen to Hartlib, 7 Feb. 1643, HP 37/118A: 'Ich meine aber in kurtzen seinen zweiten offen ins werck zu richten vnd ein theil medicamenten dadurch zu machen'.

55 Ibid.: 'hab [...] mit meiner haußfrau ihme 2 Kinder auß der tauffe gehoben'.

56 'an vielen Orthen außtrucklich sagt/ Kompt alle zu mir/ die ihr muheseelig vnd beladen seit/ ich will euch erquicken/ etc. Vnd ist Christus für alle vnd nicht allein für die Catholische/ Luterische/ Arminianische etc. sondern auch für alle Iuden/ Turcken vnd Heyden vollkomlich gestorben/ vnd ihnen den Himmel erworben' - *Glauberus Ridivivus*, 79.

57 'Ihm in der Natur ein zimblich liecht auffgangen ist' - Moriaen to Hartlib, 5 June 1658, HP 31/18/28A.

58 Appelius to Hartlib, 5 Sept. 1644 HP 45/1/13A.

59 Appelius to Hartlib, 26 Aug. 1647, HP 45/1/33A. Moriaen's report of 27 Aug. 1647, HP 37/121B, is almost identical. Appelius evidently liked practising his English in his letters to Hartlib, but never quite mastered an idiomatic style.

60 *Glauberus Ridivivus*, 70.

61 *Glauberus Ridivivus*, 12.

62 Wittop Koning, 'Glauber in Amsterdam', 2; Gugel, *Glauber*, 24; Link, *Glauber*, 35.

63 Moriaen to [Worsley?], 4 March 1650, HP 37/142A.

64 Brun to Hartlib, 13 June 1649, HP 39/2/9B.

65 Moriaen to Hartlib, 29 April 1650, HP 37/153A.

66 Moriaen to Hartlib, July 1650, HP 37/163A.

67 Moriaen to Hartlib, 7 Oct. 1650, HP 37/160A.

68 *Glauberus Ridivivus*, 67-8.

69 Ibid., 67.

70 Link, *Glauber*, 35.

71 Moriaen on 7 Oct. mentioned having received a letter from him from Wertheim and that he was now settled there (HP 37/160A).

72 *Glauberus Ridivivus*, 52.

73 Moriaen to Hartlib, 7 Oct. 1650, HP 37/160A: 'Er [hatt] ein offentlich Laboratorium auffrichtet transmut*atio*nem metallorum publice zue docirn hatt sonsten ein Bergwerkh daselbst*en* funden'.

74 According to a letter almost certainly from Moriaen and quoting a letter from Glauber, HP 63/14/8A.

75 Link, *Glauber* 35-6; Gugel, *Glauber* 20; basing their accounts on *Glauberus Ridivivus*, 68.

76 Unattributed copy letter of 28 July 1651, HP 63/14/9A. The document is filed together with other extracts definitely from Moriaen.

77 *Glauberus Ridivivus* and *De Tribus Lapidibus, passim.*

78 Link, *Glauber*, 36-7, Gugel, *Glauber*, 21. Gugel dates the move late 1652/early 1653, but Glauber had decided to leave at the end of June 1651 (HP 63/14/9A), and after changing his mind yet again about his next destination, which was initially to have been Hanau or Frankfurt (both much closer to Mainz), had arrived by 8 September 1651 (Moriaen to ?, HP 63/14/10A).

79 *Glauberus Ridivivus*, 48.

80 Part 1 had appeared before the move, by March 1651, when Moriaen obtained a copy (HP 63/14/5A).

81 The exact details of the agreement are in some doubt, but both men refer to such a vow. Fahrner in his *Ehrenrettung* (1656) cited a contract he had himself drawn up offering half his entire worldly possessions as surety, but it is not certain this was ever ratified. See Gugel, *Glauber* 22-5, and Link, *Glauber* 39-42, for fuller accounts.

82 'mit welchem stuck wan du mir glauben gehalten hättest [...] wir beyde al vnsere Kinder in kurtzen [hätten] reichlich versorgen können' ... 'in Metallicis ein guth Stück zu weisen/ welchen ich nicht habe zeugen konnen oder wollen' - *Glauberus Ridivivus*, 15.

83 'Glauber selbst hat [...] wiederholt darauf hingewiesen, ihm selbst sei nie eine solche alchimistische Verwandlung gelungen' - Gugel, *Glauber*, 8.

84 Moriaen to Hartlib, 5 Oct. 1657, HP 42/2/22A, and 20 July 1659, copies at HP 16/1/15A-16B and 16/1/17A-18B.

85 *Glauberus Ridivivus*, 74, 49, 50, 21 and 52 respectively.

86 See Link, *Glauber* 41, esp. n.168, citing Glauber's *Apologia* (1655), 19-30, and Fahrner's *Ehrenrettung* (1656), 44.

87 'durch welche Invention daß gantze Menschliche Geschlacht/ große ergetzlichkeit vnd labe/ bey Alten vnd Krancken erlangen werden/ welches ich vielleicht nicht gethan/ wan es der Gottloser Farner nicht durch seine Vntreu Lügen vnd Schmeheschrifften/ von mir außgetrieben hette/ Farner aber wirdt einen Lohn bekommen wie Iudas Ischariot' - *Glauberus Ridivivus*, 99.

88 Besides writing four works explicitly against Fahrner, Glauber peppered all his subsequent publications with parenthetical attacks on him and denunciations of his

211

'Farnerish lies' ('Farnerischen Lügen').

89 Moriaen to Hartlib, 2 Feb. 1657, HP 42/2/1B: 'der zanck mit Farner ist freÿlich nicht rühmlich vnd machen sich nur beide zueschanden damit, vnderdeßen kommen auch gute dinge an den tage die sonsten dahinden geblieben weren'.

90 'weilen ich dan gesehen/ daß ich leichtlich mit einen hauffen Trunckenen Pöltzen in action kommen möchte/ [...] habe ich getrachtet die meinigen an ein sicher Orth zu bringen' - *Glauberus Ridivivus*, 71.

91 Hartlib to Boyle, 15 May 1654, Boyle, *Works* VI, 91.

92 *Glauberus Ridivivus*, 105, and see Link, *Glauber*, 43-4.

93 *Glauberus Ridivivus*, 82; and Moriaen to [Hartlib?], 16 Oct. 1654, HP 39/2/18A: 'Er dann erstes tages für seine person nach Cölln kommen muß zu dem Churfürsten'.

94 Ibid.

95 'nun bin ich allhier zu Amsterdam vnd wohne auff der Keysers Grafft/ an einem bekanten Ort/ vnd in keinem Winckel/ hastu oder ein anderer etwas zu sagen/ so komb hieher vnd thun [*sic*] es/ werde dir redt vnd antwort geben' - *Glauberus Ridivivus*, 11-12.

96 Moriaen to Hartlib, 5 Oct. 1657, HP 42/2/22A.

97 Moriaen to Hartlib, 15 Feb. 1658, HP 31/18/4B, and 12 March 1658, HP 31/18/13B.

98 Moriaen to Hartlib, 24 Aug. 1657, HP 42/2/19A.

99 'mein sal mirabile nicht allein die Metallen sondern alle steine und Beine ja die kohlen welche sonsten durch kein corrosiv zue solvirn, radicaler solvirt [...] von welcher wunderbahren solution ich ein groß Buch machen könde' - Glauber, *De Natura Salium*, 94.

100 It is quoted verbatim in Moriaen to Hartlib, 26 May/5 June 1658, HP 31/18/27B. J.R. Partington also singles the passage out for quotation (*A History of Chemistry* II, 355).

101 'will mit gewalt aus Amsterdam' - Moriaen to Hartlib, 2 July 1658, HP 31/18/39A.

102 'Herrn Glaubers Laboratorium publicum & Secretum ist nun hier angangen, und sind viel freunde beÿ ihm, insonderheit der gute alte H joh Morian von Arnheimb; mit welchem ich etliche mahl zusammen gewesen [...] logiret beÿ H. Glaubern selber im hause, und wird vielleicht, Meinem hochgeehrten H. ein mehrers, alß ich, von H. Glaubers dingen überschreiben' - Kretschmar to Hartlib, Dury, Clodius and Brereton, 1 Aug. 1659, HP 26/64/3B.

103 In a long letter to Monsieur Bautru, Chevalier de Sègre, 13 July 1660. This is published in *Relations, lettres et discours de Mr. de Sorbière sur diverses matières curieuses* (Paris, 1660), and rather more accessibly in P.J. Blok, 'Drie Brieven van Samuel Sorbière over den Toestand van Holland in 1660', *Bijdragen en Nededeelingen van het Historische Genootschap* 22 (1901), 1-89; passage relating to Glauber 74-89.

104 'les Panacées, l'Alkaest, le Zenda, Parenda, l'Archaec, l'Enspagoycum, le Nostoch, l'Ylech, le Trarame, le Turban, l'Ens Tagastricum, et les autres visions que Van Helmont et ses confrères nous débitent' - Blok, 'Drie Brieven van Samuel Sorbière', 79.

105 'Par tout ce discours, Monsieur, je ne prétends point offencer Glauber, ny aucun de ceux qui mettent comme luy la main à la paste, ausquels plustost je voudrois donner courage [...] Il est sans doute le plus excellent ou le plus noble de tous' - Ibid., 80-1.

106 The exact date of Sorbière's visit is not known, but it was evidently some time before July 1660 (the date of his letter about it), so Glauber cannot have been over 56.

107 Serrarius to Hartlib, 3 Feb. 1662, HP 7/98/1B.

108 '[il] ne travaille plus, & n'a point de fourneaux' - Balthasar de Monconys, *Les Voyages de M. Monconys* II (Paris, 1695), 353, dated 28 Aug. 1663.

109 'nun mehr aber man dehren nicht länger von nöthen hat/ [...] den begehrenden gegen ein billiges überlassen werden' - *Glauberus Concentratus, oder Laboratorium Glauberianum* (Amsterdam, 1668).

110 Cf. Link, *Glauber*, 99, n.358. Link assesses the output of his last decade as representing 19 percent of the total in terms of number of pages.

111 *De Tribus Lapidibus*, 19.

112 *De Signatura Salium*, 13-15. Cf. Link, *Glauber*, 118-122, for a fuller discussion of Glauber's various notions of 'signatures' discernible not only in the physical makeup of things but in the words and symbols used to denote them.

113 *De Tribus Lapidibus*, 19.

114 Appelius to Hartlib, 7 June 1644, HP 45/1/6A.

115 Appelius to Hartlib, 16 Oct. 1641, HP 45/1/28A.

116 Moriaen to Hartlib, 30 March 1657, HP 42/2/5A, and see Link, *Glauber*, 178, and Bruckner, no. 232.

117 Moriaen to Hartlib, 15 Feb. 1658, HP 31/18/4B.

118 Sadler declared himself eager to meet Hartlib to discuss Glauber and other matters (4 Oct. 1648, HP 46/9/25A), and asked Hartlib to give him an extract of 'Glaubers 4th part' (probably of *Furni Novi*, possibly of *Miraculum Mundi* or *Pharmacoepia Spagyrica*: Glauber wrote nothing else in more than three parts) (n.d., HP 46/9/11A).

119 Kinner to Hartlib, 23 July 1648, HP 1/33/41A.

120 Child to Hartlib, 2 Feb. 1652, HP 15/5/18A.

121 Child to Hartlib, 29 Aug. 1652, HP 15/5/14A-15B.

122 Jenney to Hartlib, 29 Sept. 1657, HP 53/35/3A-4B, and Winthrop to Hartlib, 16 March 1660, HP 7/7/1A-8B.

123 Brun, for instance, charged that 'Gl in Metallicis hath transcribed the best things out of Erker his booke vom Berg-wercke [ie. Lazarus Ercker, *Beschreibung Allerfürnemisten Mineralischen Ertzt vnnd Bergwercks arten* (Prague, 1574)]. Hee excels only in der Scheide-kunst [*chemistry*]' (*Eph 48*, HP 31/22/8B). In fact, Glauber openly acknowledged in *Operis Mineralis* that he had taken a great deal from Ercker: cf. Link, *Glauber*, 51.

124 *Eph 54*, HP 29/4/27A.

125 *Eph 55*, HP 29/5/6B.

126 Moriaen to Hartlib, 25 March 1650,. HP 37/146B.

127 'A fundamentall & true Description how good tartar may be extracted out of wine-lees in greate quantitie. Found out, written & brought to light for *the* good of his Country By Iohn Rudolph Glaubers [*sic*] 1654'. The work has been split into three for some reason and occurs at HP 55/17/1A-4B, 16/1/85A-88B and 8/24/3A-14B in that order. These three fragments have not previously been recognised as forming a whole.

128 HP 31/8/1A-6B.

129 The title page gives 1651 as the date of publication, but each individual part is dated 1652 (cf. Link, *Glauber*, 247).

130 French, 'Preface' to *A Description of New Philosophical Furnaces* (London, 1651/2).

131 Besides a number of shorter works, he translated the entire text of and annotations to the 1637 Dutch Bible into English, and the first three books of *Paradise Lost* into German (cf. Barnett, *Theodore Haak* (The Hague, 1962) 71-5, 114-119, 168-86).

132 Moriaen to Hartlib, 7 Nov. 1641, HP 37/93A: 'wan H. Haak H. Paths [*sic*: Moriaen repeatedly made this mistake] subterraneal Treasure de agricultura Teutsch mach*en* vnd vbersend*en* wolte so würd Er sich vmb vnsere landsleuthe woll verdienen vnd H. Merian wills gern druckh*en*' ('if Mr. Haak wished to translate Mr. Plattes' *Subterraneal Treasure of Agriculture* into German and send it over, he would do a service to our countrymen, and Mr. Merian is eager to print it'). Moriaen was apparently confusing Plattes' *Subteranneal Treasure*, a treatise on mining and metallurgy which has nothing to do with agriculture, with his *Discovery of Hidden Treasure*.

133 *Eph 52*, HP 28/2/42B.

134 They came out either in 1651 or 1652 (see above, n. 129), and even if it was the very end of the latter, they could hardly have been translated and printed in less than a month.

135 Culpeper to Hartlib, 7 Sept. 1647, HP 13/186A. This can hardly refer to any other part of *Furni Novi*, as the second book had not yet been published even in German. Clucas is mistaken in assuming Culpeper to be the author of the partial English translation mentioned by French ('Correspondence of a XVII-Century "Chymicall Gentleman"' *Ambix* 40 (1993), 147-70, 168, n.59).

136 Culpeper to Hartlib, 11 March 1647. Culpeper, an idiosyncratic speller even by seventeenth-century standards, calls the other translator 'Pettit', but this (or 'Petit' or 'Petite') is how he refers to Petty in contexts where no one else can possibly be meant, eg. HP 13/225A (to Hartlib, 6 July 1648) on his 'Agricultural engine' and HP 8/31/1A (25 Jan. 1647) and 13/206A (22 Dec. 1647), both on his double writing and modifications to the inventions of Harrison.

137 Appelius to Hartlib, 26 Aug. 1647, HP 45/1/33A.

138 5? Aug. 1647, HP 13/182/5A; 7 Sept. 1647, HP 13/186A; 20 Oct. 1647, HP 13/196B.

139 5? Aug. 1647, HP 13/182/5A.

140 Appelius to Hartlib, 6 Nov. 1647, HP 45/1/37B.

141 The engravings are reproduced in F.S. Taylor and C.H. Josten, 'Johannes Banfi Hunyades 1576-1650', *Ambix* 5 (1953-6), 44-52, 44-6; cf. also the same authors' 'Supplementary Note' to the article, correcting some erroneous conjectures including the date of death, *Ambix* 5 (1953-6), 115. Jan Jonston mentioned him to Hartlib on 1 March 1633 as a mutual friend, clearly implying he was in London (HP 44/1/1A).

142 Dedication to Hunniades, dated 12 Dec. 1644, of *Anglicus, Peace, or no Peace* (London, 1645), cit. Taylor and Josten, 47.

143 Appelius to Hartlib, 22 April 1643, HP 45/1/45A.

144 Taylor and Josten, op. cit.

145 *Eph 40*, HP 30/4/51B, probably in the first half of the year.

146 'A Memoriall for the advancement of Vniversall Learning', HP 48/1/2A.

147 HP 47/15/2A-B.

148 HP 45/1/37A.

149 Moriaen to Hartlib, 27 Feb. 1648, HP 37/131A.

150 'ne nous fit point d'excuses de sa mauvaise latinité' - 'Drie Brieven van Samuel Sorbière', 81.

151 As is evident from his relations with Worsley: see below, p. 220.

152 *Eph 48*, HP 31/22/2A-B.

153 *Eph 56*, HP 29/5/92B: again, Boyle himself is given as the source.

154 Child to Hartlib, 2 Feb. 1652, HP 15/5/18A, and 8 April 1652, HP 15/5/10A.

155 Jenney to Hartlib, 29 Sept. 1657, HP 53/35/3A-4B.

156 Moriaen to Hartlib, 24 Aug. 1657, HP 42/2/19A.

157 Horn to Hartlib, 24 March 1649, HP 16/2/23A.

158 Culpeper to Hartlib, 1 Nov. 1648, HP 13/247A. Culpeper invoked Wheeler on several occasions as an archetype of the dishonest projector.

159 Culpeper to Hartlib, 14 Aug. 1649 HP 13/260A.

160 'Glauber, meine ich, thut grose sunde, das er solche Sachen andern zu lehren unterstehet, die er selbst nicht weis.' - Rasch to Hartlib, 25 July 1658, HP 26/89/19A.

161 Rasch to Hartlib, 26 Jan. 1656, HP 42/9/1A.

162 Probably the related *Tractatus de Signatura Salium*, which appeared the same year (1658).

163 'Auff der gleichen weiße hatt Er mich nun lange zeit vertröstet und auff die Spize des bergs Pisga gefuhret, ob nun noch einmal etwas daraus werden soll und was es guttes sein wird, daß er mitbringen will muß die zeit lehren, rechnung darff ich nicht mehr darauff machen, weil ich nun so offt und lang mich betrogen finde' - Moriaen to Hartlib, 26 May/5 June 1658, HP 31/18/28A.

164 Glauber to Moriaen, 2 (probably meaning 12) July 1658, quoted in a letter from Moriaen, HP 31/18/40A.

165 'ich vernehme noch zur zeit nichts davon mittler weil laufft die saatzeit mehrentheils fürüber' - Moriaen to Hartlib, 26 April 1658, HP 31/18/17B.

166 Moriaen to Hartlib, 23 July 1658, HP 31/18/42B.

167 'kombt noch etwas von ihm dz wird wunder sein, dan seines gleichen in unbeständigkeit seines furnehmens ist mir noch niemand fürkommen' - Moriaen to Hartlib, 5 June 1658, HP 31/18/28A.

168 Moriaen to Hartlib, July 1657, HP 42/2/14A.

169 Moriaen to Hartlib, 20 July 1659, HP 16/1/15A-16B.

170 'Der H wisse, dass H Morian itzt nicht mehr so viel von Glauber halte als vor diesem, den er überzeuget ist, dass das jenige gelbe metal, welches sein vermeintes aurum putabile [*sic*] gemachet, kein wahres golt, noch in allen proben bestehen könne, welchs mir ein vertrawter freundt gesagt, der dem H Morian solchs ex veris fundamentis demonstrirt, vnd H Morian ihm auch hat müssen recht geben' - Poleman to Hartlib, 17 Oct. 1659, HP 60/4/194A.

171 The letter is another plea for co-operation with the same quadrumvirate approached by Kretschmar in August 1659 (Hartlib, Clodius, Dury and Brereton: see above, pp. 161-2) and the style is not dissimilar. It survives only as a copy so the hand cannot be compared.

172 'Ich hoffe ich hab es mit Gott meistens recht, die Öfen hab ich auch wunderlich bekommen, vngeachtet er das Laboratorium feste zugeschloßen helt, nach dem sie nun gebawet sind, vnd keinen Menschen hinein lest. Es kostet mich alle mein armuth, vnd kan nun nichts mehr thun, als daß ichs ihnen hiermitt alles treulich offenbahre, vnd nochmahls umb Gottes willen bitte, es in höchster verschwiegenheit zu halten gegen iederman, sonderlich gegen H. Morian, daß ichs ihnen vbergeschrieben, vnd daß es ja Glauber nicht erfahre' - [Kretschmar?] to Hartlib, Dury, Clodius and Brereton, c. 1660, HP 31/23/30B.

173 *Glauberus Refutatus* (s.l., 1660).

174 *Sudum Philosophicum* (s.l., 1660). See Link, 106. The 'Autoris Anagramma' is 'Hai soo muß ich ja berechnen! was deß Glaubers Facit macht?' The first sentence is a perfect (if somewhat contrived) anagram of Iohannes Ioachimus Becher, and though

Link leaves the question open I do not think there can be much doubt of the ascription. There are several mentions of Becher in the Hartlib Papers, relating to his perpetual motion machine and 'new argonautical invention', but no direct reference to his controversy with Glauber. On Becher, see Partington, *History of Chemistry* II, 637-52.

175 *Gründliche Widerlegung etlicher Johan-Rudolff Glaubers zu Amsterdam herausgegebener Schrifften von Verbesserung der Metallen* (Leipzig, 1661). Fuller titles of this and the two texts mentioned above in Link, *Glauber*, 276-7.

176 'hat auch der filius Sendivogii dem Glaubero selbst grundlich [...] erwiesen, dz Er in vera Philosophia ein grosser Ignorant sey in seinem Ludo Philosophico, welches izt alhier gedruckt wird' - Poleman to Hartlib, 29 Aug. 1659, HP 60/4/111A. 'Ludo' is evidently a misreading by Hartlib (the extract is a copy in his hand) of 'Sudo': Hartlib was doubtless thinking of the Paracelsian 'ludus'. Cf. Poleman to Hartlib, 19 Sept. 1659, HP 60/10/2B, reporting that Hartprecht's work was shortly to be printed, and referring to a mention, presumably by Hartlib, of two others (obviously Becher and Montendon) who planned to write against Glauber.

177 Link, *Glauber* 106.

178 'Monsr Charle de Montendon von Yserton auß Saphaÿen, ietzt beÿ mir alhier sich aufhaltende' - HP 31/23/28A.

179 I owe this suggestion to Inge Keil.

180 'in Glauberi stinkenden vermeinten Alkahest sudelt vnd der gestalt darin sich vergriffen, dz es Ihme bey nahe sein leben gekostet' - Poleman to Hartlib, 15 Aug. 1659, HP 60/10/1A.

181 'eckelt mich auch der Glauberianischen betrugerey nun mehr zu gedencken' - Poleman to Hartlib, 6 Sept. 1659, HP 60/10/1B.

182 Poleman to Hartlib, 29 Aug. 1659, HP 60/4/111A.

183 'Was aber Glaubers grillen sein, ist solches warhaftig nicht werth, dz man doch nur eine viertel-stunde damit zubringe sich darin aufzuhalten, dan es lauter betrugerey vnd grosse-sprechereyen sein' - Poleman to Hartlib, 5 Sept. 1659, HP 60/10/1B.

184 'ich [habe] für meine person keine vrsache ihn für einen betrieger zu halten, sonsten veracht er andere, vnd andere verachten ihn, wie aller artisten gebrauch ist, da niemand nichts lobet als seine eigene wahre' - Appelius to Hartlib, 2 Aug. 1648, HP 45/1/39B.

185 Hartlib to Winthrop, 16 March 1660, HP 7/7/3B.

186 Ibid.

187 Poleman to Hartlib, 7 Nov. 1659, HP 60/4/190B.

188 'keine Arcana darin mit solchem klaren verstand begriffen, dz sie einiger mensch darauss solte machen können. Vnd dz ist die wahrhafftige wahrheit drumb man sie auch sicherlichen publiciren kan' - Poleman to Hartlib, 9 Jan. 1660, HP 60/4/191A.

189 'der vnbedachtsame Mann verrathet sich eben hiermit selbst: den so sein aurum potabile ein solch wunderthätig sache were, wie er es ausschreÿet, so dörffte er sich nicht bemühen um die Mineram cupri zu schmeltzen, vnd dieselbige für geldt aussszubieten' - Poleman to Hartlib, 17 Oct. 1659, HP 60/4/194A.

CHAPTER SEVEN

The Dawn of Wisdom

'spero [...] ut Lux oboriatur mundo tam in naturalibus quàm divinis: ita auroram jam videre mihi videor' ('I hope light will rise on the world, as well in things natural as in things divine: indeed it seems to me I can already see the dawn') - Moriaen to Benjamin Worsley, 19 May 1651, HP 9/16/5A.

Benjamin Worsley's Alchemical Mission to the Netherlands

This chapter traces the personal collaboration of a small group within the Hartlib circle on a quest to attain spiritual enlightenment through practical experiment. It is the story of an entirely serious attempt to master the techniques of transmuting metals. As such, it shows just how seriously these thinkers were committed to the idea that the physical world is not so much the object as the medium of human perception rightly understood. All the preconceptions and preoccupations discussed in the foregoing chapters come to the fore in this episode, this attempt to open the 'gate of things' and gain a view of a reality beyond the material. The correspondence between the protagonists, their reflections on the undertaking and their reaction to its ultimate and inevitable failure, supply a great many insights into their understanding of the relationship between matter and spirit, of the operation of God in the created world, and of the nature and function of knowledge itself.

In 1647, at the same time Hartlib was canvassing the possibiliy of bringing Glauber to England to teach chemistry, Benjamin Worsley[1] was preparing for a visit to the Netherlands. Little has previously been established about the nature and purpose of this expedition, which lasted from the beginning of January 1648 to autumn 1649.[2] Hartlib's papers reveal much, though by no means everything, about the undertaking. The main prize Worsley hoped to bring home with him was a detailed knowledge of Glauber's chemical equipment and operations, though there was a good deal else on his agenda besides. The idea of recruiting Glauber for Gresham College perhaps reflected a hope of obviating the need for this, but if Glauber would not come to England, England would have to send to Glauber.

From at least August 1647, Hartlib was busy assessing the prospects for such an expedition, sending specific queries to Moriaen and Appelius, his principal sources on Glauber.[3] Moriaen promised to arrange an introduction, which he was confident would prove useful.[4] Appelius considered that Glauber would probably be prepared to put Worsley up during his stay.[5] Both pointed out that there was no chance of obtaining anything from Glauber unless he were offered a suitable financial recompense. Appelius thought £100 (roughly the sum he and his friend had paid some years earlier) would be enough.[6] Moriaen was somewhat more emphatic about this point, though given Glauber's reputation, it was advice which can hardly have come as much of a surprise.

This prerequisite was to be supplied by, or by means of, Cheney Culpeper, who had already pledged his support for the Office of Address scheme, and whose imagination had been fired by his labours on the translation of *Furni Novi Philosophici*. Culpeper was

> soe muche taken, with very many of his [Glauber's] ingenuities, that (yf Mr Worsley will take soe much trouble vpon him,) as (in the trade of soe much ingenuity and knowledge) to become the Factor, & to goe ouer to Glauberus, & to purchase his ingenuities of him), I shall willingly become a marchante venturer in the busines, & shall be glad to finde others to that number, as that the voyage may be vnder taken.[7]

Worsley (c.1618-1677) was evidently a man of considerable charm, with an acute brain and eclectic imagination. Together with Boyle, he was a prime mover of the 'Invisible College' in the 1640s.[8] Had he become a member of the Royal Society, his writings would probably have attracted a great deal more attention and respect than they have.[9] His 'Physico-Astrologicall Letter', for instance, was until recently misattributed to Robert Boyle, among whose papers it was found after his death.[10]

Biographical details are scarce, and a fuller investigation of his life and thought would present a very interesting and valuable field of study. He appears in the *DNB* only by default, as the incompetent Surveyor of Ireland replaced by the much more efficient William Petty in 1658, in the teeth of support for Worsley from 'the fanatical or Anabaptist section of the army'.[11] Hartlib's papers present a rather more appealing picture both of the man and his abilities. He was probably Hartlib's personal favourite among all his many associates, certainly among those of the younger generation. Though Hartlib was never stinting of praise where he thought it due, his comments on Worsley are exceptionally warm. He used him as a yardstick of personal merit: long before any enmity between Worsley and Petty had arisen, Hartlib described the latter to Boyle as a fine linguist, very learned and 'of a sweet natural disposition and moral comportment', but for all that 'not altogether a very dear *Worsley*'.[12] He was proud to tell Boyle that this 'noble and high soaring spirit'[13] had 'resolved, for time to come, to look upon me no more as a private friend, but as a father'. Hartlib accordingly took to referring to him as 'my philosophical son'.[14] Boyle too obviously entertained the warmest affection for him.[15]

Worsley's formal education seems to have been limited, if not so severely as Glauber's. The clearest indication of his lack of a scholarly background is supplied by the shortcomings of his Latin. In a letter almost certainly to Worsley, Moriaen apologised for not being able to translate a message from Glauber into English,[16] and later clearly indicated that he felt obliged to write English to Worsley: 'May he [Worsley] excuse me for not writing to him in person; I cannot write English so readily'.[17] Again in 1657, Moriaen apologised for not being able satisfactorily to translate a German enclosure for Worsley, and asked Hartlib to do so.[18] Since there is no question of Moriaen's competence in Latin, this can only mean that Worsley did not understand the language well. The ten letters from Moriaen to Worsley which are in Latin, all dating from 1651,[19] were presumably intended to be translated by someone for the recipient. It is clear that Worsley replied in English.[20]

This social and scholarly disadvantage did not prevent Worsley from becoming an autodidact of some distinction. He was also something of an entrepreneur. In the mid-1640s, when his association with Hartlib began, he was busy promoting a scheme for producing saltpetre by a method more profitable and less inconvenient than the usual[21] - an interest Glauber strongly shared. In about 1640 or 41 he had been an army surgeon in Ireland, and he was studying medicine in 1647,[22] but though he later took to calling himself 'Dr Worsley', it seems he never obtained a degree.[23] In August 1649, shortly before his return from the Netherlands, he announced that he was thinking of giving up formal study. He envisaged instead going out to Virginia to help establish new plantations there or improve existing ones. Alternatively, he hoped to obtain some public office in Britain or Ireland through the influence of Dury, Hartlib, Culpeper and Sadler.[24] This plan bore fruit. It was almost certainly on Hartlib's recommendation that he was appointed Secretary to the short-lived Council of Trade (1650-51), following which he spent most of the rest of his life in a succession of other official secretarial and administrative posts related to trade and economics.[25]

Worsley's mission to the Netherlands ran into difficulties before it had even started. On 17 November 1647, Culpeper withdrew his offers of support both for Hartlib's Office of Address and Worsley's Dutch expedition. As a result of a family quarrel arising from Culpeper's support of the Parliamentary faction, he had been largely dispossessed, and was not in a position to contribute as he had hoped.[26] Nevertheless, Worsley set out, in December 1647 or January 1648, in a Micàwberish trust that funds would somehow materialise in the course of the journey. Culpeper, perhaps feeling a little embarrassed, remarked in March that 'I am extremely sorry for Mr Woorsly whome (to deale freely with you) I must judge somewhat erroneous, that wowlde not see him selfe well bottomed before hee vndertooke his journy. For my selfe I continue in my late condition'.[27]

Worsley was certainly well supplied with an assortment of commissions, and received more during his stay, but whether he was being paid for them is not clear. His first task was to try to find out what had become of the drainage mill William Wheeler had been granted a Dutch patent for in 1639. Dorothy Dury, who was thinking of taking up the production of 'cordiall waters', wanted an account of the distilling techniques practised in the Netherlands, and Worsley duly sent her (via Hartlib) a long and detailed account of various processes.[28] For her husband he investigated the charges made by Menasseh ben Israel for the productions of his Hebrew press in Amsterdam and the theory being put about in Menasseh's and Serrarius's circles that the native Americans were the lost tribes of Israel.[29] He also promised to supply intelligence to Robert Child, though exactly what about is unclear.[30] But he did not forget the principal object of the exercise: 'The next opportunity I send once more to Glauberus, and then I shall be able to give you a more full account of things'.[31] At the bottom of his copy of a letter from Dury to Worsley, Hartlib scribbled a quotation from Isaiah 60:17 which is very suggestive of the hopes invested in Worsley's intelligence-gathering expedition: 'For brasse j will bring gold, and for iron j will bring silver, and for wood brasse and for stones iron'.[32]

Worsley reached Amsterdam on 25 February 1648, having been in the Netherlands about a month and a half, and made his first personal contact with

Moriaen.[33]   Here another disappointment was in store, for Glauber had written - presumably from Arnhem - to declare himself unwilling to put Worsley up in his house, as Helena Glauber was again in childbed, and Glauber himself was taken up twenty-four hours a day with a new experiment. Worsley found this very demoralising, and it would seem to have discouraged him from proceeding to Arnhem, though Glauber had offered to find him other accommodation there. At the end of May he was still with Moriaen in Amsterdam, experimenting on some exotic seeds supplied from America through the agency of Hartlib.[34] Moriaen was especially concerned about the language barrier, highlighting again that neither Glauber nor Worsley had a very good command of Latin:

> Glauber understands Latin if it is pronounced in the German manner, but he will not want to speak Latin: this will dampen his spirits and make him unwilling to converse.[35]

The prospects for technical and scholarly communication can hardly have looked bright.

Moriaen did his best to keep Worsley's spirits up and to help him find his feet in Amsterdam, just as he had earlier done for Rittangel and Pell, and this time with rather more success. Language problems notwithstanding (they presumably communicated in English, in which Moriaen was less than comfortable), the two became good friends. Brun, after his visit to Amsterdam the following year, reported: 'I hear that he [Moriaen] thinks very highly of Mr Worsley and lets him walk at his right hand', adding darkly and somewhat mysteriously,

> which is not well looked upon by many, and indeed not without reason, for Herr Moriaen is a man of a goodly age, and expert in many arts and sciences.[36]

What impropriety was seen in this age gap (about twenty-six or twenty-seven years) is unclear. The implication is perhaps that Worsley was suspected of trying to obtain the older and presumably frailer man's hard-won secrets by coercion or deception. As will become apparent, Moriaen did indeed later come to believe that Worsley was guilty of giving rather less than he gained in their alchemical exchanges.

Appelius, who was living nearby in Purmerent at the time, spoke in May of unspecified 'hinderances' to Worsley's undertaking,[37] and at the beginning of August sent a more detailed and not very encouraging report of his doings (though making it clear that by this time he had at least met Glauber, who by this stage had returned to Amsterdam):

> Mr Worsley's business proceeds slowly: Glauber does not appreciate that the time and expense is a burden on him; they waste much time on compliments and do not say roundly what they want or how they want it, in what way or manner a thing is to be agreed or accepted; many fear that Glauber will be unable to fulfil his side of the agreement.[38]

Some sort of negotiations were clearly in progress, and some suggestion will be given below of what they were about, but the details remain vague and uncertain. Most regrettably, hardly any letters survive from the whole period of the Dutch trip from either of the two men who were in a position to shed most light on such matters, Worsley himself and Moriaen.

Whatever the hindrances Worsley had to overcome, Culpeper was delighted to find him 'very intentiue in frawghtinge himselfe with riche ladinge', having been sent (through Hartlib) details of a 'very pretty' experiment relating to one of his favourite topics, the 'nature & vse of cold'.[39] Culpeper went on: 'yf hee meete with more in that nature, hee shall muche oblige me by them', and added once again that if he could bring his financial affairs into order he would willingly 'venter a share' in the enterprise.[40] At the end of July, though still prevaricating about the question of money to be supplied by him (apparently another source of funding had been secured by Hartlib[41]), he was eagerly hoping 'that Mr Woorsly wowlde make himselfe *master* of all Glauberus his furnaces'.[42]

Glauber, however, was very far from being Worsley's only new contact in the Netherlands. Kuffler and his wife visited Amsterdam in the summer of 1648, and were introduced to Worsley by Moriaen.[43] Culpeper thanked Worsley for communicating 'Dr Kuffler's wife's experiments, especially concerning harty chocks [artichokes]'.[44] Worsley also discussed schemes for draining the English fens with various Dutchmen, principally Moriaen's 'cousin' Jacob Pergens.[45] Dutch achievements in land reclamation were the envy of the world, and even the standard anti-Dutch topos that the Netherlands were only a bog that ought by rights to be under water reveals a grudging admiration.[46] Worsley had hopes of persuading Pergens and his friends to invest both money and expertise in the fens, but met once again with a dispiriting response. Pergens promised to spread word of the suggestion, but warned that uncertainty about or antipathy to the new regime in England was likely to discourage Dutch investors, and moreover 'many of the cheife of the Dutch, and of his owne freinds, had beene themselves dreyned by having a hand in our fenns already'.[47]

The inventor Caspar Kalthof was in Amsterdam at the same time, intending to demonstrate one of his perpetual motion machines,[48] and Worsley made his acquaintance too. The device was burned down the night before the planned demonstration - by 'the dutch boores [i.e. peasants]', according to Worsley's report, though Brun (who was something of a gossip) relayed a rumour that Kalthof had set fire to it himself, having realised it would not live up to his claims.[49] Worsley put Kalthof in touch with Petty, who planned to collaborate with him on a mine drainage scheme, or so at least Worsley thought.[50] In view of their later bitter dispute, there is a rather sad irony in Worsley's fervent admiration at this juncture for Petty, whom he apparently saw as an exemplar of the 'free and generous communication of secrets' that was the whole Hartlib circle's ostensible goal:

> you could not [...] easily haue given mee greater cause, passionatly to loue you, then you haue in that generous offer of yours, to conjoine your enedeauors with Mr Kalthofs [...] there being nothing amongst great or peeral witts, more frequent, tho nothing lesse manly, then æmulation,

> envy and detraction [...] and consequently nothing more rare or to bee
> admired then to find the contrary disposition.[51]

In fact there is some doubt as to whether Petty ever really did intend to
'conjoin his endeavours' with Kalthof, and was not merely, à la Clodius,
taking advantage of the other man's research to further his own. At least four
months before Worsley's letter, Hartlib had noted that Petty 'will also within a
few day's perfect Kalthof's Invention and will now not joine with him'.[52] In
April or May the same year, so still before Worsley's letter, Petty was
apparently convinced that

> Kalthof will finde himself deceived as to this application or vse. Hee
> [Petty] conceives that hee can doe more in his way then Kalthof himself
> [...] as himself [Kalthof] shall bee made sensible of by his owne letter to
> him, which hee sends enclosed in Mr Worslys.[53]

There was some disparity, it would seem, between what Petty was telling
Hartlib and what he was telling Worsley. At all events, no such collaboration
ever did take place.

Worsley was particularly taken with the productions of the mechanic
Fromantil or Fremantil, especially his microscopes.[54] These were a revelation
to Worsley, unveiling to him an unimagined diversity in created matter. Far
from confirming micro-macrocosm analogies, they brought home to him the
individuality and disparity of the component parts of Creation:

> wee may say not every man only but evey [sic] beast or fowle of the
> same, species, yea, every sand is knowne by its name [...] I beleeve it
> would imploy many yeares, & fill a good volume, to discover to the
> world this little Atlantis, or Vnknowne part of the Creation, hitherto not
> well looked after by Any.[55]

This moved Worsley to take up lens-grinding himself (probably with help and
encouragement from Moriaen), and to declare 'Optikes' to rank alongside
'Chymia' as the most excellent branch of knowledge available to man. This
passionate interest in optics remained with him for the rest of his life, and after
his return to England, he became one of the best customers for the telescopes
and microscopes of Wiesel sent into England by Moriaen.

From these musings, Worsley proceeded directly to declare that he had
'abdicated much reading of Bookes, vulgare received Traditions & common
or Schoole opinions', and had 'divided knowledge into Divine & humane'.[56]
It is highly suggestive of the intellectual and cultural climate in which
Worsley's thought had been formed that he could so brashly suppose the idea
of distinguishing secular from divine knowledge to be an original one, when
Comenius a decade earlier had been taken to task precisely for failing (or
refusing) to make such a distinction. He believed no other 'divine'
knowledge to be

> the necessary Rule of fayth but what the spiritt of god hath sett doune
> plainely, in symple & univocall tearmes & easy to the understanding of
> any, looking vpon all poynts controverted, as the opinions but at best, if
> not the Inventions & pryde of men [...] thinking it no shame to be

ignorant of many places of Scripture I meane the infallible sensce of them.[57]

Such an attitude effectively declared comprehensive exegetical methods such as Dury's *Analysis Demonstrativa* wholly redundant. But neither was Worsley prepared to admit the other radical Evangelical standby of personal revelation as a certain means of Scriptural illumination: if it were, he pointed out, 'wee should have no difference of opinion among good men, which we see to *the* contrary'.[58] Indeed, on the face of it, this seems like a complete rejection of the sort of chemico-religious enlightenment that was the hallmark of the 'Chemical Philosophy'. The impression could be given of Worsley as moving towards a wholly areligious conception of experimental learning. It is quite clear that, having established 'his' division of knowledge, he himself was a good deal more interested in the 'human' than the 'divine' department. But it would be a mistake to view Worsley's philosophy through the filter of eighteenth-century rationalism. It was certainly not his intention to dismiss God from the laboratory altogether.

In a much later letter, probably to Hartlib, on 'Vniversal Learning', Worsley asserted the interdependence of all subjects, singling out the disciplines of astrology, medicine, chemistry and divinity.[59] All four, he insisted, were bound up with each other, and no one of them could properly be understood without reference to the others, especially the fourth. Worsley was far from dismissing human knowledge as a means of gaining insight into the work and the ways of God, and was still firmly committed to the pansophic notion that all disciplines are interrelated, and that all are ultimately comprehended within the study of divinity in the broadest sense. He still saw all learning, as Comenius did, as a means to raise men's minds to the contemplation of God. In the same letter about the microscopes in which he proclaimed the division of human and divine knowledge, he also affirmed that this discovery of infinite variety in the microscopic world 'more setts out the immensity of the wisedome of God then any other, & proves that nothing was done by chance or occasion'.[60]

The 'divine learning' that Worsley wanted to distinguish and exclude from his physical, chemical and astrological studies was not divinity in its broadest sense, but the specific discipline of Scriptural exegesis. All his somewhat dismissive comments on 'divine learning' refer to the interpretation of the Bible, not to the understanding of God. Indeed, he very much implied that the understanding of God would be a good deal better promoted by the study of Nature than that of Scripture, with all its ambiguities and obscurities. Worsley's thought had already been developing in this direction for some time. The earnest young student John Hall, whom Hartlib cultivated as a contact at Cambridge and put in touch with Worsley, early in 1647 expressed to the latter his doubts concerning the question 'Whether the Scripture bee an adequate Iudge of Physical Controversies or no?'[61] Hall was frank about the derivativeness of his thoughts on this subject. The case against is that Scripture 'dos expresse some th*ings* contrary to the received Tenents of Nature' and is consequently, in such cases, interpreted by 'Men of great Authoritie' as being merely figurative. The arguments in favour are that, as Comenius points out in the 'Preface' to his *Physica*, 'Man can but teach one thing at a time G*od* who is infinit all th*ings* at once', and that Moses' description of Creation 'questionles hath an End meant by the Holy Spirit'. Clearly conditioned to favour faith over reason, Hall found the latter view more convincing, but still had reservations.

What is interesting about this document, and makes it illustrative of the intellectual climate of the times and of the conceptual problems facing the promoters of 'experimental philosophy', is not the rather flimsy argumentation put forward for either side, but the fact that a young scholar such as Hall, evidently struggling to establish his own intellectual orientation, saw this as a crucial point to be determined. It is significant too that Hartlib obviously thought the exchange worth preserving and (presumably) distributing: two copies each of Hall's letter and Worsley's reply are preserved in his papers.[62] Worsley's substantial and considered response also testifies to the seriousness with which he took the question, and contains arguments of rather more intrinsic interest. It would be presumptuous, Worsley opined, 'to affirme what primitive or materiall Truths the Scripture conteineth not',[63] but it was already quite clear to him that, with regard at least to 'Physical Controversies', any such truths were expressed in Scripture in a manner that mankind in its fallen state was not capable of comprehending. Indeed, in an intriguing insight into a Protestant scholar's idea of Heaven, he envisaged Biblical study as a feature of the afterlife, suggesting that 'it is not absurd to thinke. It shall be part as well of our happinesse, as of our imployment in the other lyfe, to find that in it [Scripture], which the whole Ages of the world came short of discovering'.[64]

In the meantime, however, humankind was thrown back on its own resources of practical observation and experiment to supply those revelations about the nature of things that in holy writ were couched too obscurely, if at all, for mere mortals to comprehend. He neatly turned the literalist argument on its head, suggesting that the sin of presumption lay not with those who preferred the evidence of their merely human senses above the divine authority of Scripture, but with those who preferred their merely human interpretation of Scripture above the evidence of their God-given senses:

> if any upon a probable phrase of scripture, shall build an axiome in physickes without thinking himselfe afterwards obleiged (for the satisfaction of others) to hold strictly a Correspondency with the rules and lawes of Reason, and experience. I should not conceive my selfe tyed, by any any rule or law in Scripture, to believe or give creditt to his Assertion: neither should I confound his allegation of Scripture, with the authority of Scripture, where any evidence of Reason or demonstration from experience did oppose him. As apprehending it much more safe, to bend the words of Scripture to truth, then to writhe truth so, as it may speake to such or such a sense of Scripture. For truth will ever, admirably cleere, open, and illustrate Scripture, whereas the Scripture it selfe, very oft, concealeth what Truth that is, it conteineth.[65]

All this is very reminiscent of the argumentation 'by the light of Nature' that Moriaen commended in Adam Boreel - who was another new contact Worsley made in Amsterdam, presumably through Moriaen.[66] The remarks on Scriptural exegesis are very similar to Moriaen's repeated insistence that to commit oneself to a particular elucidation of any point of detail, or to expect such commitment from others, could only lead to schism and dissent, whereas freedom of conscience encouraged fraternity and union. While it should be stressed that Worsley is dealing only with 'Physical Controversies', and not with moral precepts, prophecies or divine matters, his argument goes a stage further, bringing out what is at most only implicit in Moriaen's and Boreel's stance. The light of Nature is to be used not only to demonstrate but actually to interpret Scriptural truth. What Worsley was effectively saying was that, at least as far as our current imperfect condition goes, Scripture is ambiguous, that it may be necessary to 'bend the words of Scripture to truth'.

Worsley had plenty to keep him occupied, then, but the principal object of the exercise, the investigation of Glauber's laboratory and techniques, does not seem to have been achieved until Worsley had been in the country for nearly a year and a half. On 11 June 1649, however, Moriaen wrote that he and Worsley were at long last preparing 'to set to work with Herr Glauber on this and that, that Mr Worsley may not have come over in vain or expended so much time to no purpose'.[67]

Worsley's attitude to the project was highly ambivalent and changeable. At the beginning of July 1649, he had 'no heart at all to come over' to England, evidently seeing brighter prospects in the Netherlands, unless he could be found 'a place or settled imployment in England'.[68] So at least he told Hartlib: the following month he flatly contradicted this in a letter to Dury, declaring that 'For my Coming over/ As to my naturall Appetite, It is there already;/ This place not perfectly agreeing with my health, & as little, or lesse, with my affection'.[69] However, his hopes were rising of a profitable outcome from the Dutch venture: 'some thing is <still> further <expected> in our metallicke Busynesse; which if I may speake my owne thoughts in/ I lesse despayre about than ever/'.[70]

It is not at all clear when Worsley finally did leave the United Provinces. By the middle of August 1649, both Dury and Culpeper were expecting him any day,[71] and according to Appelius, he had already left, or was about to, by late September, in a state of high dudgeon:

> Mr Worsley is returning home. I cannot say how perplexed I am as to why Glauber has held him up for so long and yet now lets him return home empty-handed after the expense of so much time and money. Glauber repeats that it is not so much his fault as Mr Worsley's, and yet they do not understand one another; it amazes me that Glauber judges so harshly of him, having shown himself so resolute and generous towards him at the outset.[72]

Yet a month later, Henry More was still speaking of his arrival in England in the future tense.[73] Perhaps he had left Amsterdam but was engaged on other business on the Continent.[74] What is clear, however, is that he and Glauber parted on very bad terms. The following March, Moriaen sent over something he described as Glauber's 'declaration', evidently a proposal of some sort, but Worsley was no longer interested: 'I thought to delight him [Worsley] greatly with Herr Glauber's proposal, but it has all turned out wrong; he [Worsley] has formed such a bad opinion of him that he puts the worst possible interpretation on everything'.[75] In his usual even-handed way, Moriaen tried to act as peacemaker, at once blaming Glauber's coarse and overly forthright manner and Worsley's melancholy and over-sensitivity for the falling out. He also tried to clarify the terms of the offer, which he thought Worsley had misunderstood.[76] His intervention seems to have mollified Worsley sufficiently for him to respond offering his own terms for the proposed deal, since the next month Moriaen wrote that Glauber was willing to accept Worsley's conditions.[77]

This proposal or 'declaration' sent by Glauber via Moriaen to Worsley was, I believe, an offer to reveal a process of extracting gold from tin scoria (i.e. the residue of the ore after tin has been extracted from it). This is described in the usual vague terms in a document attributed to Glauber and preserved in Hartlib's papers, which sets the charge for a full revelation at 2000 ducats (in the region of £1400). Together with it is an account of another method of extracting silver and gold, this time from lead ore, valued at 1000 ducats. This document is presented in Appendix Three. The strongest evidence that this is indeed the project under discussion is Moriaen's remark in his letter accompanying the proposal, 'you may consider if this will serve the Commonwealth of England as I hope it will. For a great store of this matter of Tin must needs be there to no vse at all'.[78]

It was at just this time that Glauber made his abrupt departure from Amsterdam to escape his creditors, and, temporarily abandoning his wife and children, disappeared into Germany. It may well be that this strategic withdrawal was financed by the sale of this secret to a small alchemical consortium including Moriaen, Worsley, Johann Sibertus Kuffler and a very shadowy figure going by the suggestive name of 'Aurifaber' ('Goldmaker'). For in 1651, despite being in two different countries, these four were engaged collaboratively on a variety of ambitious projects to transmute metal, including this very process, the extraction of gold from tin.

Moriaen and the 'Great Work'

Moriaen and Worsley had almost certainly come to an agreement, either formally or informally, to pursue the 'metallicke Busynesse' in their separate countries after Worsley's return to England, and to pool the results of their experiments. Ten letters from Moriaen to Worsley, dating from 1651, deal almost exclusively with alchemical experimentation, and feature detailed accounts of the work Moriaen was engaged on and repeated requests for information and materials from Worsley. Among the materials requested, there is specific mention of English tin scoria.[79] The letters are an excellent example of how linguistically precise alchemists could be, when it suited them, in their private correspondence. Here are no dragons, white doves of Diana or black crows' bills: substances are named by their names, quantities specified, processes described in detail and the type and intensity of heat required specified as accurately as possible. The only limitation on full and clear communication is that imposed by language itself, by the boundaries of the experimenter's own knowledge and the capacity of contemporary instruments to give precise readings - limitations, of course, that apply to the scientific discourse of any period.

Moriaen was himself conscious of the linguistic limitations he was confronted with. He promised to explain an operation to Worsley 'insofar as this can be done in writing, for indeed the greatest part of its explanation lies in method and manual dexterity'.[80] Describing one of his transmutational projects, he repeatedly stressed the need to obtain the 'right sort' of ore as a raw material, a goal he attained only by oral communication concerning 'the place, yea the very mine (for in one and the same place there are different sorts) in which the right sort of antimonial mineral, suitable for our work, is to be found'.[81] Given the tone of the rest of the letter, it is highly unlikely Moriaen would have concealed the exact nature of this mineral from Worsley if he had himself known what it was and been able to express it. Like Clodius when enquiring 'what sort' of silver Kretschmar was making gold from,[82] Moriaen had the technical knowledge to discern a difference between two similar substances, but lacked the vocabulary to define it.

Glauber was back in Germany by this point, making alcahest, aurum potabile and artificial wine in Wertheim. Moriaen's main collaborators in Amsterdam were Kuffler (who paid regular visits from Arnhem to take part in the experiments) and the mysterious 'Aurifaber'. This is a somewhat surprising pseudonym for an alchemist, given that its German translation 'Goldmacher' was a stock term of derision for mercenary or false adepts, but perhaps the pejorative connotations were deemed to be expunged by use of the more dignified Classical tongue. Another figure who was originally intended to feature in the business was Moriaen's brother-in-law Peter von Zeuel, from whom he received the vital information about where to obtain the mineral, but von Zeuel died in 1651 shortly after passing on this piece of knowledge.[83]

Very little is known of 'Aurifaber' except that he lived in Amsterdam and was rich. Besides mentions in Moriaen's letters, there are only three references to him in Hartlib's papers, all from the *Ephemerides* of 1650 and 1651, and all citing Worsley as informant. Worsley was evidently rather more impressed by him than by Glauber: 'The Aurifaber at Amst*erdam* is the best mechanical man that ever hee [Worsley] met withal i.e. purely mettalical'.[84] According to another entry, his real name was 'Gralle',[85] but this appears to be a mistake by either Worsley or (more probably) Hartlib. 'Aurifaber' was the Antony Grill whom Moriaen twice mentioned by name,[86] and from whom Moriaen sent an extract on Swedish copper mines for Worsley.[87] The identification occurs in a letter from Moriaen to Worsley describing the two processes being used in the tin experiment: 'one [way] we will call Kufflerian, the other Grillian' ('Unam Kufflerianam, alteram Grillianam appellabim*us*'). After a long account of Kuffler's method, he then proceeded to 'the other way, which is Aurifaber's' ('Altera qu*æ* est Aurifabri via').[88] However, nothing else whatsoever seems to be known about this Antony Grill.

Moriaen was highly impatient to receive, in return for the extensive reports he was sending, details of an experiment Worsley and an unnamed nobleman ('nobilis') had conducted to fuse gold and mercury indissolubly. Moriaen also wanted some of the materials sent to him. It is not possible to identify this 'nobleman' conclusively. Culpeper is an unlikely candidate: it is very doubtful whether his imaginative enthusiasm for alchemical theory was matched by his practical expertise, as also whether he had access to the material resources necessary to carry out many of the processes mentioned. Worsley's collaborator apparently knew more even than the forty-two medical preparations of antimony Moriaen himself laid claim to.[89] A more likely suggestion is Brereton, or Worsley's close friend Boyle. But another possibility is that there was a misunderstanding, and that Worsley had employed some such formulation as 'noble spirit', which Moriaen had taken to mean someone of noble birth. If this was indeed the case, the American alchemist George Starkey, though he was not nobly born, becomes a candidate. William Newman, the leading expert on Starkey, concludes that there was little or no contact between Moriaen and Starkey beyond one letter from the latter, but he was not aware of the references to this mysterious 'nobleman'. I would stress, however, that the suggestion is purely speculative. But even if Starkey was not himself directly involved in the project, he certainly supplied part at least of the inspiration for it.

Starkey had come to London in 1650 and been welcomed into the Hartlibian fold, and in 1651 was working as Boyle's assistant-cum-collaborator.[90] Just eleven days after Moriaen's first reference to this 'nobleman',[91] Starkey was persuaded by the circle to contact Moriaen with a view to the pooling of their antimonial wisdom.

Starkey made his overture to Moriaen on 30 May 1651, in a long and florid Latin letter which represents an early stage in Starkey's elaborate programme of self-mythologisation.[92] Reworking a legend current in alchemical circles about the early seventeenth-century magus Michael Sendivogius (one of Culpeper's favourite authors), Starkey portrayed himself as an eager student of the hermetic art and the disciple of an unnamed 'Cosmopolite' he had known in America, from whom he had received a number of priceless manuscripts and a small quantity of the true elixir. Starkey, however, had squandered this through his incomplete knowledge of the processes to be applied to it, and found himself plunged into poverty.

Starkey related this story to many correspondents besides Moriaen, and also in his published works. The myth went through various refinements between 1651 and 1654, with the 'Cosmopolite' fading gradually into a mysterious distance and becoming the author of works that were in fact by Starkey himself, principally *George Riplye's Epistle to King Edward Unfolded* and *Introitus Apertus ad Occlusum Regis Palatinum*. This strategy offered a number of advantages: it conferred great value and authority on the manuscripts, while at the same time relieving Starkey himself of the onus of actually performing everything he claimed was possible. Yet it also recommended him as an initiate who had progressed a good way down the path of wisdom, and deserved support and patronage to enable him to complete the journey. As Newman puts it, he perhaps 'realised that it was far too uncomfortable to *be* an adept, and just as useful to have one for a friend'.[93] So successful was Starkey's self-projection that not only were Hartlib and his friends completely taken in, but attempts to identify the 'Cosmopolite' continued until 1990 when he was finally established as Starkey's fictional creation, and his works as Starkey's own.[94]

Starkey's letter to Moriaen retails the story of the lost elixir in some detail, and also speaks of some 'sophic mercury' given him by the fictitious adept, who at this early stage appears in relatively concrete guise as 'a certain young friend, still living'.[95] This too he lost in an unsuccessful attempt at 'multiplying' it. 'Aflame with desire of imitating that mercury', Starkey had subsequently succeeded, after great expense of time, money and pains, in extracting from antimony something he was not confident to call true sophic mercury, but which came very close to it. By means of this he had further produced 'the mercury of life of the great Paracelsus' ('*mercurij* vitæ

Paracelsis magni'), with which he could cure gout, consumption, paralysis and other supposedly incurable diseases.[96] Though no specific terms are mentioned, the general aim of this extremely obscure and convoluted letter was plainly to arouse Moriaen's interest in a collaboration or trade of alchemical lore, for by this juncture, Moriaen and his associates in Amsterdam had added to their projects the transmutation of antimony, the very substance that was supposed to be the source of Starkey's 'sophic mercury'. In 1651, probably in late April or early May, so just before Starkey sent Moriaen his letter, Hartlib noted that

> Mr Dury saw Stirky really to extract silver out of Antimony, which was in weight equal to Gold, and out of Iron Gold of a most high colour as your Rosenobles are. Hee may easily make of it 300. lib. a year. Mr Dury.
> Worsley, Morian and Aurifaber vndertake to turne that Antimonial silver into Gold. Also to extract Gold out of Tinne (for which they have set up their great Work) and Gold out of Iron in great quantity. [...]
> Stirke is now pidling and toiling for smal quantities, wheras if hee joine, hee cannot but bee a vast gainer by them. Worsly.[97]

Moriaen was obviously impressed by Starkey's approach. From this point on, antimony rather than tin became his favourite subject, and it was from this project that he hoped for the greatest rewards. On 30 June, in the first letter he sent after receiving Starkey's, he specifically mentioned that 'the other work concerning tin' ('alterum opus [...] ex Iove') was also proceeding successfully, but that he was so taken up with his work on antimony that he barely had time to attend to it.[98] It seems likely that the 'right sort' of antimony he had at last obtained did indeed contain traces of gold, for Moriaen was entirely certain he was extracting gold at the rate of one pound per hundredweight, and that once he had learned to 'lead the material on to greater maturity' ('si materia [...] ad majorem maturitatem perducatur'), the yield would be greatly increased.[99] In June and July, Moriaen was positively ecstatic about his success in transmuting metals, particuary antimony, and even more excited about the prospect of revelations from Worsley concerning mercury, which may relate to the 'sophic mercury' of Starkey.[100]

No letters from Moriaen to Starkey survive, but he wrote effusively to Worsley about the new contact, lauding Starkey's exceptional learning and generosity, hoping he would prove himself worthy of such a contact, and telling Worsley that he would 'have a poor nose indeed if he could not smell the recommendations of his friends' behind this desire on Starkey's part to take him into his confidence.[101] This was not in fact particularly perceptive of him, since Starkey had specifically told him it was Worsley who had brought Moriaen's 'truly heroic virtues' to his attention.[102] However, Moriaen rather pointedly added that the reward Worsley could expect from communicating his secrets would be the satisfaction of helping Moriaen live up to the commendations Worsley had himself given.[103] This strongly suggests that Moriaen thought Worsley was failing to match his own candour and forthcomingness in their exchange of arcana, and was trying to set a price on the knowledge he was acquiring. Worsley for his part perhaps felt that he was making better progress than his colleagues in Amsterdam, and deserved a more tangible recompense for imparting his results than news about less successful experiments.

Moriaen's letters chart a growing disillusion with Worsley, as requests for information and material were repeatedly ignored. The tin scoria he had asked for in January 1651 had still not materialised by the beginning of August.[104] Neither had the 'miraculous silver fused with mercury' which Worsley had apparently also promised.[105] Some information Worsley had sent him about oils he considered to be 'common knowledge'.[106] It was evidently not God's will, Moriaen observed with lugubrious predestinarian irony, that he should be able to rely on Worsley.[107]

Late 1649, the date of Worsley's disgruntled return home, was precisely the time of Moriaen's bitterly lamented financial crash. This may help to explain the sudden overt enthusiasm for an alchemical process with obvious implications of vulgar financial gain. Repeated mentions of specific projected profit levels and considerations of the likely return on a given outlay suggest that while he probably did not contemplate so blatantly commercial a project as many of Glauber's were, the thought that the pious labour might incidentally provide some material relief was becoming more of a consideration.

This is not to suggest that the spiritual dimension had ceased to matter. The frequent and lengthy outbursts of thanks to God, and attribution to His personal intervention of any success the experiments were having, were not mere pious rhetoric. Worsley's 'nobleman' apparently criticised Glauber's mercenary attitude (again this is consistent with the suggestion that this means Starkey, who in his letter to Moriaen roundly upbraided Glauber for precisely this fault[108]). Moriaen agreed: 'The nobleman's judgment of Glauber is certainly correct; commercial considerations are unseemly in this undertaking'.[109] Just as in the later case of his dye-works, however, Moriaen saw nothing wrong with making money provided it was being made for the right reasons, 'to serve the good of many'. As in all Moriaen's accounts of his labours in natural philosophy, delight in experimentation and discovery shines through his reports, and the very fact that he was so frank about hoping to make a profit confirms his good faith in rejecting the profit motive as the be all and end all of the enterprise. The real excitement was akin to that engendered in Comenius by his supposed discovery of perpetual motion: by demonstrating transmutation, Moriaen was confirming the metaphysical basis of his whole world-view, proving that man could indeed comprehend the universal, harness cosmic forces, and discern the true pattern, the divine method, underlying Creation itself.

But the project - rather predictably - was a failure. Two years later, the *Ephemerides* record that

> Mor*ian* disbursed once 12 thou*sand* Rixdollars upon one Experim*ent*, in which he miscarried, his wife knowing nothing of it. Upon another Exper*iment* he spent 2 or 3 t*housand* Gil*ders*, which yet hee hath to shew of Gold and Antim*ony* of which he might get back some ounces of gold, but in hope that some will yet be found to transmute the rest of the Antim*ony* into Gold he wil not doe it.[110]

These two financially catastrophic experiments are surely the tin-transmuting project probably inspired by Glauber, and the antimony-transmuting project probably inspired by Starkey. It would obviously be rash to assume that the figures quoted are entirely reliable, but given the quantity and nature of the materials referred to by Moriaen in his letters to Worsley, they do not seem excessive. There is talk in these letters of importing three hundred pounds of ore from Hungary, of casting tin in quantities of a hundred pounds at a time, and antimonial ore by the hundredweight, with an unspecified admixture of silver. There can be little doubt that these alchemical undertakings, which Moriaen had so hoped would restore his prosperity, in fact turned financial decline into disaster.

Moriaen's money problems at the time raise in turn the question of how he had obtained funds for experimentation on this scale. Kuffler can hardly have invested much, for he was himself in difficulties by this date and already in debt to Moriaen.[111] Nor had Worsley much to spare after his emotionally and economically exhausting visit to the Netherlands. Grill was certainly a major contributor. Moriaen told Worsley that Grill was spending 12,000 guilders (about £1200) on buying or building a house near Moriaen's, which was to be equipped with no less than six laboratories for the perfecting of the 'great work'.[112] This information also found its way into the *Ephemerides*: 'Aurifaber [...] hath gotten an estate of 60. th*ousand* lb. Now hee adventur's 12. hund*red* lb. vpon an Exp*eriment* of Tinne and something else in w*hich* Mr Mor*ian* hath also an Adventure and is a very promising busines'.[113] But some sponsorship at least, and it was probably a substantial amount, had come from that tireless supporter of lost causes, Comenius's patron Laurens de Geer.

Six years after the alchemical debacle, with Moriaen still in deep financial difficulties, and Kuffler making no headway with the promotion of his inventions in England, Hartlib suggested that Comenius petition de Geer for fresh support for Moriaen. Comenius duly made the representation, but met with little sympathy:

> I recently read him [de Geer] your letter and what you wrote about Moriaen and his unhappy lot, and how he might be helped if God would arouse the sympathy of my Patron L.D.G.; to which his only response was: 'He has caused his own downfall, or ruined himself, with alchemical nonsense'.[114]

The reasons for de Geer's sudden and uncharacteristic coldness are revealed in a later letter from Comenius's son-in-law Petr Figulus to Hartlib:

> Mons de Geer may bee will write unto you what hee resolues to doe about your projects. But all what I saye and endeavour to encline him to some resolution about yours & Mr Morians &c publicke Concernements, hee seemes to haue some secret feare & doubtings of all the like Inventions and Endeavours. And as a child that hath burnt himselfe feareth the fire. For hee seemeth to haue beene engaged in the like promotion both with Mr. Morian & especially with Glauberus, but all his moneyes lost: & hee neuer bene able to see any the least effect of all their Inventions. Glauberus having prooued to bee a deceiuer, & neuer meaning uprightly to reveale any thing.[115]

Figulus repeatedly tried to reassure de Geer about Moriaen's probity and to arrange a meeting, presumably in the hope of persuading him to renew his patronage, but seemingly without success.

Neither personal profit nor transcendent enlightenment had resulted from Moriaen's involvement in the 'great work'. Just as with the pansophic scheme - to use an analogy he was himself fond of - he had climbed like Moses to the summit of Mount Pisga and beheld the Promised Land, but it had not been granted him to enter into it.

The Gate of Things

Understandably enough, Moriaen's enthusiasm for Glauber cooled somewhat in the immediate aftermath of this debacle. There may well be a personal twist to Hübner's report the following year that 'Herr Moriaen told me in confidence that Glauber had done himself no little harm by accepting large sums for certain supposed secrets of art which, however, he has never tested himself and found to be true, for which reason he has many times been put to shame.[116] Another two years later, Hartlib told Boyle that 'Mr *Morian* writes no more of him [Glauber], or his other promised magnalia'.[117] However, Moriaen did not lose faith in alchemy, and if he did fall out with Glauber they were later reconciled. It says much either about Moriaen's good nature or his gullibility that by 1657 he was once again prepared to give Glauber the benefit of the doubt, and to suggest that those who failed to replicate Glauber's processes should not automatically condemn the author, but consider whether the error did not perhaps lie with themselves.[118]

Fahrner subsequently claimed that Glauber had sold De Bra (Moriaen's brother-in-law) a worthless recipe for making vinegar for 1000 guilders and also swindled a certain 'Herrn Mörian'.[119] But Moriaen obviously came to the conclusion that he had not been cheated, and two years after the publication of Fahrner's attack was back on friendly terms with Glauber. Indeed, it was Fahrner he considered to be the liar when it came to alchemical claims: 'Fahrner gives out that he can extract 12 loth of silver from 100 pounds of lead, but if it were true and profitable, he would surely keep [the method] secret and perform it himself'.[120]

It might be pointed out that the same strictures could be applied to Glauber: if he was so confident of his tin experiment, why did he not conduct it himself instead of selling the process to Moriaen and his friends? The explanation would probably have been - and it is not implausible - that he lacked the necessary capital. It would in any case be unfair to convict Glauber of bad faith without more conclusive evidence. The kindest interpretation is that he thought it likely the process would work, but preferred to see others risk their money on finding out for sure, making do for his part with the smaller but more certain profit of selling his secret rather than applying it. By 1657, some six years after the collapse of the tin and antimony ventures, Moriaen was awaiting letters from both Glauber and 'Aurifaber', and planning to visit Glauber at his new house in Amsterdam to discuss 'everything' with the two chemists.[121] Whether this represents a projected new collaboration is unclear, though if so nothing seems to have come of it. At all events it is obvious the three were again on good terms.

Worsley responded similarly to the affair. At first, he was plunged into deep disillusion, and for a while would seem to have lost faith in the very notion of transmutation. Moriaen, who in turn was out of sorts with Worsley at the time, put this down to the instability of Worsley's character. He himself was not to be shaken from belief in a truth he had seen proven with his own eyes simply because he had lost twelve thousand Imperials by it: 'that Mr Worsley refuses to believe any longer in transmutation is to me a sign of his unsteadiness of character, but for all that [...] the truth will still remain true'.[122]

However, Worsley subsequently revised this jaundiced view, and in later life exhibited an even stronger interest in alchemy. Some five years after his return from the Netherlands, he took to declaring himself an adept, and making grandiose alchemical declarations entirely typical of the most committed 'Chemical Philosophers'. He invoked a favourite topos: just as in the Puritan view of Scriptural understanding, no amount of human endeavour and learning could lead to true insight without the spark of enlightenment that could only be imparted by divine grace. The failure of his undertakings during and just after his alchemical mission, he decided, were due not to any inherent error in the processes he had learned, but to the fact that God had not yet seen fit to bless him (or, presumably, Moriaen) with the means of understanding them. Subsequently, it was granted him to see what before he had only looked at:

> I further professe honestly to you, that upon a deepe consideration of some of Glaubers writings & other discourses, I mett with when I was in Holland, it pleased god to discover *the* thing [ie. the art of transmutation] so clearly to me, that I sett downe *the* very thing in my Adversaria [personal note-book], as a matter to be weighed & experimented, & yet understood it not.[123]

Worsley cast his younger self in the role of a competent technician who had not received insight into the hidden mysteries of his own knowledge. He explicitly compared his subsequent alchemical enlightenment to the imputed grace of Calvinist theology:

> nor should [I] have beene ever able to have applyed any of these hynts, so as to have made any vse of them vnlesse God had (as he did) further as it were imposed the consideration of it upon me, by bringing my observation to a non plus, upon a kinde of fortuitous experiment made by me, which I speake even to this End to shew; that the Lord hath his seasons, & that it is not of him that wills, or of him that runnes, but of God only who in this as in more higher things enlightens whom he will.[124]

This retrospective self-image of a man granted knowledge but denied understanding strikingly parallels the response to Glauber within the Hartlib circle, insofar as a consensus can be defined. Glauber burst onto the scene with his great promises of a 'secret philosophic fire' a 'menstruum' for extracting the 'principles', and something at least approximating to the universal solvent. Eye witness accounts from Moriaen and Appelius vouched that there really were extraordinary physical and technological achievements on show in Amsterdam to support such claims. On closer inspection, however, the innovations were found to be merely technical. Glauber had made genuine progress in manipulating the outward, physical body of Nature, but when it came to penetrating her soul, he had provided no new insights. If anything, his exaggerated or bogus claims were positively counter-productive. He did not know how to apply his own expertise to the deeper mysteries.

An anonymous Dutch contact of Clodius's exemplifies this attitude. This individual, described as one who 'hath all manner of Arcanas [sic] and is an Adept', and so was obviously qualified to comment, considered that Glauber had indeed discovered 'the true Alcahest'. Unfortunately, however, he did not know what to do with it: 'if Glauber himself knew how to vse it by it great things might bee done'.[125] Moriaen himself expressed the same opinion. As early as 1650 he asserted that 'it is most certain that others finde more in Mr Glaubers Book's, which are already published then hee knoweth himself or is able to put in practise',[126] and he repeated eight years later, in almost the same terms, 'I still believe as before that he has been granted a considerable insight into Nature, but he does not know how to profit by it'.[127]

This ambivalence towards Glauber finds its clearest and most fully worked out expression in the letters of Culpeper. Culpeper distinguished more clearly than any other commentator represented in Hartlib's papers between the merely utilitarian and the 'philosophical' aspects of Glauber's work - between the chemical and the alchemical, in the contemporary sense of those words suggested in Chapter Five. In complete contrast to later progressivist historians who have either derided Glauber because of, or admired him in spite of, the alchemical component in his works, Culpeper became increasingly concerned that they were not nearly alchemical enough. For all the initial excitement inspired by his work on translating *Furni Novi*, he became more and more suspicious in the course of Worsley's visit to the Netherlands that Glauber had failed to probe beyond the mere external shell of created matter in his chemical investigations.

From his gleanings from Lull, Sendivogius and (above all) Nuysement,[128] Culpeper had concluded that to attain an 'excitation of the spirit of nature', some impurity had to be introduced, since matter in its natural state had no cause further to perfect itself: 'without an apposition of impurity (rightly chosen) there can nothinge be done in that woorke'.[129] What Culpeper seems to have had in mind, though he would obviously not have understood the comparison, was something akin to the practice of innoculation. By being infected with a judiciously chosen trace of a given disease or 'impurity', the body is stimulated to enhance its own innate powers, to attain a higher level of perfection. Following Nuysement, Culpeper fused this account of transmutation theory with his understanding of theology, and considered the necessary impurity or infection to be analogous to sin, the imperfection in humanity that was a prerequisite for the operation of grace which transmuted the human soul.

In the midst of Worsley's alchemical mission, Culpeper sent him a long letter full of citations from hermetic authors and his own abstruse reflections on the 'exaltation of the Spirits of Nature'. Among the extremely diverse and somewhat rambling meditations that comprise the letter is the following prime example of analogical thinking, an indissoluble alloy of practical experiment, alchemical allegory, micro-macrocosm theory and religious metaphor. Culpeper had been brewing some beer, and found that low temperatures slowed the process down. This, he declared, in a characteristic leap from the mundane to the metaphysical,

> agrees with what Nicholas Flammell saith (viz.) that when the 2. dragons
> have siezed upon one another they never cease from fightinge if the cold
> hinder them not) till they bee all on a gore blood, and till that in the end
> they have killed one another, and out of these putrified carcases arises our
> puissant King; I pray yf from my scriblinge you now apprehend me try
> whether Glauberus can and will give an Answer what this Canaanite is
> that exercises our spirits of Nature, and what that is in Nature, which like
> sinne to a gracious soule, serves to encrease repentance and all the other
> graces for thus (by the mercifull and wise God) doe the sinnes worke
> where the Spirit of grace hath taken roote, & thus if my Philosophy faile
> not) doth something in nature (analogicall to sinn) worke upon the Spirit
> of nature.[130]

Culpeper was firmly convinced of the general principle behind all this, but
what he was not at all sure about, as the confusion of his terminology
abundantly bears out, was the exact physical nature of this necessary
impurity, and this more than anything was the question he hoped Worsley
would resolve for him:

> now what this Sulphur externum, this Agent [...] this Ignis contra
> naturam, these feces grossieres or impurités, this Ignis non de materia, is.
> This is my question, which if Glauberus either cannot or will not
> understand; I say againe that you may expect other pretty or vsefull
> experiments from him; but he will proove to seeke in the greate
> worke.[131]

There was a parallel here not only with the operation of grace but also with
the Paracelsian notion that poisons correctly treated and administered were
conducive to increased health and vigour in the human body. It was precisely
such parallels that appealed to Culpeper's analogical imagination. Separating
substances into their constituent parts was, Culpeper thought, a trivial
occupation: mere chemistry, that would produce no 'exaltation' but leave
nature essentially what it had been in the first place: 'this wrackinge of nature,
is not the helpe that shee expectes from us, but onely a putting her into
reiterated newe motions'.[132] Glauber failed to provide the enlightenment, the
vistas onto infinity, that Culpeper had hoped for. Re-reading the first part of
Furni Novi, he declared that in it

> I finde a ready way to more discoueries of nature by outwarde fire onely,
> than hathe beene heeretofore helde forthe by any, but, in philosophy as
> well as Christianity, it is the inwarde fire or Spirit, to which wee ought
> principally to looke & this inwarde spirit yf excited into motion, will
> make life to diffuse from the center to the outwarde parts; Oh where
> wowlde this divinity & philosophy ende, this other of Glauberus is, but
> to discouer, not to exalte, what wee finde in nature.[133]

This identification of 'divinity & philosophy' is a logical extension of the
world-view that begat Comenius's Pansophy. The dissatisfaction with
Glauberian chemistry is in turn illustrative of the metaphysical unease that
inspired Pansophy. It represents a refusal to conceive that the universe might
be reducible to a collection of physical phenomena and their interreaction, that

235

everything might be explicable in terms of the so-called 'secondary causes'. The true investigation of matter had to entail the revelation of its spiritual and divine components.

Glauber's chemistry was altogether too practical for Culpeper's tastes. His style, so plain and direct by the standards of the day, failed to supply the spiritual nourishment Culpeper relished in Sendivogius and Nuysement. Though there are pious invocations enough in Glauber's writing, they are extraneous to the experimental details. What Culpeper wanted was a chemical Epiphany, an exact analogy of the 'inward fire of the spirit' that was so crucial to Puritan theology, and a fully worked out scheme of sin, grace and redemption reflected in the human manipulation of nature.

Culpeper was expressing these reservations about Glauber in the early years of the latter's career, the years that saw the publication of what his progressivist admirers have considered his most important work, *Furni Novi Philosophici* (1646-49), which of all Glauber's writings was the one based most directly on his laboratory practice and most fully describing his technological innovations. It is rich in 'pretty or usefull experiments', but decidedly short on 'inwarde & centrall fire' and 'operation of the spirit of grace'. His only other production during the period was *De Auri Tinctura* (1646). There is, unfortunately, no evidence available of Culpeper's, Worsley's or Moriaen's reaction to Glauber's work after Hartlib's death in 1662, the work which dismissed his earlier merely physical studies and turned wholly to mystic spiritualism and alchemical prophecy. The spirit of these late works seems much closer to their notion of attaining the metaphysical through the *Janua Rerum*, the Gate of Things, than his earlier and more empirical productions.

It is a measure of how similarly alchemical and Scriptural texts were interpreted by the more devoted 'chemical philosophers' that the former as much as the latter were frequently invested with prophetic significance. One great enthusiasm of Glauber's last years was the interpretation of Paracelsus's supposed prediction that the hidden mysteries of Nature would shortly be revealed by a mystic figure called 'Elias Artista', acting as a latterday John the Baptist to usher in the Second Coming of Christ.[134] This was a prospect that greatly excited many alchemists of the day, some of whom even claimed to be Elias.[135] Glauber resolved the prophecy by relating it to his lifelong obsession with salt. 'Elias Artista', he realised, was an anagram of 'et artis salia' ('and the salts of [the] Art'): 'ein Herrlicher/ Glorioser, vnd Triumphirender Monarch ist/ ELIAS ARTISTA, wenigen bekant, ET ARTIS SALIA, Vielen genant' ('a splendid, glorious, and triumphant monarch is ELIAS ARTISTA, known to few, ET ARTIS SALIA, named by many').[136]

Worsley, after his initial disillusion with alchemy had been overcome, became a great enthusiast of the Elias prophecy, which he took a good deal more literally than Glauber. The obscure oracle stated that the unfolding of Nature would occur in 'the fifty-eighth year'. There were various interpretations of what was meant by 'the fifty-eighth year': earlier it had been widely seen as 1602, the fifty-eighth year after Paracelsus's death, but this had had to be readjusted. By the early 1650s, there was an obvious appeal in reading it as meaning simply 1658, an interpretation that also accorded well with many predictions of the date of the millennial dawn. On 4 Feb. 1659 (i.e., as he pointed out in his own dating of the letter, the end of 1658 in the old style by which the year began in March), Worsley declared with the greatest confidence that 'The Devill [...] shall shortly fall before the greate Elias & his ministry which is suddainly to surprize part of *the* world' and even claimed to be personally acquainted with 'some that are really (at this present) of *the* said schoole of the said Elias Artist *the* great'.[137] Culpeper too was very taken with the prospect of Elias's advent. Writing in 1645 with regard to attempts to secure a patent for the Hartlib-backed inventor Pierre le Pruvost, he suggested that there was not much point in holding out for a patent of over fourteen years: 'truly yf others had my faithe concern*ing* the change that will be in the worlde before 59: they wowld not muche seeke for a perpetuity in any thinge but heauen'.[138]

Stephen Clucas suggests that 'For Culpeper, chemistry seems largely to have been a literary experience'.[139] It is certainly true that he almost invariably supported his chemical speculations not with any original or even second-hand experimental evidence but with a barrage of rather tenuously connected citations from his favourite chemical authors. The linguistic jumble of the terms to be found in his alchemical musings results from his citing them directly from a range of English, Latin and French tracts, principally those of Nuysement, Lull and Sendivogius (or 'Zengiuode', as Culpeper regularly called him in perhaps the most imaginative piece of spelling in the whole Hartlib archive). It is also true that imagination played a much greater role than logic, either inductive or deductive, in the establishment of his world-view. At least, this is true if 'imagination' is used in the modern sense of a faculty clearly distinguishable from the 'rational' or 'logical'. Comenius would have called Culpeper's approach 'syncretism', and would not have regarded it as in the least illogical. I would suggest that Culpeper, and a great many others of his day, Comenius and Moriaen among them, simply did not distinguish between a 'literary' and a 'scientific' response to the world about them. When thinkers of this period speak of Nature as the 'book of God's works', it is a mistake to take them over-metaphorically. Just as words were supposed to be symbols by which a single, definable, extra-linguistic 'meaning' was represented, so things were symbols representing the ideas of God, which mankind was capable of reading. God was the author of Creation - and it is significant that the Latin term 'auctor', meaning 'creator' in any sense, has in all modern Romance languages, in English and even in German, come specifically to mean 'writer'. Mankind was in the somewhat ambivalent position of being at once part of the text and the intended readership. Looking in nature for sin, repentance and the operation of grace, Culpeper was not so much inventing his own metaphors as interpreting God's.

Clucas further draws attention to the fact that Dury's 'analytical method', his pansophic system of Scriptural exegesis, was taken up by chemical philosophers such as Culpeper and applied to their subject: 'It is interesting that although the *methodus Duræus* was essentially a tool for scriptural analysis, it became applicable to *any textual corpus*.'[140] I have to quibble here with the letter, though not the spirit, of Clucas's analysis. What Culpeper was asking for was probably fresh commentary by Dury on the alchemical texts Culpeper favoured rather than application to them of the specifically theological exegesis Dury had proposed in the *Analysis Demonstrativa*.[141] However, it is reasonable to assume that what Culpeper expected from Dury was a very similar type of analysis. Alchemical texts were viewed as scarcely less sacred than the Bible itself, and their apparent obscurities were supposed, like the Bible's, to contain a simple, fundamental, underlying truth. Dury's talent for minute, detailed exegesis was seen as appropriate for the elucidation of both. Whether Dury's method was regarded as applicable to 'any textual corpus' whatsoever is debatable, but it was certainly deemed applicable to any divinely sanctioned corpus, and hence to the writings of any true alchemist.

Clucas proceeds to argue that 'Culpeper's urge to apply the analysis to chemistry was symptomatic of a wider secularization of the methods of theological systemizers.'[142] I would suggest, however, that to practitioners such as Culpeper and Dury, this represented not so much a secularisation of theological method as a theologisation of experimental learning. It exemplified the pansophic conviction that demarcations between disciplines are arbitrary and artificial, that all things are related and mutually illuminating, that all subjects fall into the category of 'divinity' in its widest sense, and that 'right method' is therefore universally applicable, its ultimate aim in all parts of learning being to lead men to God.

The intellectual histories of Worsley and Moriaen, the two main protagonists of the alchemical tragicomedy recounted in the previous section, were dominated by trends that have become something of a refrain in this study: disillusion with Scriptural analysis, withdrawal from confessional allegiance, commitment to seeking transcendental enlightenment not in verbal formulations but in the practical study and physical manipulation of Nature. They became, if anything, more religious as they became less religiose.

It should be stressed that while Culpeper, Worsley and Moriaen were certainly highly individual, they were by no means eccentric or unrepresentative. A host of other thinkers who have featured in this study, such as Brun, Rasch, Kretschmar, Glauber, Hartprecht, Poleman, Clodius and Starkey, were engaged on a similar synthesis of divinity with philosophy, practical experiment with theosophic enlightenment. However violent their personal differences and their disagreement on matters of detail, they were all guided by the same profound conviction.

The whole purpose of their intellectual - or, as they saw things, their spiritual endeavour was to attain a truer, more direct, more universal understanding of God than had proved possible through the old orthodoxies they were rejecting. The driving impulse behind their alchemical thought was precisely the same as that behind Pansophy: the fear of relativism, the fear of losing control and comprehension of the world through sheer overload of knowledge, the unfathomable complexity of the universe. This was countered by a determination to find in micro-macrocosm analogies and the notion of man as the divine image an underlying unity, harmony and pattern in all things.

In alchemy as in Pansophy it was 'right method' that would provide the key to unlock the 'Gate of Things'. Nowhere is this more apparent than in Worsley's reconversion to alchemical faith in the late 1650s. His letter of 1657 on 'Vniversal Learning' asserts once again the interconnection of all subjects and concludes by proclaiming all human knowledge to be but a shadowing of spiritual understanding. From the pansophic 'Temple of Wisdom' to the alchemical 'Shut-Palace of the King', the vision is barely altered. Worsley's declaration could have been penned by Comenius himself.

It provides an apt summation of the underlying faith he shared with Moriaen, Hartlib and Culpeper, the faith that sustained them even as, in personal, political and philosophical terms, their world fell apart around them:

> he that knoweth any thing in the lawes, course, & motions, of nature itselfe, & seeth not a harmony, Image & resemblance between these & the lawes, mysteryes, Revelations, & discoveryes of things spirituall; either doth not know them at all, or doth but yet thinke he knoweth them, yet he knoweth them not comprehensively, analytically, originally & exemplarly: for if he did he would in all things see one face, viz. Constancy, simplicity, Identity, Homogeneity, Vnity.[143]

Notes

1. On Worsley, see below, and also Charles Webster, 'Benjamin Worsley: engineering for universal reform from the Invisible College to the Navigation Act'; *SHUR*, 213-35; Antonio Clericuzio, 'New light on Benjamin Worsley's natural philosophy', *SHUR*, 236-46; J.J. O'Brien, 'Commonwealth Schemes for the Advancement of Learning', *British Journal of Education Studies* 16 (1968), 30-42. A handy summary of the known facts about his career, with an extensive list of sources, is provided by G.E. Aylmer, *The State's Servants: The Civil Service of the English Republic 1649-1660*, (London, 1973), 270-2.

2. Webster suggests late Feb. 1647 as the date of Worsley's departure (op. cit., 223), but this is far too early. He was still in England on 10 Dec. 1647, when Culpeper was trying to locate some recipes his wife had lost, and asked Hartlib to 'doe me the kindnes to search diligently at yourselfe & Mr Woorsly for them' (HP 13/206B). Clucas, on the other hand, situates the visit 'some time in the summer of 1648' ('The Correspondence of a XVII-Century "Chymicall Gentleman"', *Ambix* 40 (1993), 147-70, esp. 152): Worsley was indeed in the Netherlands that summer, but had been there since at least January. A letter to Hartlib dated The Hague, 14 Feb. 1648 (HP 36/8/1A-6B), gives a detailed account of Worsley's recent contacts and activities. He mentioned having arrived at The Hague on 'the 27th', presumably of January, before which he had spent some time in Rotterdam.

3. Hartlib's letters do not survive, but it is obvious from the replies that they were full of detailed queries about Glauber.

4. Moriaen to Hartlib, 3 Feb. 1648, HP 37/127A. Worsley was already in the Netherlands by this date but had not met either Moriaen or Glauber.

5. Appelius to Hartlib, 26 Sept./6 Oct. 1647, HP 45/1/37A.

6. Appelius to Hartlib, 26 Sept./6 Oct. 1647, HP 45/1/37B.

7. Culpeper to Hartlib, 20 Oct. 1647, HP 13/197A. The illogical bracketing is Culpeper's. On Culpeper's offer of funding for the Office of Address, see Hartlib to Boyle, Nov. 1647, Boyle, *Works* VI, 76.

8. See Webster, 'New Light on the Invisible College', *Transactions of the Royal Historical Society* 24 (1974), 19-42; also *Great Instauration*, 59-67.

9. As Charles Webster remarks, 'Benjamin Worsley: engineering for universal reform', *SHUR*, 213-35, esp. 225.

10. 'General History of the Air', Boyle, *Works* V, 638-44. For the reattribution, see Clericuzio, 'New Light on Benjamin Worsley's natural philosophy', *SHUR*, 238-9.

11. *DNB* XLV, 113, under Petty; see Webster, op. cit., for a reappraisal of this harsh and superficial judgment. Webster is to supply an entry on Worsley for the next edition of the *DNB*.

12   Hartlib to Boyle, 16 Nov. 1647, Boyle, *Works* VI, 76. Hartlib later became extremely disillusioned with Petty: see his bitterly humorous account to Boyle of 10 Aug. 1658, Boyle, *Works* VI, 112-113.

13   Hartlib to Boyle, 28 Feb. 1654, Boyle, *Works* VI, 79.

14   Hartlib to Boyle, 27 April 1658, ibid., 104-5. Hartlib was about eighteen years Worsley's elder.

15   Cf. Webster, 'Benjamin Worsley', 220, and *Great Instauration*, 59-60 and the letters cited there.

16   HP 37/142A.

17   'Er [Worsley] wolle mich excusiren das Ich an ihn selbst*en* nichts schreib bin im Englisch*en* nicht so fertig' - Moriaen to Hartlib, 15 April 1650, HP 37/152A. Cf. also Moriaen to Hartlib, 25 March 1650, HP 37/146A: writing to Worsley 'fält mir [...] zue schwehr vnd langsam' ('is too difficult and slow for me').

18   Moriaen to Hartlib, 22 June 1657, HP 42/2/10B-11A.

19   HP 9/16/1A-13B and 63/14/13A-B (all holographs, so they cannot have been translated into Latin).

20   Worsley's letters are lost, but in one of his replies Moriaen quoted Worsley back to him in English, though Moriaen's own text is in Latin (Moriaen to Worsley, 26 May 1651, HP 9/16/6A).

21   See his proposals for the saltpetre project at HP 71/11/1A-B and 17/11/12A-13A; a similar unascribed document at HP 53/26/6A-B is probably also by Worsley. See also Webster, *Great Instauration*, 378-80, and 'Benjamin Worsley: engineering for universal reform', 215-17.

22   Moriaen, before getting to know him, twice referred to him as 'candidatus medicinæ' (HP 37/122A and 37/123A), this evidently being the description Hartlib had provided.

23   Aylmer, *The State's Servants* (London and Boston, 1973) 271; Webster, 'Benjamin Worsley', 213.

24   Worsley to Dury, 27 Aug. 1649, HP 33/2/3A-4B.

25   Fuller details in Aylmer, loc. cit.

26   Culpeper to Hartlib, 17 Nov. 1647, HP 13/204A. During a severe illness in 1641, which he expected to prove fatal, Culpeper had signed over the control of his estates to his father, Sir Thomas Culpeper. Sir Thomas was supposed to return control to his son in the event of the latter's recovery, but, outraged by Cheney's support of Parliament at the outbreak of civil war, he refused to do so. Furthermore, Sir Thomas's own debts were charged to the revenue of the estates he had taken over from his son. In the course of 1646-47, with the estates now apparently again under his control, Culpeper was trying to get the fine imposed on them reduced, and succeeded in having the charge cut by about a third, but was still confronted in Nov. 1647 with a bill for £844 1/-. He was consequently in financial straits throughout the rest of his life, and was heavily in debt at his death. For fuller details, see 'Introduction' to M.J. Bradwick and M. Greengrass (eds.), *The Letters of Sir Cheney Culpeper (1641-1657)*, Camden Miscellany XXXIII (Cambridge, 1996), 118-23

27   Culpeper to [Hartlib?], 29 March 1648, HP 13/214B.

28   Worsley to Hartlib, 22 June/2 July 1649, HP 26/33/1A-3B.

29   Dury to Worsley, 14 March 1648, HP 1/2/1A-B and 12 July 1649, HP 26/33/4A-5B, and Worsley to Dury, 27 July 1649, HP 33/2/18A-19B. On this theory and its ramifications, see above, p. 43 and the literature cited there.

30   Worsley to Hartlib, 14 Feb. 1648, HP 36/8/6A.

31   Ibid. On 10 Feb. Moriaen mentioned having forwarded a letter from Worsley (then in Rotterdam) to Glauber (HP 37/129A).

32   HP 1/2/1B.

33   As Moriaen wrote to Hartlib two days later, HP 37/131A.

34   Moriaen to Hartlib, 28 May 1648, HP 37/133A.

35   'Glauber verstehet woll Latein wans auff hoch teutsch außgesprochen wird aber Er wird nicht Lateinisch reden wollen [...] das wird Ihme unlustig und die conversation zue wieder machen' - Moriaen to Hartlib, 27 Feb. 1648, HP 37/131A.

36   'Ich höre dz Er [Moriaen] Herrn Worslÿ sehr ehret vndt auf der Rechten handt läßet gehen, welches Ihm aber von etlichen nicht zum besten wird aufgenommen, vnd zwar nicht ohne vrsach, dan H. Morian ist ein zimlich betagter Man, in vielen Künsten vndt wißenschafften erfahren' - Brun to Hartlib, 13 June 1649, HP 39/2/9A.

37   Appelius to Hartlib, May 1648, HP 45/1/47A.

38   'Mr Worsleys werck geht langsam fort, Glauber fühlt nicht dz ihm die zeit vnd kosten schwer fallen, man bringt viel zeit mit complementen zu, vnd sagt nit rund aus was vnd wie man ein ding begehrt, was oder wie man ein ding zusagt, vnd auf sich nimt: etliche förchten Glauber werde seiner zusage keinen genügen können thun' - Appelius to Hartlib, 2 Aug. 1648, HP 45/1/39B.

39   Culpeper to Hartlib, 5 April 1648, HP 13/215A. On Culpepper's interest in this subject, see above, p. 166.

40   Ibid.

41   Culpeper to Hartlib, 25 July 1648, HP 13/231A: 'I vnderstande from yourselfe that hee is (for the presente) otherwise supplied'. I can find no hint as to what this alternative source might have been.

42   Ibid.

43   Cf. Worsley to ?, 22 July 1648, HP 42/1/1A, recounting that he had dined with the Kufflers at Moriaen's.

44   Culpepper to Hartlib, 5 April 1648, HP 13/217B.

45   On this subject, see H.C. Darby, *The Draining of the Fens* (Cambridge, 1940).

46   Schama, *The Embarrassment of Riches* (Berkeley, Los Angeles and London, 1988) 257-88.

47   Worsley to Hartlib, 22 June/2July 1649, HP 26/33/1A.

48   Kalthof (or Calthof) aroused much interest in Hartlib for his work on drainage and perpetual motion. He was co-recipient of patents for perpetual motion machines from the states General in 1642 and from the States of Holland in 1653 (Doorman, 144, G432, and 179, H72).

49   Worsley to Petty, 15 June 1649, HP 8/50/1A, and Brun to Hartlib, 13 June 1649, HP 39/2/9A.

50   Worsley to Petty, 15 June 1649, HP 8/50/1A-2B.

51   Worsley to Petty, 15 June 1649, HP 8/50/1A.

52   *Eph 49*, HP 28/1/3B.

53   *Eph 49*, HP 28/1/17A, giving Petty himself as the source.

54   Fromantil is a thoroughly obscure figure who appears to have been an all-round inventor. There are numerous mentions in the *Ephemerides* of 1649 on, and Hartlib's papers include a list of 'Ahasverus Fremantils Mechanical Vnder takings in his owne hand' (n.d., HP 71/19/1A-B), in all probability sent or brought over by Worsley. These include various clocks, an engine for levelling river beds and various engines for raising weights or water. He also invented a fire engine (HP 53/35/5A), an instrument for measuring the concentration of liquids in compound, and an 'art of

making notches in Iron-wheels', perhaps meaning cog wheels (*Eph 49*, HP 28/1/32B and 35A). Worsley is the only correspondent to mention his microscopes. He is surely identical with, or at least related to, the Assuerus Fromanteel of the Dutch Reformed Church in London who in 1645 had joined the Anabaptists and was consequently excommunicated from the Dutch church the following year: see O.P. Grell, *Calvinist Exiles in Tudor and Stuart England* (Aldershot, 1996), 90-1.

55 Worsley to ?, 27 June or July 1648, HP 42/2/1A. Hartlib was obviously circulating this very interesting letter, which constitutes something of a manifesto for natural philosophy, as there are three copies in his papers, HP 42/2/1A-2A, 8/27/2B-7B and 8/27/9A-13B. The second of these is dated June, the other two July.

56 Worsley to ?, 27 June or July 1648, HP 42/2/1B.

57 Ibid.

58 Ibid.

59 HP 42/1/7A-8B, 14 Oct. 1657. By 'astrology', Worsley meant not the art of divination but the study of the physical effects (direct or indirect) of celestial bodies on sublunary matter and motion, as he explained in his 'Physico-Astrologicall Letter' of c. July 1657 (copies at HP 26/56/1A-4B and 26/56/5A-8B; Latin translation at 42/1/18A-25B). Cf. Clericuzio, 'New light on Benjamin Worsley's natural philosophy', *SHUR*, 236-46, esp. 242.

60 HP 42/2/1A.

61 Hall to Worsley, 5 Feb. 1647, HP 3/6/1A-B.

62 Hall's letter at HP 3/6/1A-B and 36/7/2B-3A; Worsley's (16 Feb. 1647) at HP 36/6/3A-8B and 36/7/3A-6B.

63 HP 36/6/4B.

64 HP 36/6/4B.

65 HP 36/6/5B-6A.

66 E.g. Dury to Worsley, 2 May 1649, HP 4/1/26A-B, thanking Worsley for obtaining from Boreel or Moriaen a catalogue of Menasseh's Hebrew books, and sending regards to both. Dury also hoped Boreel could learn from Menasseh or another rabbi whether there were any Jewish refutations of Islam to be had.

67 'mit H Glaubern ein vnd anders ins werkh zuestellen damit H Worsleÿ nicht vergeblich herkommen oder so lange zeit vnnüzlich zuegebracht habe' - Moriaen to Hartlib, 11 June 1649, HP 37/137A.

68 Worsley to Hartlib, 22 June/2 July 1649, HP 26/33/2B.

69 Worsley to Dury, 27 July/6 Aug. 1649, HP 33/2/19B (misdated '27 July 165?' in the HP transcript: though the MS gives no year, the letter is obviously a reply to Dury's of 12 July 1649, HP 26/33/4A-5B).

70 Ibid.

71 Dury to ?, 8 Aug. 1649, HP 1/31/1B; Culpeper to Hartlib, 14 Aug. 1649, HP 13/260A-261B.

72 'D. Worsley zeügt wieder nach haus [...] ich kan nicht genug verwundern, woher es komt, dz er von Glauber so lang aufgehalten worden, vnd nun auch mit lehrer hand nach haus reiset, nach dem er so lange schwehre kosten gethan [...] Glauber sagt alle zeit, es mangele an ihn nicht so [*word missing*] auch H Worsley, vnd gleichwol verstehen sie ein ander nicht, es wundert mich dz Glauber so hart [*word missing*] gegen ihn ist, da er sich doch so resolut vnd liberal gegen ihn vor [sic] anfang erzeigt hat' - Appelius to Hartlib, 20 Sept. 1649, HP 45/1/41A.

73 More to Hartlib, 21 Oct. 1649, HP 18/1/35A. Moriaen later mentioned that Worsley had intended to observe the solar eclipse of 4 Nov. with him (HP 37/146A), but

whether it was his departure or something else that prevented him from doing so is not stated.

74   The first clear indication of his being back in England does not occur until late January 1650, when Moriaen sent his regards and More expressed a hope of visiting Worsley and Hartlib in London - Moriaen to Hartlib, 21 Jan. 1650, HP 37/140A, and More to Hartlib, 29 Jan., HP 18/1/25A. Moriaen also mentioned in this letter that he had written several times to Worsley, who was apparently complaining that he had not heard from Moriaen, but whether Moriaen had been writing to him in England or not is not specified.

75   'Ich hab gemeint mit H Glaubers furschlag ihn [Worsley] sehr zueerfrewen aber es falt ganz wiederartig aus seine einbildung die Er von Ihm hatt ist so ganz schlecht das Er alles zum argsten auffnimbt' - Moriaen to Hartlib, 25 March 1650, HP 37/146A.

76   He stressed in particular that Glauber's method had been tested using large quantities of material (for the greater the quantity experimented on, obviously, the greater the reliability of the results: this distinction between operations effected in bulk and those only tested on small samples is regularly drawn in chemical texts of the period).

77   Moriaen to Hartlib, 29 April 1650, HP 37/153A: 'berichte das Glauber die conditiones von Mr W. annimbt'.

78   Moriaen to Worsley, 4 March 1650, HP 37/142A. This is not a holograph so it is unclear whether the English is Moriaen's own or a translation from German or Latin. Worsley is not cited as the addressee, but the internal evidence is overwhelming.

79   Moriaen to Worsley, 27 Jan. 1651, HP 9/16/1B.

80   'quoad fieri per literas potest, namque maxima eius ratio in methodo et manuali dexteritate posita est' - Moriaen to Worsley, 26 May 1651, HP 9/16/6A.

81   'quo in loco, imo cujus in fodinâ (nam in uno eodemque loco illæ differunt) debita et ad opus nostrum idonea minera antimonij invenienda sit' - Moriaen to Worsley, 16 June 1651, HP 9/16/8A.

82   See above, p. 162.

83   Moriaen to Worsley, 9 June 1651, HP 9/16/7A.

84   *Eph 51*, HP 28/2/15A.

85   *Eph 50*, HP 28/1/49B: 'The Refiners name at Amsterdam worth 10 thousand lb. is Gralle. Hee is the Aurifaber of which hee [presumably Worsley or Moriaen] speakes in his Letters.'

86   HP 37/161A and 42/2/9A.

87   HP 42/2/10B-11A.

88   Moriaen to Worsley, 26 May 1651, HP 9/16/6A.

89   Moriaen to Worsley, 19 May 1651, HP 9/16/5A.

90   On Starkey, see William Newman's excellent biography, *Gehennical Fire: The Lives of George Starkey, an Alchemist of Harvard in the Scientific Revolution* (Harvard, 1994). Newman has also written a number of valuable shorter studies on specific aspects of Starkey's career: 'Prophecy and Alchemy: the Origin of Eirenæus Philalethes', *Ambix* 37 part 3 (Nov. 1990), 97-115; 'Newton's *Clavis* as Starkey's *Key*', *Isis* 78 (1987), 564-74, and 'George Starkey and the selling of secrets', *SHUR*, 193-210. See also Turnbull, 'George Stirk, Philosopher by Fire', *Publications of the Colonial Society of Massachusetts* 38 (1959), 219-51, and R.S. Wilkinson, 'George Starkey, Physician and Alchemist', *Ambix* 11 (1963), 121-52, though both these have been largely superseded by Newman's work.

91   Moriaen to Worsley, 19 May 1651, HP 9/16/5A.

92   Starkey to Moriaen, 30 May 1651, HP 17/7/1A-2B. This is summarised and
      analysed in detail by Newman, 'Prophecy and Alchemy', 101, and my account here is
      based largely on Newman's.

93   'Prophecy and Alchemy', 111.

94   E.g. R.S. Wilkinson, 'The Problem of the Identity of Eirenæus Philalethes', *Ambix*
      12 (1964), 24-43. Newman's 'Prophecy and Alchemy' provides the conclusive
      identification. 'Eirenæus Philalethes' is a pseudonym subsequently applied to
      Starkey's fictional adept, though not one he used himself.

95   Starkey to Moriaen, 30 May 1651, HP 17/7/1A: 'quodam amico juvene [...] adhuc
      vitali'.

96   Ibid., HP17/7/2A.

97   *Eph 51*, HP 28/2/18A. The names '*Dury*' and 'Worsly' appended to the entries
      indicate that these were the sources of Hartlib's information. Precise dating of entries
      in the *Ephemerides* is seldom possible, but the previous entry but one to this refers
      to events of 23 April, so it is certainly later, but probably not much later, than that.
      The next mention of a specific date is 26 July, several pages later (HP 28/2/23B).

98   Moriaen to Worsley, 30 June 1651, HP 9/16/9A.

99   Ibid.

100   Especially the letters of 30 June (HP 9/16/9A-B), 2 July (9/16/10A-B) and 9 July
      (9/16/11A-12B).

101   30 June 1651, HP 9/16/9B: 'obesæ naris sim si amicorum commendationes non
      suboleam'.

102   Starkey to Moriaen, 30 May 1651, HP 17/7/1A: 'virtutis vestræ verè Heroicæ'.

103   30 June 1651, HP 9/16/9B: 'operæ pretium fuerit eum, quem commendare non
      erubuistis, vestro consilio et auxilio juvare ut aliquo modo virum se præstare possit
      ne aliquando commendationis vestræ vos pudeat'.

104   Moriaen to Worsley, 4 Aug. 1651, HP 9/16/13A.

105   Moriaen to Worsley, 7 July 1651, HP 9/16/11B: 'Lunam vestram mirabilem unam
      cum mercurio anxie desidero' ('I anxiously desire your miraculous silver fused with
      mercury'); and 4 Aug. 1651, HP 9/16/13A: 'de non missa luna nullam video
      excusationem' ('I can see no excuse for not having sent the silver').

106   Moriaen to Worsley, 4 Aug. 1651, HP 9/6/13A: 'illud vulgare esse existimo'.

107   Ibid: 'Ego ulterius non Urgebo, sed in voluntate Divinâ acquiescam' ('I shall press
      [you] no longer, but acquiesce in the will of God').

108   HP 17/7/1A: 'Venalia nulla secreta habeo, quod et abominor, eoque solo nomine,
      Magister Iohannes Glauberus (vir sane inclytus) mihi vituperandus censetur'.

109   Moriaen to Worsley, 2 July 1651, HP 9/16/10A: 'judicium Nobilis, de Glaubero
      prorsus rectum est. [...] Turpis ex hoc negotio mercatura est'.

110   *Eph 53*, HP 28/2/64B: no source is given for the information.

111   Moriaen to Worsley, 4 Aug. 1651, with reference to 'debitor meus Kufflerus' ('my
      debtor Kuffler'), HP 9/16/13A.

112   Moriaen to Worsley, 31 March 1651, 9/16/4A.

113   *Eph 51*, HP 28/2/15A.

114   Comenius to Hartlib, 10 August 1657, HP 7/111/23A: 'legi nuper illi epistolam
      Tuam etiam qvæ de Moriano, illiusque misera sorte, & qvomodo illi subveniri
      posset, si Patroni D. L. de G. animum excitaret Deus, scripsisti: ad quæ ille nihil,
      nisi Er hat sich mit Alchymisterey gestürzt, vel ruiniret'.

115   Figulus to Hartlib, 6 Nov. 1650, HP 9/17/45A-B, also in Blekastad, *Figulus Letters*,
      236.

116 'Von Glaubern sagte H. Mor*ian* mir im vertrawen das Er damit sich nicht wenig shaden [*sic*] gethan hätte, das er sich grosses geld fur gewisse vermeinte kunst-stucklein geben lassen, die er doch selbst niemals versuchet, vnd sie in der that also befunden, dannenhero er dan ettliche mahl mit shanden [*sic*] bestehen mussen' - Hübner to ?, 24 March 1652, HP 63/14/21A. The letter exists as a copy in Hartlib's hand, and this idiosyncratic German spelling ('sh' for 'sch') is a distinctive quirk of Hartlib's, probably reflecting how Anglicised he had become.

117 Boyle to Hartlib, 8 May 1654, Boyle, *Works* VI, 86.

118 Moriaen to Hartlib, 24 Aug 1657, HP 42/2/19A.

119 Christoph Fahrner, *Ehrenrettung* (1656), 75; cf. Link, *Glauber*, 33.

120 'Farner gibt fur wie Er aus 100 lb ble ÿ 12 lot Silber bringen könne gieng es aber mit nuz zue wurde Ers woll schweigen und selbst practisiren' - Moriaen to Hartlib, 24 Aug. 1647, HP 42/2/19A.

121 Moriaen to Hartlib, 4 May 1657, HP 42/2/7B: 'de qvibus cum Aurifabro & Glaubero agendum mihi est nihil dum rescribere possum qvosq*ue* illorum responsa recepero. Glaub: hoc ipso tempore de domo in domum migrat, qvo facto ad aliqvot dies me convenire consituit, qvando opportuna dabitur de omnibus colloqvendi occasio Deo benè juvante'.

122 'das H W keine transmutation mehr glauben will, ist mir ein zeichen seines wanckelbahren gemuehts, darumb wird [...] warheit doch woll warheit bleiben' - Moriaen to ?, 3 May 1652, HP 63/14/20A.

123 Worsley to ?, 14 Feb. 1655/6, HP 42/1/5A.

124 Ibid., citing Romans 9:16. This is an unascribed copy letter, but the style, the subject matter, the autobiographical details and the fact that it is from Dublin leave virtually no doubt of Worsley's authorship.

125 *Eph 59*, HP 29/8/5A.

126 30 Dec. 1650, HP 31/8/1A. This letter, a copy in Hartlib's hand which to judge by the numerous manuscript corrections is probably a translation, is unattributed, but there is much internal evidence to suggest Moriaen's authorship.

127 'bin noch d*er* meinung wie vor diesem das ihm in d*er* Natur ein zimblich liecht auffgang*en* ist dz Er Ihm aber selbst*en* nicht zue nuz mach*en* kan' - Moriaen to Hartlib, 26 May 1658, HP 31/18/28A.

128 For a summary of Nuysement's chemico-religious doctrines and their direct influence on Culpeper, see Clucas, 'Correspondence of a XVII-Century "Chymicall Gentleman"', *Ambix* 40 (1993), 147-70, esp. 153-4.

129 Culpeper to Hartlib, 14 Aug. 1649, HP 13/260B.

130 Culpeper to Worsley, 9/19 May 1648, HP 13/219B-220A; the illogical parentheses are again Culpeper's.

131 Culpeper to Worsley, 9/19 May 1648, HP 13/219A. Whether the writers he was citing here were indeed, as Culpeper maintained, all talking about the same thing is a moot point.

132 Culpeper to Hartlib, 14 Aug. 1649, HP 13/260A.

133 Culpeper to Hartlib, 4 July 1649, HP 13/155A.

134 The prophecy occurs in the *Liber Mineralium* which is probably not in fact by Paracelsus.

135 Pagel, 'The Paracelsian Elias Artista and the Alchemical Tradition', *Kreatur und Kosmos: Internationale Beiträge zur Paracelsus-Forschung*, ed. Heinz Dillinger (Stuttgart, 1981); Newman, 'Prophecy and Alchemy', 97-9.

136 From the full title of *Miraculum Mundi Ander Theil* [in fact the fifth part] *Oder Dessen Vorlängst Geprophezeiten ELIÆ ARTISTÆ TRIUMPHIRLIcher Ein Ritt. Vnd auch Was der ELIAS ARTISTA für einer sey?* (Amsterdam, 1660).

137 Worsley to ?, HP 33/2/16A-B.

138 Culpeper to Hartlib, Dec. 1645, HP 13/112A: Culpeper goes on to cite the 'Paracelsian' prophecy verbatim.

139 'Correspondence of a XVII-Century "Chymicall Gentleman"', 154.

140 Ibid., 157-8.

141 Culpeper wished that Dury would 'give me an hower or two of his analiticall thowghts upon my Chymicall quotations, Oh that I cowld but sometimes injoy an hower with him about his Analisis in which I see enough to rayse but not enough to satisfy my desires' - to Hartlib, 17 Feb. 1646, HP 13/128A.

142 'Correspondence of a XVII-Century "Chymicall Gentleman"', 158.

143 Worsley to [Hartlib?], 14 Oct. 1657, HP 42/1/7A-B.

Conclusion

The focus of this study has been deliberately narrow. Its main aim is to render more accessible an invaluable body of source material for the intellectual history of the seventeenth century by summarising and contextualising Moriaen's correspondence. Correspondence such as Moriaen's, sifted, edited, transcribed and disseminated by Hartlib or at Hartlib's behest, initiated no new ideas, but played an essential role in broadcasting new ideas and stimulating discussion and reassessment of them. To borrow the mercantile imagery so often employed by members of the circle, he was not a producer of 'ingenuity and knowledge' but he was a major trader in it. It has not been my purpose to challenge or champion any particular interpretational orthodoxy, but rather to supply details of specific research which I hope will inform broader theoretical debate. As a conclusion, therefore, I am more concerned to suggest future lines of enquiry and to proffer a few frankly personal and subjective responses than to venture any wider analysis or definitive statement.

There is an unavoidable danger, in the assessment of any historical period, that a skewed picture will be presented on the basis of fortuitously preserved fragmentary evidence. The very existence of Hartlib's papers, or at any rate a substantial part of them, is at once a boon and a pitfall for the historian. On the one hand, they present an enormous fund of primary evidence about the intellectual life of the period. On the other, they present only one person's individual collection of contemporary documentation, and as such represent an inevitably partial view. The task is to assess the extent to which they can be regarded as representative, and what exactly they can be regarded as representative of. It is virtually a truism that the discovery of this archive has entailed the rewriting of the history of the period, but it should always be borne in mind how different that rewriting might be if it were someone else's papers - Moriaen's, for instance, or Hübner's, or Glauber's - that had been discovered instead. For Hartlib's papers to be assessed as a document of their time, it is necessary to determine whether they chart an individual obsession or are a random jackdaw selection of interesting tidbits, whether they were collected purely for the sake of being collected or serve a particular agenda, whether they document an individual or a society, or a given group within a society.

It is, therefore, of some significance that Hartlib can be shown to have been recognised by a particular group of people as their organiser and spokesman. The term 'Hartlib circle' is not merely a convenient tag. It was, however, a very large and diffuse group which cannot be reduced to any such simplistic formulation as 'Puritan', 'experimental', 'hermetic', 'Baconian' or the like. As the foregoing study illustrates, there were radical differences of approach and priority, and sometimes bitter conflicts of opinion within the circle. But there was a circle, and its members were conscious both that they belonged to it and that Hartlib was its centre. Moriaen's first surviving letter to Hartlib vividly conveys both Hartlib's centrality and the sense of community among his supporters. Urging his new friend to take at least some thought for himself and not to pay for the promotion of Comenius with his own financial ruin, Moriaen provided a neat vignette both of Hartlib's discreet but crucial role in the operation and the sense of community among his supporters: 'You oblige the rest of us and do quite enough by directing the work, initiating and maintaining correspondence, and providing and sending out each man's portion: as for the costs, they should be borne jointly by the devotees of the project'.[1]

Given that the group existed, a more difficult task is to define it, in terms both of its membership and its ideology. Obviously, no rigid demarcation is possible. At its nexus, it was an association of personal friends. Hartlib and Dury were the two key figures: Comenius, despite their best efforts, always remained a cause they were supporting rather than a fellow co-ordinator. Around them were Hübner, Haak, Pell, Moriaen, Rulice, Hotton and Appelius, later to be joined by Sadler, Culpeper, Worsley, Boyle and Clodius. But as soon as one looks any further than this from the centre, the lines of communication begin to branch and cross, threading their way into the entire intellectual community of Europe and America. It is a circle with a definable centre but an almost infinitely extendable periphery. For this reason, no wholly satisfactory methodological framework for the study of the group has yet been constructed. Perhaps it is a mistake to try to construct one.

Charles Webster used the papers to draw conclusions about 'the Puritan world view and the rise of modern science'.[2] But although there undoubtedly is a Puritan and Calvinist bias in Hartlib's milieu, there was nothing denominationally exclusive about his undertaking, and indeed the rejection of confessionalisation was itself characteristic of many figures in the circle. As often as not, of course, 'rejection of confessionalisation' simply means expecting everyone else to accept one's own. But I hope I have shown that figures such as Moriaen, Worsley and Hartlib himself did promote an approach that was genuinely anti-denominational without being in the least atheological.

Hugh Trevor-Roper, in depicting Hartlib, Dury and Comenius as the 'philosophers of the Puritan revolution', accepted the notion of a unifying Puritanism to serve a very different agenda. By going on to trivialise their thought, he set out to imply that the 'Puritan revolution' did not have much of a philosophy at all. Though it is overstated, over-simplified, and transparently inspired by a sense of personal antipathy across the centuries, Trevor-Roper's approach should perhaps not be wholly dismissed. It is undeniable that, with the exception of Robert Boyle, there was no individual anywhere near the centre of Hartlib's circle possessed of intellectual gifts comparable to those of Descartes or Hobbes, and Boyle's forte was practical chemistry, not political philosophy. More debatable is whether the engineers of the revolution really did set so much store by them, or for that matter by any other individuals. That Cheney Culpeper and John Sadler were committed supporters and promoters of Hartlib and his schemes is beyond dispute, but their personal influence was not vast. When it came to putting things into practice, there is precious little evidence of real commitment from Parliament as a whole beyond a modest and irregularly-paid private pension for Hartlib himself. Durham College sank without trace within a few years of its foundation. Funding was never found for Comenius, or Kuffler, or

Rittangel, or Chelsea College, or the College of Jewish Studies, or the Office of Address, or a host of other Hartlib-inspired projects. Hartlib was not without influence in the inter-regnum Parliament, but he was hardly the revered guru Trevor-Roper makes him out to have been.

More recently, Richard Popkin has attempted to define a 'Third Force' in seventeenth-century thought that 'seems to be neither rational, nor empiricist, but combines elements of both with theosophy and interpretation of Biblical prophecy'.[3] This arose and took on definition, he argues, in response to the sceptical crisis of the seventeenth century, to the revival of Pyrrhonism, the deductivism of Descartes and the materialism of Hobbes. It was heavily inspired by Jacob Böhme, and its principal exponents were all members of the Hartlib circle: Dury, Comenius, Joseph Mede, William Twisse, Henry More. But whatever the uses of Popkin's new category for the broader analysis of seventeenth-century thought, the Hartlib circle refuses as usual to accommodate itself to the pigeonhole. While many in the group were certainly interested in Mede, Twisse and More, these can hardly be described as core members, and More in particular positively cold-shouldered some of Hartlib's advances. Hartlib himself, for that matter, together with many of his friends, was also very interested in Descartes and Hobbes.

What the archive supplies is a fragmentary but panoramic view of the European intellectual landscape at a particular historical moment. It does not, on its own, provide the material for an account of any definable philosophical or ideological trend. Hartlib's papers are a ragbag, which is precisely what makes them so interesting and valuable historically.

I have no wish to debunk or disparage Popkin's work, which displays great scholarship and insight, and has been a major stimulus to my own thinking. But by locating within the Hartlib circle the origins of an anti-sceptical, anti-materialist 'Third Force', 'neither rational nor empiricist' but combining elements of both, he seems to me to put the cart before the horse. He perceptively identifies the metaphysical unease that informed all the multifarious (and often mutually contradictory) beliefs, ideas and ideals of the group, but analyses it in anachronistic terms. It is true that there is precious little evidence to be found in their writings of fully-fledged philosophical rationalism, scepticism or materialism - but then, where are these to be found in the early and middle seventeenth century? These systems of thought, which were to gain ascendency in the decades following Hartlib's death, were, however, in the process of gestation. The epistemological uncertainties of Dury and Descartes, the spectacular results of the new universal algebra championed by Pell, the atomism of Gassendi, the elevation (championed by Boreel and Worsley) of experimental learning over textual exegesis of Scripture, would all in due course feed in, directly or indirectly, to more fully worked-out formulations of those philosophies in the last decades of the century. But if any of the thinkers close to Hartlib were conscious at all of such a gestation, they would have been utterly horrified to foresee what they were giving birth to. If they did indeed have such an inkling, they were not so much reacting against these philosophies as trying to abort them before they came to term.

The principal unifying characteristic of the figures at the core of the circle was a fundamental and slightly hysterical optimism about the nature and value of knowledge. It was perhaps this optimism, rather than any genuine methodological debt, that was most authentically 'Baconian' in their outlook. They expected the increase of knowledge to alleviate man's lot in every respect, from the most mundane to the metaphysical: by improving living conditions, by producing wealth, by curing disease, by promoting consensus, by bringing humanity closer to God and by preparing for the Millennium. But did they not perhaps protest too much? Did the endlessly reiterated assertions of faith in method really reflect confidence in such a culmination, or were they a prophylactic mantra against the conception of an unorganised, unguided, and ultimately unknowable universe?

Their guiding ideals in all their undertakings were unity and universality. Dury laboured to be 'all things to all men', Comenius to 'teach all things to all people in all ways'. Warning against Pell's projected involvement with Descartes and his parabolic lenses, and in favour of his pursuing instead the study of analytical method, Moriaen urged:

> what he [Descartes] seeks is still uncertain, and, besides, only a point of detail. But what he [Pell] knows and can perform already in elaborating [Vieta's] Universal Logic is altogether certain, and moreover a universal labour from which countless particularities will follow of their own accord.[4]

The image of a key, or of an opened door, recurs significantly in their own writings and their favoured texts in all their fields of interest, from Comenius's pansophic *Janua Rerum* (*Gate of Things*) through Mede's chiliastic *Clavis Apocalyptica* (*Key to the Apocalypse*) to Starkey's alchemical *Introitus Apertus in Occlusum Regis Palatinum* (*An Open Entrance to the Shut-Palace of the King*). Entry to the citadel of wisdom was to be gained not by siege but painlessly and peacefully, by finding the key to it. Finding the key required great labour and diligence, but once it was found, the search would be over once and for all.

This well-nigh obsessive harping on unity and universality was symptomatic of a profound sense of disunity and fragmentation. This was a period of unprecedented division and diversity of opinions and ideologies in all fields, the religious, the political, the philosophical and the scientific. Christianity had always had its schisms, but never had it shattered so quickly into so many distinct and mutually antagonistic groups as between the mid-sixteenth and the mid-seventeenth century. Nor had there ever been a conflict as widespread or as destructive as the Thirty Years War. In intellectual matters, the rise of specialisation, so abhorrent to Comenius, threatened to hedge in every intellect with an impenetrable mass of detail. Mankind - or so it seemed to these thinkers - was in danger of being left like so many people trapped in a maze, each gazing down a different blind alley and unable to communicate with the others, while an overview would - or must? - discern the one true path that would lead them all out of it.

Both Moriaen and Hartlib provide classic examples of personal intellectual histories that appear, superficially, to represent a progressive secularisation of interests. However, as this study has striven throughout to make plain, doctrinal non-specificity is not to be confused with secularisation, and the notion of 'scientific' enquiry as a distinct field from religious study is rarely if ever appropriate to the thought of this period. The Latin 'scientia' does not mean 'science' in the modern sense, it simply means 'knowledge'. All these different lines of enquiry represent different routes to the same goal, the discovery of the true method that would, quite literally, make sense of everything. The notion of pansophic method and that of the Philosophers' Stone have much in common. Both have more than a whiff of the miraculous about them. Both were deemed attainable only by divine grace: 'it is not of him that wills, or of him that runnes, but of God only who in this as in more higher things enlightens whom he will'.[5] Both were quite explicitly presented as the means to restore humankind to its prelapsarian state, perfectly understanding Nature and exercising dominion over it. Both were articles of faith clung to with perceptibly mounting desperation as what we now call relativism, materialism and scepticism began to take on definition within Western thought. They were expressions of a beleaguered faith in universal harmony, order and purpose, in providential guidance of the universe by an ultimately benevolent deity. They were envisaged as a sort of *deus ex machina* to close the final act of the human comedy.

This genuine and passionate belief in a transcendental quick fix is perhaps the hardest aspect of these people's thought for a modern sensibility to take seriously. Many of their ideas have become so exclusively the province of placard-bearing cranks and brainwashed cults that it is difficult to imagine how so many sane, intelligent, educated people could organise their whole existence around them. But they undeniably did so. They seriously expected to master the transmutation of metals and the cure of all diseases, to gain access to all knowledge and to unite the entire human race in one faith, and all in a matter of years. All they had to do was formulate the right method. That is not to say that anyone thought finding the right method would be easy. But once it was found, everything else would follow. This outlook was tenable only in the context of an equally profound faith in an omnipotent God who intervened personally in the destiny of mankind, who would himself provide the illumination that would make all this possible, and would appear himself in glory when the providential plan was accomplished.

Like so many of their specific projects, this exalted unifying faith of Hartlib and his comrades fizzled out as a damp squib. Thirty years of bloodshed in Germany ended not in the overthrow of Antichrist but in a settlement that left the overall balance of religious power pretty well the same as it had been at the outset. The visionary new Commonwealth of England, instead of building a New Jerusalem, aborted itself after twelve years and handed back the reins of power to the family it had so painfully wrested them from. No panacea or Philosophers' Stone materialised. 1658 came and went without any verified sighting of Elias Artista. The Jews remained obstinately Jewish. Comenius died without completing his Pansophy, and the Second Coming began to seem less and less imminent.

The increase of knowledge, in which the Hartlib circle had undoubtedly played an important role, exacerbated the fragmentation of learning rather than healing it. It did indeed, in due course, contribute to a rise of scepticism and to a secularisation of both learning and society. Whatever their intellectual and ideological significance in the broader historical perspective, on their own terms Hartlib and his friends failed utterly.

They had believed themselves to be living in the last days, when 'many shall run to and fro, and knowledge shall be increased' (Daniel, 12:4). They had paid less heed to the warning of Ecclesiastes 1:18: 'In much wisdom is much grief: and he that increaseth knowledge increaseth sorrow'.

Notes

1   'Der herr obligirt vnß andere doch vnd thut eben genug daß er das werckh dirigirt die Correspondentz pflanzet vnd erhält vnd einem Ieden das seinige verschafft vnd zuesendet was die kost*en* belanget die behören von den Liebhabern gesambter hand getrag*en* zue werden' - Moriaen to Hartlib, 13 Dec. 1638, HP 37/2B.

2   Webster, *Great Instauration*, 484-520.

3   Richard Popkin, *The Third Force in Seventeenth Century Thought* (Leiden, 1992) 90.

4   'was Er suchet ist noch vngewiß vnd darzue nur ein particular stuckh. Was Er aber bereit weiß vnd *præ*stirn kan in elaborando Logistica speciosa das ist ganz gewiß darzue ein Uniuersal werckh dareus [*sic*] dergleich*en* vnzehliche particularia von sich selbst*en* entspring*en* werd*en*' - Moriaen to Hartlib, 14 Nov. 1639, HP 37/47A

5   Worsley to ?, 14 Feb. 1655/6, HP 42/1/5A.

APPENDIX

1. Copy in Heinrich Appelius's hand of Glauber's 'Furni Novi Philosophici Utilitates' (Amsterdam, 1643)
HP 63/14/48A-49B.

[63/14/48A]
Furni Noui *Philosophici* Utilitates oder Beschreibung der eigenschafften eines sonderbaren new erfundenen[*altered*] *Philosophischen* distillir ofens, auch was für Sp*iritus*, olen, flores vnd der gleichen bisshero vnbekante Vegetabilische, Animalische vnd Mineralische medicamenten damit können zugericht vnd bereit werden. Der warheit vnd spagyrischen kunst liebhabern an tag geben durch Iohannem Rudolphum Glauberum, itziger zeit wohnhafft in Amsterdam.
Zu Amsterdam gedruckt beÿ Broer Ianß. Anno 1643.
    Furni *Philosophici* a Ioh. Rudolpho Glaubero primum inuenti utilitates.
1. Die Nutzbarkeit dieses ofens ist diese, nemlich dz alles das sonsten durch retorten oder andere gewöhnliche vnd bekante glaserne oder erdene instrumenta destillatoria mit ~~grossem~~ <vielen> kosten grossen fewern, vnd langer zeit mus ausgetrieben werden kan in diesem mit wenig kosten vnd muhe, kleinem fewer vnd kurtzer zeit, sehr compendiosé gethan werden.
2. Dann in einer stund kan alhier mit 4 oder 5 lb Kohlen ein lb sp*iritu* salis gemacht werden, da doch sonsten durch die gemeine weiß per retortam solches in 30. oder 40 stunden kaum mit einem grossen sack voll geschehen kan.
3. Desgleichen kan mit 3 oder 4 lb kohlen in j stund j lb Antimonij in schöne flores sublimirt werden welches auf die bekante manier in etlich tagen nicht kan gethan werden.
4. Auch mag man in d*istil*liren vnd sublimiren aufhören vnd nachlassen, auch wiederumb anfangen wann man will, hindert nichts in der destillation, Dann es kan kein retort oder recipient brechen, auch kan man alle stund einen besondern spiritum d*istil*liren, also dz man in einem tag vnterschiedliche sp*iritus* Olea vnd flores mit einem ofen machen kan. [63/14/48B]
5. Vnd alle Bergarten, nicht allein die bekanten mineralia vnd metallen oder alle lapides als Cristallen, Granaten, Kißling vnd dergleichen, sondern auch Talcum, zwitter, spath, Alabaster vnd ihres geschlechts, die sonst fast von allen Chymicis bißhero für fix vnd fewerbestendig seind gehalten worden, können in herrliche vnd nützliche sp*iritus*, olea, flores, so wol zur Alchymia als zur Medicin dienstlich, in vnd eüsserlich zugebrauchen, destiilirt oder sublimirt werden.
6. Auch kan der flüchtige vnd volatilische sp*iritus* aller salien als Vitrioli, salis communis, salis armoniaci etc wie auch aller mineralien vnd metallen sp*iritus* sulphureus subtilissim*us* gefangen ~~werden~~ vnd behalten werden, welches bißher von wenig laboranten erkant worden, dieweil an ihnen als ein vnsichtbarer geist durch ihr lucken entflogen ist, vnd sein corpus als einen spiritum acidum im recipienten hinterlassen hat.
7. Deren vnd noch viel mehr andere gute <vnd> nützliche vortheilen im d*istil*liren werden alhier in diesem ofen gefunden.

8. Wer dann solchen hat, vnd den rechten gebrauch desselben weiß vnd verstehet; der kan dadurch gar leicht schöne vnd köstliche medicamenta erlangen, damit wunder ding in der medicina konnen gethan werden. Als zum exempel etliche derselben sollen angezeigt vnd verrichtet werden. wie folget.

9. Aus allen Vegetabilibus, als kräuter, wurtzeln, vnd höltzen gantz geschwind ein grosse quantitet Aceti oder spiritus acidi mit wenig kohlen zu distilliren also compendiosé, dz man auch in j tag viel lb aceti oder spiritus ligni. Hebeni, quercini, Iuniperi buxi, Quajaci oder dergleichen, nun mit j lb kohlen distilliren kan, dz auch die spiritus nit mehr kosten als das holtz oder kraut selbsten daraus der Spiritus gemacht werden.

10. Aus den Animalibus, in sonderheit Menschenhaar, hiernschetel, röhren, knochen etc. auch hirschhörner, Elephantenbein, Elandsklawen [etc] Spiritus vnd olea in grosser quantitet gar geschwind zu distilliren.

[catchword: 11.] [63/14/49A]

11. Alle olea Vegetabilium vnd Pinguedines animalium[1] so subtil machen, dz sie auch den Sulphur[2] oder Tinctur der Mineralien Metallen et lapidum extrahirn. [right margin, H: 10 Rthl[3]]

12. Aus den Metallen vnd mineralien ihr Elementum Igneum in forma spiritus subtillissimi zumachen mit welchem grosse dinge können gethan werden.

13. Ein sauren vnd scharffen acetum per se ohne addition aus dem Antimonio, wie auch aus andern mineralien vnd metallen zu distillirn.

14. Alle Metallen et Mineralien per se in spiritus, flores et salia zu sublimirn.

15. Alle lapides in flores zu zu sublimirn.

16. Aus den silicibus, cristallis alijsque lapidibus ein spiritum et oleum <zu distilliren.>

17. Aus dem Talco ein oleum zu distilliren.

18. Aus dem Bezoartico[4] minerali oder Antimonio diaphoretico fixo, flores zu sublimiren.

19. Aus dem Antimonio, sulphure alijsque mineralibus flores zu sublimiren, welche sich in alle liquoribus soluiren vnd keine vomitus machen.

20. Sal tartari, auch tartarum Vitriolatum vnd andere salia fixa in spiritus zu distilliren.

21. Aus Vitriolo, Antimonio wie auch aus all andere mineralien vnd metallen ein liebliches vnd süsses roth oleum zu distilliren. [right margin, H: 10.]

22. Ein Menstruum welches der mineralien vnd metallen tincturam extrahiret vnd mit sich vbern helm führet.[5] [right margin, H: 20.]

23. Ein Menstruum in welchem die Mineralia et Metalla in einem tag putrificiren vnd schwartz werden, den andern tag aufwachsen als ein baum mit wurtzeln, stam vnd vielen nesten,[6] vnd zweigen, wunderbarlicherweis. [right margin, H: 30 oder 40[7]]

24. Ein spiritus oder Menstruum welches die olea distillata aromatum in liebliche Balsama coagulirt, die nimmer mehr ranzucht[8] oder zeh werden, vnd sich in wasser, wein auch all andern liquoribus soluirn lassen. [right margin, H: 10.]

25. Ein spiritus welcher die silices, cristallos oder andere harte stein in wenig stunden zu einem klaren wasser auf soluiret vnd solche mit sich vbern helm führet, auch sich wiederumb von den cristallis scheidet, dz die[altered from sie] selbe per se in forma olei seu liquoris bleiben. [right margin, H: 20.]

[catchword: 26.] [63/14/49B]

26. Alle Metalla vnd Mineralia astralisch machen, & purum ab impuro separare solo igne secreto Philosophico [left margin, H: 100.]

27. Aqua Vitæ Philosophorum, damit in 1 oder 2 stunden der sulphur oder tinctur fast aller mineralien, metallen vnd lapidum kan extrahirt werden. [left margin, H: 20.⁹]

28. Balneum siccum Philosophicum, mit welchem der mehrentheil Krankheiten nur von außerhalb des leibs applicirt wunderbarlicher weiß können curirt werden. [left margin, H: 100]

29. Spiritum Vini¹⁰ also zu dephlegmiren vnd stercken, dz er nicht allein tincturas Vegetabilium, animalium et mineralium extrahirt, sondern auch silices, cristallos, talcum vnd der gleichen harte ding soluirt. [left margin, H: 10.]

30. Solche vnd dergleichen noch viel vnzehlige gute medicamenta können in diesem ofen gemacht werden, welche vmb der kurtze willen vnvermeldet bleiben, auch ist es nicht möglich alles zuerzehlen, was damit kan gethan werden, dann es finden sich noch alle tag noch mehr vnd mehr newe ding so man damit laboriret, vnd ist gleichsam einen vnausschöpfflichen brunnen ~~gleich~~ zu vergleichen, aus welchem zu allen zeiten vnauffhörlich frisches wasser heraus laufft, vnd dennoch nicht aufhöret zu rinnen.

31. Also habe ich Gott zuehren vnd dinste meines nächsten diese meine newe inuention wollen bekant machen, vnd vermeine dadurch vielen vrsach zugeben, hinfort die verborgene heimlichkeiten der Natur desto leichter zuergrüblen; gäntzlicher zuversicht, es werde manchem frommen medico wol damit gedient sein: vnd ob schon der ofen sampt dem modo destillandi nicht gesetzt, soll er gleichwol dem liebhaber darumb nicht gewegert sein.¹¹

Item er hat noch ein Menstruum, welchs man an allen orten ohne einige destilland haben kan, zeücht der metallen sulphura gar seltzam aus, vnd kan sie verbessern. für 40 Rtt.

NB. Er hat nur einen ofen erwehnet; hat aber doch zween, einen grossen vnd einen sehr kleinen, alle beide samt aller gesetzter sachen operation will er zeigen fur 30 Rthl: ausgenommen etliche stücke beÿ welchen ihr pretium absonderlich gesetzt, vnd bedeuten alles Rthl.

2. Copy extract in Hartlib's hand, Charles de Montendon to ?, 4 March 1661.
HP 15/9/19A-B

[15/9/19A]
   Leipsigk. March 4. 1661
 Glauber is fallen vpon mee at the Altenburg-Court, where hee charges mee that I have beene the only cause, why his busines did not proceed having gotten the 24. Processe which I had entrusted to the Electoral Delegats of Mentz which I imparted to the Delegates from Altenburg, least [deletion?] <Hee> should have gotten the Monies which were promised, which indeed would have beene the highest Injustice, and therfore those of Altenburg had separated themselves from his Schoole, going away without taking their leaves, and keeping the Monies, which they also made the Bavarian to doe amounting to 4000. Rixd. All this I confesse I have done. by which meanes I have saved such Monies out of the Impostors claw's. Nor doe I care to attest

this Truth[12] and to maintaine it, which also the Court hath approved. I am glad therfore that I have exercised myselfe in the Germane - Language, so that now I need not to put out my Refutation of Glaubere in the French ~~Language~~ <Tongue> which otherwise I should have beene necessitated to doe. For having found the Deceivers (Glaubers) deceits by my owne losses, which <now> I know to bee nothing else but falshood and cousenage, I have [count.?] it my duty to warne [others.?] for their good by a Treatise on purpose entituled - A needful Refutation of Glaubers hitherto divulged Vn-Truths. I confesse I have beene somwhat sharp and passionat calling <him> Villaine Knave and Theefe yea the great and impudent Arch-Cheater. I have also certain writings vnder his owne hands, so that I shall bee able [*15/9/19B*] to enter into a course of Law with him[*altered from* them] either to performe what hee hath vndertaken and promised or to recover the Monies, which hee hath had from ~~mee~~ a Friend of mine. the fore-said Treatise is here printed and will bee ready against the Mart.[13] Thus far Charls de Montendon from Leipzigk concerning his Purpose and Booke against Glauber.

3. Glauber's 'undertaking', or offer of alchemical secrets for sale, undated: partial English translation and copy of German original
HP 67/15/1B and 3A

[*67/15/1B*]
[*Hartlib:*]
   The trial of the Tin-scoriæ or refuse
Note that by the Tin-scoriæ is vnderstood that matter which at the Mines is thrown away, when the Tinn is no more in it.

When the Scoriæ are reduced with a good flux the hunderd weight yields from 25. to 30 lb. a kind of vnformed blackish and impure Tinne. But if the said Scoriæ bee first fixed (which may bee done within 3. or 4. days the Hundred weight requiring about 10. or 12. gilders ~~char~~ for charges) they yeeld ~~in~~ afterward in the melting of it ~~from~~ no such vnformed Tin; but from 2. to $2\frac{1}{2}$ loth of good Gold. And when all the required charges for fixing melting ~~ete~~ and ~~taking of~~ <drieing out> from $2\frac{1}{2}$ loth of Gold are deducted there remaines richly of every hundred weight 1 loth gold, which is to bee accounted for the gaine of it. And both [*67/15/2A*] as well fixing melting as drieing out may bee performed in great with many hundreds of weight at once, so that the profit will bee ~~very rich~~ considerable. For this Art after j ~~had~~ haue shown it in great quantity I demaund the sume of 2. thous*and* Ducats./

[*16/15/3A*]
[*another hand:*]
   Gethane prob über das Bleÿ Erz aus Engell*and*.

Erstlich das Erz, nach dem kleinen Zentner-gewicht versucht, gibt der Zentner wan es genaw gesucht wird über 60 lb bleÿ doch nicht recht geschmeÿdig, So mans aber so genaw nicht außschmelzt, so gibt der Zentner 50 biß auff 56 lb geschmeÿdig vnd gutt bleÿ, vnd der Zentner von diesem Bleÿ hält 6 Loth Silber

<*left margin:* NB> So man aber diß Erz zuevorn cimentirt od*er* figiert so gibt der Zentner Erz 48 oder 50 lb Bleÿ, 5 loth Silber vnd ein halb Loth Goltt. Die vnkosten so auff dießes Stößen oder figirn an kolen vnd zuesaz erfordert werden, kommen auff j zentner vngefähr 2 oder auffs höchste dreÿ gülden. vnd läst solche figirung sich so groß thun als man will. Vnd wans figiert ist auch so leichtlich schmelzen in großer quantitet gleich ein Iedweder gemein Bleÿ Erz. Vnd so es begehrt wird soll eine prob oder etliche so viel nötig sein wird von 10, 20 oder mehr pfunden dauon gemacht werden Fur die communication derselben wißenschafft soll mir ein Tausend ducat*en* bezahlt werden

Prob vber die Zinnschlacken *

<* Nota <u>Zinnschlacken</u>/ Ist die materia die man auff den bergwercken hinweg wirfft was das Zinn heraus ist.>

Wan solche schlacken mit einem guten fluß reducirt wird so gibt der Zentner zue 25 biß auff 30 lb vnartig, brüchig, schwarzlicht od*er* vnsauber Zinn. So man aber zuevorn dieselbe schlacken figiret (welches innerhalb 3 oder 4 tagen geschehen kan) vnd der Zentner vngefähr 10 oder 12 gulden vnkosten darzue von nöthen hatt,) So gibt Er hernach im schmelzen kein vnartig Zinn mehr sondern zue 2 biß auff $2\frac{1}{2}$ Loth gutt Goltt. Vnd wan alle angewandte Kosten, auffs figirn, schmelzen vnd abtreiben von den $2\frac{1}{2}$ Loth goltt abgezogen sein So bleibt reichlich von Iedwederem Zentner j Loth goltt welches fur gewin gerechnet wird. Vnd läst so woll das figiren als schmelzen vnd abtreiben sich im großen thun mit viel Zentnern zuegleich also das es reiche außbeut geben kan. Darfur Ich begehre 2 Tausend Ducat*en* wan Ich solche Kunst ins große zue thun gezaiget hab.

Iohan: Rudolph: Glauber

Notes

[1]   'vegetable oils and animal fats'.

[2]   In the Paracelsian sense of 'sulphur' as one of the three 'principles'.

[3]   These marginal notes of the prices are taken from Appelius's letter to Hartlib, 6 Nov. 47, HP 45/1/37A-B, though Hartlib's notes do not always correspond exactly to what Appelius told him.

[4]   Bezoar, a term possibly derived from Persian and meaning 'counter-poison', applied to a range of supposed mineral remedies in the early modern period. See Partington, *History of Chemistry* II, 98.

[5]   I.e. the 'tincture' (or sulphurous 'principle') is distilled together with the 'menstruum' by passing over the helm, i.e. the head of the retort.

[6]   *Sic*: surely a mistake for 'aesten'? The Latin gives 'cum stirpe, radicibus, ramis et frondibus multis' ('with a trunk, roots, many branches and much foliage').

[7]   Unambiguously 'XXX thl' on Appelius's list.

[8]   Not a word I have encountered anywhere else. It apparently means 'dry' or 'dessicated': the Latin is 'ut nunquam exsiccentur aut tenacia evadent'.

[9]   Only 10 according to Appelius.

APPENDIX

10   I.e. alcohol.
11   This clearly marks the end of Glauber's advertisement; what follow are Appelius's own remarks.
12   I.e. nor do I have any objection to attesting this truth.
13   I.e. the Frankfurt Book Fair.

Bibliography

The following bibliography is in four sections: (I) manuscript sources, (II) reference works and bibliographies, (III) primary printed sources and (IV) secondary printed sources. Reference works are listed alphabetically by compiler, or by title in the case of multiple collaborations. Primary printed sources are listed alphabetically by original author. The author's name is given in square brackets in the case of translations, compilations of miscellaneous extracts and works reproduced within the work of a later writer. Compilations of correspondence or of other writings by more than one hand, if not clearly focussed on a given individual, are listed alphabetically by editor. Works by the same author are listed chronologically by date of composition, with compilations and collections of correspondence appearing last.

Prepositions appearing as separate words within surnames (eg. de, von) are ignored for the purposes of alphabeticisation: thus E.G.E. Van Der Wall appears under W, not V.

I: Manuscript Sources

British Library:
> Birch MS 4279, Fols. 147-8: Moriaen to Pell, 30 March 1652, and Moriaen to Jan
>   Abeel, 5 Aug. 1658
> Sloane MS 649 fol. 212: Moriaen to Hartlib, 13 June 1653

Gemeendearchief Arnhem:
> RA 513: Procuratie de Anno 1656 Tot 1653

Herzog August-Bibliothek, Wolfenbüttel:
> Cod. Guelf. 56 Extrav.: correspondence of J.V. Andreæ
> Cod. Guelf. 65.1 Extrav.: letters of J.V. Andreæ to Herzog August the Younger of
>   Wolfenbüttel
> Cod. Guelf. 149.6 Extrav.: letters of J.V. Andreæ and Herzog August to Georg Philip
>   Hainhofer
> Cod. Guelf. 236.1-236.2 Extrav.: letters of Herzog August to J.V. Andreæ and copy
>   letters, Herzog August to Georg Philip Hainhofer
> Cod. Guelf. 98 Novi fol. 308: Wiesel to Moriaen, 17 Dec. 1649
> Cod. Guelf. 74 Noviss. 2^O: letters of J.V. Andreæ to Georg Philip Hainhofer
> Cod. Guelf. 15 Noviss. 8°: letters of Herzog August to J.V. Andreæ

Sheffield University Library:
> The Hartlib Papers

Staats- und Universitätsbibliothek Hamburg:
> Sup. Ep. 100, 60-63: Hartlib to J.A. Tassius, 10 Aug. 1638
> 98.19-22: Joachim Morsius to Joachim Jungius, 26 Aug. 1643
Universiteitsbibliothek Amsterdam:
> N65a-h: letters of Moriaen to Justinus Van Assche

II: Reference Works and Bibliographies

Aa, A.J. Van Der: *Aardrijkskundig Woordenboek der Nederlanden* (Gorinchem, 1844)

BIBLIOGRAPHY

Allgemeine Deutsche Biographie (Leipzig, 1875-1912)

Biographie Générale (Paris, 1852-66)

Bruckner, J.: *A Bibliographical Catalogue of seventeenth-century German Books Published in Holland* (The Hague and Paris, 1971)

Catholic Encyclopedia, The (New York, 1907)

Dictionary of National Biography (London, 1885-1903)

Dictionary of Scientific Biography (New York, 1970-80)

Dictionnaire d'histoire et de géographie ecclésiastiques (Paris, 1988)

Doorman, G.: *Patents for Inventions in the Netherlands during the 16th, 17th and 18th Centuries* (abridged trans. Joh. Meijer, The Hague, 1942)

Dünnhaupt, Gerhard: *Personalbibliographien zu den Drucken des Barock* (Stuttgart, 1990)

Duveen, Denis I.: *Bibliotheca Alchemica et Chemica* (London, 1949)

Elias, Johan E.: *De Vroedschap van Amsterdam* (Amsterdam, 1963: first ed. Haarlem, 1903-5)

Encyclopædia Judaica (Jerusalem and New York, 1972)

Faber du Faur, Curt von: *German Baroque Literature: A Catalogue of the Collection in the Yale University Library* (Yale, 1958)

Ferguson, John: *Bibliotheca Chemica* (Glasgow, 1906)

Fortsetzung und Ergänzungen zu Jöchers allgemeinem Gelehrten-Lexicon, angefangen von Johann Christoph Adelung (Leipzig, 1784-1897; photolithograph Hildesheim, 1960-61)

Fürst, Julius: *Bibliotheca Judaica* (Leipzig, 1849-63)

Graesse, J.G.Th. and Friedrich Benedict: *Orbis Latinus oder Verzeichnis der wichtigsten lateinischen Orts- und Ländernamen* (Berlin, 1909)

Grosses vollständiges Universal Lexicon aller Wissenschaften und Künste ('Zedlers Universal Lexicon') (Halle and Leipzig, 1732-54)

Jöcher, Christian Gottlieb: *Allgemeines Gelehrten-Lexicon* (Leipzig, 1750-51; photolithograph Hildesheim, 1960-61)

Kumpera, Jan: *Jan Amos Komensky: Poutník na Rozhraní Veku* (Ostrava, 1992).

Müller, Joseph: 'Zur Bücherkunde des Comenius: Chronologisches Verzeichnis der gedruckten und ungedruckten Werke des Johann Amos Comenius', *Monatshefte der Comeniusgesellschaft* I (1892), 19-53

Nationaal Biografisch Woordenboek (Brussels, 1964-74)

Neue Deutsche Biographie (Berlin, 1953-94)

Nieuw Nederlands Biografisch Woordenboek (Leiden, 1911-37)

Partington, J.R.: *A History of Chemistry* II (*1500-1800*) (London, 1961)

Recke, J.F. von and K.E. Napiersky: *Allgemeines Schriftsteller- und Gelehrten-Lexikon der Provinzen Livland, Esthland und Kurland* (Mitau, 1827-32)

Scholem, Gershom: *Bibliographia Kabbalistica* (Leipzig, 1927)

Thieme, Ulrich and Felix Becker: *Allgemeines Lexikon der bildenden Künstler, von der Antike bis zur Gegenwart* (Leipzig, 1907)

Thorndike, Lynn: *A History of Magic and Experimental Science* V-VIII (*Sixteenth and Seventeenth Centuries*) (New York, 1941-58)

Toepke, G. (ed.): *Die Matrikel der Universität Heidelberg von 1386 bis 1662* (Heidelberg, 1886)

Woodcroft, Bennet: *Titles of Patents of Invention* (London, 1854)

Zibrt, Cenek: *Bibliografie Ceské Historie* (Prague, 1912)

Primary Printed Sources

Andreæ, Johann Valentin: *Chymische Hochzeit Christiani Rosenkreutz Anno 1459* (first pub. 1616), *Quellen und Forschungen zur Württembergischen Kirchengeschichte* VI, ed. Richard Van Dülmen (Stuttgart, 1973)

260

BIBLIOGRAPHY

- *Reipublicæ Christianopolitanæ Descriptio* (Strasbourg, 1619)
- [-] *Christianopolis*, English translation of the above by Felix Held (New York, 1916)
- *Christianæ Societatis Imago* (Tübingen, 1620)
- *Christiani Amoris Dextera Porrecta* (Tübingen, 1620)
- [-] George Turnbull, 'Johann Valentin Andreæs Societas Christiana', *Zeitschrift für deutsche Philologie* 73 (1954), 407-432 (introduction and Latin text of Andreæ's *Christianæ Societatis Imago* and *Christiani Amoris Dextera Porrecta*, q.v., transcribed from the Hartlib Papers) and 74 (1955), 151-85 (John Hall's English translation of the above, first pub. 1647)
- *Amicorum singularium clarissimorum Funera* (Lüneburg, 1642)
- [-] *Selbstbiographie* (translation from the manuscript of *Vita ab ipso conscripta* by David Christoph Seybold, Winterthur, 1799)
- [-] *Johann Valentin Andreæ - ein schwäbischer Pfarrer im Dreißigjährigen Krieg*, ed. Paul Antony (Heidenheim an der Brenz, 1970). Selected writings in German translation.
- Anon.: *Fama Fraternitatis des löblichen Ordens des Rosenkreutzes* (first pub. 1614), *Quellen und Forschungen zur Württembergischen Kirchengeschichte* VI, ed. Richard Van Dülmen (Stuttgart, 1973). The edition attributes this and the following work to J.V. Andreæ.
- [Anon.]: *Confessio Fraternitatis oder Bekanntnuß der löblichen Bruderschafft deß hochgeehrten Rosen Creutzes* (first pub. 1615), *Quellen und Forschungen zur Württembergischen Kirchengeschichte* VI, ed. Richard Van Dülmen (Stuttgart, 1973)
- Anon. (ed.): *Theatrum Chemicum, Præcipuos Selectorum Auctorum Tractatus de Chemiæ et Lapidis Philosophici Antiquitate, veritate, jure, præstantia, & operationibus* (Strasbourg, 1659-60)
- Anon. (ed.): *Musæum Hermeticum Reformatum et Amplificatum* (Frankfurt am Main, 1678)
- Ashmole, Elias (ed.): *Theatrum Chemicum Britannicum, Containing Severall Poeticall Pieces of our Famous English Philosophers, who have written the Hermetique Mysteries in their owne Ancient Language* (London, 1652: reprint with an introduction by Allen G. Debus, *The Sources of Science* no. 39, New York and London, 1967)
- Aubrey, John: *Brief Lives, Mainly of Contemporaries, set down by John Aubrey*, ed. Andrew Clark (Oxford, 1898)
- Bacon, Francis: *The Works of Francis Bacon*, ed. James Spedding, Robert Leslie Ellis and Douglas Denon Heath (London, 1857-74)
- Beeckman, Isaac: *Journal tenu par Isaac Beeckman de 1604 à 1634*, ed. Cornelijs de Waard (The Hague, 1939-53)
- Bell, Henrie: *Doctoris Martini Lutheri Colloquia Mensalia, Or Luther's Last Divine Discourses* (London, 1652)
- Blekastad, Milada (ed.): *Unbekannte Briefe des Comenius und seiner Freunde 1641-1661* (Ratingen and Kastellaun, 1976)
- Böhme, Jacob: *Werke*, ed. Will-Erich Peuckert (Stuttgart, 1961)
- Boyle, Robert: *The Sceptical Chymist: or Chymico-Physical Doubts & Paradoxes, Touching the Spagyrist's Principles Commonly call'd Hypostatical; As they are wont to be Propos'd and Defended by the Generality of Alchymists. Whereunto is præmis'd Part of another Discourse relating to the same Subject* (London, 1661)
- *The Works of the Honourable Robert Boyle*, ed. Thomas Birch (London, 1772)
- *The Early Essays and Ethics of Robert Boyle*, ed. John T. Harwood (Carbondale and Edwardsville, 1991)
- Braddick, M.J. and M. Greengrass (eds.) *The Letters of Sir Cheney Culpeper (1641-1657)* (Camden Miscellany XXXIII, Cambridge, 1996)
- Browne, Thomas: *The Works of Sir Thomas Browne*, ed. Geoffrey Keynes (London, 1928, new edition 1964)
- [Campanella, Tommaso]: *La Cité du soleil* (orig. *Civitas Solis*, 1623), edited with an introduction and notes by Luigi Firpo, trans. Arnaud Tripet (Geneva, 1972)

261

BIBLIOGRAPHY

Cardilucius, Johann Hiscius (ed.): *Magnalia Medico-Chymica, oder Die höchste Artzney-und feurkünstige Geheimnisse, wie nemlich mit dem circulatio majori oder dem universal aceto mercuriali [...] die herrlichsten Artzneyen [...] zu machen*, etc (Nürnberg, 1676)

[Comenius, Jan Amos]: *Der Labyrinth der Welt und das Paradies des Herzens* (orig. *Labyrint sveta a ráj srdce*, 1631), trans. Zdenko Baudnik (Lucerne and Frankfurt am Main, 1970)

[-] *A Reformation of Schooles* (anon. English translation of *Prodromus Pansophiæ*, 1639 and *Conatuum Pansophicorum Dilucidatio*, 1639) (London, 1642)

-   *Opera Didactica Omnia* (Amsterdam, 1657: facsimile reproduction Prague, 1957)

[-] *Comenius' Självbiografi: Comenius about himself* (reprint of *Continuatio Admonitionis Fraternæ de temperando Charitate Zelo*, 1670, with Swedish and English translations by Jan-Olof Tjäder and Agneta Ljunggren) (Stockholm, 1975)
    See also under Blakastad, Kracola and Patera.

[-] *De Rerum Humanarum Emendatione Consultatio Catholica,* (incomplete translation by A.M.O. Dobbie):
    I: Panegersia (Shipton on Stour, 1990)
    II: Panaugia (Shipton on Stour, 1987)
    IV: Pampædia (Dover, 1986)
    V: Panglottia (Shipton on Stour, 1989)
    VI: Panorthosia (chapters 19-26) (Sheffield, 1993)
    VII: Pannuthesia (Shipton on Stour, 1991)

[-] John Sadler: *Comenius* (London, 1969). English translations of selected writings, with an introduction.

[-] R.F. Young: *Comenius in England* (London, 1932). English translations of selected writings, with an introduction.

[-] *John Amos Comenius on Education* (Unesco, 1957). Selected writings, trans. M.W. Keatinge and Iris Unwin, with an introduction by Jean Piaget.

Donne, John: *Ignatius His Conclave*, ed. T.S. Healy (Oxford, 1969)

Dury, John: *Considerations tending to the Happy Accomplishment of Englands Reformation in Church and State* (London, 1647)

Evelyn, John: *The Diary of John Evelyn*, ed. W. Bray (London, 1879)

Figulus, Petr: *Peter Figulus. Letters to Samuel Hartlib 1657-58*, ed. Milada Blekastad (*Lychnos, Lärdomshistorika Samfundets Årsbok*, 1988)

Gauden, John: *The Love of Truth and Peace: A Sermon Preached before the Honovrable Hovse of Commons Assembled in Parliament Novemb. 29. 1640* (London, 1641)

Glauber, Johann Rudolph: 'Briefwechsel zwischen J.R. Glauber und Otto Sperling', ed. Ad Clément and J.W.S. Johnsson, *Janus* 29 (1925), 210-33

-   *Furni Novi Philosophici Oder Beschreibung einer New-erfundenen Distillir-Kunst* (Amsterdam, 1646-49)

-   *Miraculum Mundi oder Außführliche Beschreibung der wunderbaren Natur/ Art vnd Eigenschafft deß großmächtigen Subjecti, von den Alten Menstruum Universale oder: Mercurius Philosophorum: genandt* (Amsterdam, 1653-60)

-   *Glauberus Ridivivus; Daß ist: Der von Falschen und Gifftigen Züngen ermorte/ vnd mit Lügen und Lastermaulen gleichsam begrabene/ nun aber durch Hülff vnd Zeugnis der Wahrheit wieder auffgeständene Glauber* (Amsterdam, 1656)

-   *Des Teutschlandts Wohlfart* (Amsterdam, 1656-61)

-   *Tractatus De Natura Salium: Oder Außfürliche Beschreibung deren bekanten Salien, vnterscheiden Natur, Eigenschafft/ vnd Gebrauch* (Amsterdam, 1658)

-   *De Tribus Lapidibus Ignium Secretorum* (Amsterdam, 1667)

[-] *Glauberus Concentratus oder Kern der Glauberischen Schrifften* (Leipzig and Breslau, 1715). An abridged version (editor anon.) of Glauber's complete works, with marginal comments and 'explanations' that are of some interest for an assessment of early 18th-century interest in alchemy.

BIBLIOGRAPHY

Hartknoch, Christoph: *Preussische Kirchen-Historia, darinnen von Einführung der christlichen Religion in diese Land, wie auch von der Conservation, Fortpflanzung [...] und dem heutigen Zustande derselben ausführlich gehandelt wird. Nebst vielen denckwürdigen Begebenheiten [...] Aus vielen gedruckten [...] Dokumenten [...] zugetragen* (Frankfurt am Main and Leipzig, 1686)

Hartlib, Samuel (ed.): *A Further Discoverie of the Office of Publick Addresse for Accommodations* (London, 1648)

- (ed.) *Samuel Hartlib His Legacie of Husbandry. Wherein are bequeathed to the Common-Wealth of England. not onely Braband, and Flanders, but also many more Outlandish and Domestick Experiments and Secrets* (3rd. edition, London, 1655)

- (ed.) *Chymical, Medicinal, and Chyrurgical Addresses Made to Mr Samuel Hartlib Esq.* (London, 1655)

- (ed.) *The Reformed Common Wealth of Bees. Presented in several Letters and Observations to Sammuel Hartlib Esq.* (London, 1655)

Hessels, J.H. (ed.): *Ecclesiæ Londino-Batavæ Archivum* (1887-97)

[Israel, Menasseh ben]: *The Hope of Israel* (anon. translation of *Spes Israelis*, 1650) (London, 1650)

Jungius, Joachim: *Über die Originalsprache des Neuen Testaments vom Jahr 1637, aufgefunden, zuerst herausgegeben und eingeleitet von Johannes Geffcken* (Hamburg, 1863)

[-] *Des Dr. Joachim Jungius Briefwechsel*, ed. R. Avé-Lallemant (Lübeck, 1863)

Kvacala, Jan: *Korrespondence Jana Amosa Komenského* (Prague, 1897-1902)

- *Die Pädagogische Reform des Comenius bis zum Ausgange des XVII Jahrhunderts I: Texte: Monumenta Germaniæ Pædagogica XXVI* (Berlin, 1903)

[Lodwick, Francis]: *The Works of Francis Lodwick: A Study of his Writings in the Intellectual Context of the Seventeenth Century.* Facsimile edition of Lodwick's published works and transcription of 'Of an Universall Real Character' and 'Concerning Short Writing', with an introduction by Vivian Salmon ('throughout the world', 1972).

Löhr, Rudolf (ed.): *Protokolle der hochdeutsch-reformierten Gemeinde zu Köln 1599-1754* (*Inventare Nichtstaatlicher Archive* vols. 20, 24, 27, 33) (Cologne, 1976-90)

Luther, Martin: see Bell, Henrie

[Mersenne, Marin]: *Correspondance du P. Marin Mersenne, Religieux minime*, ed. Cornelis de Waard et al. (Paris, 1945-83)

Monconys, Balthasar de: *Les voyages de M. Monconys* (Paris, 1695)

Morsius, Joachim: *COPIA Einer kurtzen eylfertigen/ doch Rechtmässiger Ablehnung oder Protestation, kegen [sic] die vnbedachtsame vnd widerrechtliche Citation Burgermeister vnd Rath der Stadt Hamburg/ in justissimâ causâ Morsiana* ('Philadelphia, PaCe DeI Internâ, nIsI paX eXterna frVaMVr' [= Hamburg?, 1634])

Paracelsus (Theophrastus Bombast von Hohenheim): *Werke*, ed. Karl Sudhoff (Berlin, 1922-33)

Patera, A (ed.): *Jana Amosa Komenského Korrespondence* (Prague, 1892)

[Pell, John]: 'An Early Mathematical Manifesto: John Pell's *Idæa of Mathematics*', P.J. Wallis, *Durham Research Journal* 18 (1967), 139-48 (first pub. London, 1638). The complete English text of the *Idæa* with an introduction and a summary of contemporary reaction in English translation.

Pepys, Samuel: *The Diary of Samuel Pepys*, ed. Robert Latham and William Matthews (London, 1970-83)

Plattes, Gabriel: *A Discovery of Infinite Treasure; Hidden since the Worlds Beginning. Whereunto all men, of what degree soever, are friendly invited to be sharers with the Discoverer, G.P.* (London, 1639)

- *A Discovery of Subterraneall Treasure, viz. Of all manner of Mines and Minerals. from the Gold to the Coale; with plaine Directions and Rules for the finding of them in all Kingdomes and Countries* (London, 1639)

BIBLIOGRAPHY

- *A Description of the Famous Kingdome of Macaria* (London, 1641)
[Poniatovská, Christina]: *The Divine Revelations of Christina Poniatowska made in the years 1627, 1628 & 1629 faithfully translated from the Bohemian language into Latin by J.A. Comenius*, English translation by W.J. Hitchens (The Hartlib Papers Project, University of Sheffield, unpublished)
Raselius, Christoph Andreas: *Trew-Hertzige Buß-Posaune, Angeblasen vber eine sehr denckwürdige zur zeit Kaysers Ludovici Bavarii vor 300. Iahren/ Anno 1322 geschehene Propheceyung/ Vom jetzt vnd zukunfftigen zustande des Teutschlands/ Kayserthumbs/ vnd andrer Stände auch des Königs in Schweden* (s.l., 1632)
Roth, Leon (ed.): *Correspondence of Descartes and Constantine Huygens* (Oxford, 1926)
Sorbière, Samuel: *Relations. lettres et discours de Mr. de Sorbière sur diverses matières curieuses* (Paris, 1660)
[-] 'Drie Brieven van Samuel Sorbière over den Toestand van Holland in 1660', ed. P.J. Blok, *Bijdragen en Mededeelingen van het historische Genootschap* 22 (1901), 1-89
Sprat, Thomas: *History of the Royal Society* (London, 1667)
Teting, Nicolaus: *Abgetrungene Kurtze/ jedoch gründliche/ vnd mit H. Schrift vnd Lutheri, Philippi Melanthonis, Pomeranii, Brentii vnd anderer Authentisierten Lutherischen Theologen mehr Wolbewehrte Verantwortung/ NICOLAI TETINGS, Auff Deß zu Lübeck/ Hamburg vnd Lüneburg Predigampts ohnlengst in Trucke außgegangenem Buche/ vnter dem Titel: Außführliches Bericht*, etc. (s.l., 1635)
Webster, Charles (ed.): *Samuel Hartlib and the Advancement of Learning* (Cambridge (Eng.), 1970). Selected writings of Hartlib and Dury.
Wheeler, William: *Mr William Wheelers Case from his Own Relation* (London, 1649)
Winthrop, R.C. (ed.): *Correspondence of Hartlib, Haak, Oldenburg and Others of the Founders of the Royal Society with Governor Winthrop of Connecticut 1661-1672* (Boston, 1878)
Wood, Anthony à: *Athenæ Oxoniensis, an exact History of all the Writers and Bishops who have had their Education in the University of Oxford* (London, 1813-20)

IV Secondary Printed Sources

Adelung, Johann Christoph: *Geschichte der menschlichen Narrheit* (Leipzig, 1785)
Åkerman, Susanna: *Queen Christina of Sweden and her Circle: The Transformation of a Seventeenth-Century Philosophical Libertine* (Leiden, 1991)
Althaus, Friedrich: *Samuel Hartlib: Ein deutsch-englisches Charakterbild* (Leipzig, 1884)
Anon. (ed.): *Die Erbe des Christian Rosenkreuz: Vorträge gehalten anläßlich des Amsterdamer Symposiums 18-20 November 1986* (Amsterdam, 1986)
Arnold, Gottfried: *Unpartheyische Kirchen- und Ketzer-Historien vom Anfang des Neuen Testaments biß auf das Jahr Christi 1688* (Schaffhausen, 1740-42)
Arnold, Paul: *Histoire des Rose-Croix et les origines de la franc'maçonnerie* (Paris, 1955)
Avé-Lallemant, R.: *Yn Gudes Namen: Das Leben des Dr. Med. Joachim Jungius aus Lübeck* (Breslau, 1882)
Aylmer, G.E.: *The State's Servants: The Civil Service of the English Republic 1649-1660* (London and Boston, 1973)
Bailey, Margaret Lewis: *Milton and Jakob Boehme: A Study of German Mysticism in Seventeenth-Century England* (New York, 1964)
Barnett, Pamela: *Theodore Haak, FRS (1605-1690): The First German Translator of Paradise Lost* (The Hague, 1962)
Batten, J. Minton: *John Dury, Advocate of Christian Reunion* (Chicago, 1944)
Berg, J. Van Den and E.G.E. Van Der Wall (eds.): *Jewish-Christian Relations in the Seventeenth Century: Studies and Documents* (Dordrecht, Boston and London, 1988)
Bethall, S.L.: *The Cultural Revolution of the Seventeenth Century* (London, 1951)

BIBLIOGRAPHY

Bircher, Martin and Ferdinand van Ingen (eds.): *Sprachgesellschaften, Sozietäten, Dichtergruppen: Arbeitsgespräch im Herzog August-Bibliothek, Wolfenbüttel, 28-30 Juni 1977* (Hamburg, 1978)

Blekastad, Milada: *Comenius: Versuch eines Umrisses vom Leben, Werk und Schicksal des Jan Amos Komensky* (Oslo and Prague, 1969)

Borowczyk, Jacques: 'Enseignement et Diffusion de l'*Algèbre Nouvelle* de François Viète', *Diffusion du savoir et affrontement des idées 1600-1770: Festival d'Histoire de Montbrison 30 Septembre au 4 octobre 1992* (Montbrison, 1992), 287-309

Brauer, Karl: *Die Unionstätigkeit John Duries unter dem Protektorat Cromwells* (Marburg, 1907)

Chomsky, Noam: *Cartesian Linguistics: A Chapter in the History of Rationalist Thought* (New York and London, 1966)

Clasen, Claus-Peter: *The Palatinate in European History 1559-1660* (Oxford, 1963)

Clucas, Stephen: 'Samuel Hartlib and the Hamburg Scientific Community 1631-66: 'Samuel Harlib's *Ephermerides*, 1635-59, and the Pursuit of Scientific and Philosophical Manuscripts: The Religious Ethos of an Intelligencer', *The Seventeenth Century* 6 (1991), 33-55. A Study in Intellectual Communications' (Hartlib Studies Seminar, Sheffield University, 5 February 1990)

-       'The Correspondence of a XVII-Century "Chymicall Gentleman"': Sir Cheney Culpeper and the Chemical Interests of the Hartlib Circle', *Ambix* 40 (1993), 147-70

-       'Samuel Hartlib's Communications with the Low Countries: The Structures of a Seventeenth-Century Intelligence' (forthcoming)

Cohen, Albert: 'Jean Le Maire and La Musique Almérique', *Acta Musicologica* 35 (1963), 175-79

Cressy, David: *Literacy and the Social Order: Reading and Writing in Tudor and Stuart England* (Cambridge, Eng., London, New York, New Rochelle, Melbourne and Sydney, 1980)

Crombie, A.C.: *Styles of Scientific Thinking in the European Tradition: The history of argument and explanation especially in the mathematical and biomedical arts and sciences* (London, 1994)

Cunningham, Andrew and Ole Peter Grell (eds.): *Religio Medici. Medicine and Religion in Seventeenth-Century England* (Aldershot, 1996)

Darby, H.C.: *The Draining of the Fens* (Cambridge, 1940)

Debus, Allen G. *The English Paracelsians* (London, 1965)

-       (ed.): *Science, Medicine and Society in the Renaissance: Essays to Honour Walter Pagel* (London, 1972)

-       'The Medico-Chemical World of the Paracelsians', *Changing Perspectives in the History of Science*, ed. Mikulás Teich and Robert Young (London, 1973), 85-99

-       *The Chemical Philosophy: Paracelsian Science and Medicine in the Sixteenth and Seventeenth Centuries* (New York, 1977)

-       *Chemistry, Alchemy and the New Philosophy: Studies in the History of Science and Medicine* (Variorum Reprints, London, 1987)

[Deursen, A. Th. Van]: *Plain Lives in a golden Age : Popular culture, religion and society in seventeenth-century Holland* (trans. Maarten Ultee, Cambridge, 1991).

Dickens, A.G.: *The German Nation and Martin Luther* (London, 1974)

Dillinger, Heinz (ed.): *Kreatur und Kosmos: Internationale Beiträge zur Paracelsus-Forschung* (Stuttgart, 1981)

Dülmen, Richard Van: 'Schwärmer und Separatisten in Nürnberg (1618-1648)', *Archiv für Kulturgeschichte* 55 (1973), 107-37

Edighoffer, Roland: 'Deux écrits de Johann Valentin Andreæ retrouvés ou le nouveau *Neveu de Rameau*', *Etudes Germaniques* (Oct.-Dec. 1975), 466-70.

Fletcher, Anthony: *The Outbreak of the English Civil War* (London, Melbourne and Auckland, revised edition 1985)

BIBLIOGRAPHY

Foster, Leonard Wilson: *Georg Rudolf Weckherlin: Zur Kenntnis seines Lebens in England* (Basel, 1944)

Funke, Otto: *Zum Weltsprachenproblem in England im 17. Jahrhundert: G. Dalgarno's 'Ars Signorum' (1661) und J. Wilkins' 'Essay towards a real character and a philosophical language' (1668)* (Heidelberg, 1929)

Gagliardo, John: *Germany under the Old Regime 1600-1790* (London and New York, 1991)

Gardiner, Samuel R.: *History of the Great Civil War 1642-1649* (London, New York and Bombay, 1897-98)

- *History of the Commonwealth and Protectorate 1649-1656* (London, New York and Bombay, 1903)

Graham, W. Fred (ed.): *Later Calvinism: International Perspectives* (Kirksville, 1994)

Greengrass, Mark: 'Samuel Hartlib: "Intelligenceur" Européen', *Diffusion du Savoir et Affrontement des Idées 1600-1770: Festival d'Histoire de Montbrison 30 Septembre au 4 Octobre 1992* (Montbrison, 1992), 213-34

- 'The Financing of a Seventeenth-Century Intellectual: Contributions for Comenius', *Acta Comeniana* XXXV (1996), 71-87 and 141-57.

- 'Samuel Hartlib and Scribal Publication', *Acta Comeniana*, 12 (1997), 89-104.

Greengrass, Mark, Michael Leslie and Timothy Raylor (eds.): *Samuel Hartlib and Universal Reformation: Studies in Intellectual Communication* (Cambridge, 1994)

Grell, Ole Peter: *Dutch Calvinists in Early Stuart London: The Dutch Church in Austin Friars 1603-1642* (Leiden, New York, Copenhagen and Cologne, 1989)

- *Calvinist Exiles in Tudor and Stuart England* (Cambridge, 1996)

Gugel, Kurt F.: *Johann Rudolph Glauber 1604-70: Leben und Werk* (Würzburg, 1955)

Guhrauer, G.E.: *Joachim Jungius und sein Zeitalter* (Stuttgart and Tübingen, 1850)

Harris, L.E: *The Two Netherlanders: Humphrey Bradley and Cornelius Drebbel* (Cambridge, 1961)

Harwood, John T.: 'Introduction' to *The Early Essays and Ethics of Robert Boyle* (Carbondale and Edwardsville, 1991), xv-lxix

Hesse, Mary: 'Reasons and Evaluation in the History of Science', *Changing Perspectives in the History of Science*, ed. Mikuláš Teich and Robert Young (London, 1973), 127-47

Hill, Christopher: *The World Turned Upside Down: Radical Ideas during the English Revolution* (London, 1972)

Holstun, James: *A Rational Millennium: Puritan Utopias of Seventeenth-Century England and America* (New York and Oxford, 1987)

Hotson, Howard: *Johann Heinrich Alsted: Encyclopedism, Millenarianism and the Second Reformation in Germany* (PhD thesis, Oxford, 1991)

Hunter, Michael: *Science and the Shape of Orthodoxy: Intellectual Change in Late Seventeenth-Century Britain* (Woodbridge, 1995)

Hutton, Ronald: *Charles II, King of England, Scotland and Ireland* (Oxford, 1989)

Israel, Jonathan: *The Dutch Republic and the Hispanic World 1606-1681* (Oxford, 1982)

[Jacobi, Jolande]: 'Paracelsus: His Life and Work', *Paracelsus: Selected Writings*, ed. Jolande Jacobi trans. Norbert Guterman, (London, 1951), 39-74.

Jardine, Lisa: *Francis Bacon and the Art of Discourse* (Cambridge, 1974)

Joly, Bernard: *La rationalité de l'alchimie au XVIIe siècle* (Paris, 1992)

Josten, C.H. and F.S. Taylor: 'Johannes Banfi Hunnyades 1576-1650', *Ambix* 5 (1953-6), 44-52

- 'Johannes Banfi Hunnyades: A Supplementary Note', *Ambix* 5 (1953-6), 115

Kayser, Rudolf: 'Joachim Morsius', *Monatshefte der Comeniusgesellschaft* 6 (1897), 307-19

Keller, Ludwig: 'Johann Valentin Andreæ und Comenius', *Monatshefte der Comeniusgesellschaft* 1 (1892), 229-41

BIBLIOGRAPHY

- 'Comenius und die Akademien der Naturphilosophen des Siebzehnten Jahrhunderts', *Monatshefte der Comeniusgesellschaft* 4 (1895), 1-28, 69-96, 133-84
Kenyon, John: *The Civil Wars of England* (London, 1988)
Kienast, R.: *Johann Valentin Andreæ und die vier echten Rosenkreutzer-Schriften* (Leipzig, 1926)
[Klein, Jacob]: *Greek Mathematical Thought and the Origin of Algebra* trans. Eva Brann (Cambridge Mass. and London, 1968)
Klemperer, Victor: *LTI: Notizbuch eines Philologen* (Berlin, 1949)
Knowlson, James: 'Jean le Maire, the Almérie, and the "musique almérique": a set of unpublished documents', *Acta Musicologica* 40 (1968), 86-9
- *Universal Language Schemes in England and France 1600-1800* (Toronto and Buffalo, 1975)
Koenigsberger, Helmut G.: 'Die Krise des 17. Jahrhunderts', *Zeitschrift für historische Forschung* 9 (1982), 143-65
Kopp, H.: *Beiträge zur Geschichte der Chemie* (Braunschweig, 1869)
Kvacala, Jan: *J.V. Andreæs Antheil an geheimen Gesellschaften* (Jurjew, 1899)
- 'Über die Schicksale der *Didactica Magna*', *Monatshefte der Comeniusgesellschaft* 8 (1899), 129-44
- *Die Pädagogische Reform des Comenius in Deutschland bis zum Ausgange des XVII Jahrhunderts II: Historischer Überblick, Bibliographie, Namen- und Sachregister: Monumenta Germaniæ Pædagogica* XXXII (Berlin, 1904)
Leslie, Michael and Timothy Raylor (eds.): *Culture and Cultivation in Early Modern England: Writing and the Land* (Leicester and London, 1992)
Lindberg, David C. and Robert S. Westman (eds.): *Reappraisals of the Scientific Revolution* (Cambridge, 1990)
Link, Arnulf: *Johann Rudolph Glauber 1604-1670: Leben und Werk* (doctoral dissertation, Heidelberg, 1993)
Lisk, Jill: *The Struggle for Supremacy in the Baltic 1600-1725* (London, 1967)
Löhr, Rudolf: 'Zur Geschichte der vier heimlichen Kölner Gemeinden', *Protokolle der hochdeutsch-reformierten Gemeinde zu Köln* (q.v.: see section III) IV, 11-33
Lovejoy, A.O.: *The Great Chain of Being: A Study of the History of an Idea* (New York, 1960)
Luhrmann, T.M.: 'An Interpretation of the *Fama Fraternitatis* with Respect to Dee's *Monas Hieroglyphica*', *Ambix* 33 (1986), 1-10
McGuire, J.E. and Robert S. Westman: *Hermeticism and the Scientific Revolution* (Los Angeles, 1977)
McLaughlin, R. Emmet: *Caspar Schwenckfeld: Reluctant Radical. His Life to 1540* (New Haven and London, 1986)
MacLeod, Christine: *Inventing the Industrial Revolution: The English Patent System 1560-1800* (Cambridge, 1988)
Merriman, R.B.: *Six Contemporaneous Revolutions* (Hamden, Connecticut, 1963: reprint of 1938 Clarendon Press edition)
Moeller, Bernd: 'Frömmigkeit in Deutschland um 1500', *Archiv für Reformationsgeschichte* 56 (1965), 5-31
Montgomery, John Warwick: *Cross and Crucible: Johann Valentin Andreæ, Phoenix of the Theologians* (The Hague, 1973)
Moran, Bruce T.: *The Alchemical World of the German Court: Occult Philosophy and Chemical Medicine in the Circle of Moritz of Hessen (1572-1632)* (*Südhoffs Archiv Beiheft* 29, Stuttgart, 1991)
- (ed.) *Patronage and Institutions: Science, Technology and Medicine at the European Court 1500-1750* (Boydell, 1991)
Mulsow, Martin: '*Sociabilitas*: Zu einem Kontext der Campanella-Rezeption im 17. Jahrhundert', *Studia Bruniana et Campanelliana* I (1995), 205-32.

BIBLIOGRAPHY

Multhauf, Robert: 'The Significance of Distillation in Renaissance Medical Chemistry', *Bulletin of the History of Medicine* 30 (1956), 329-46

Murphy, Daniel: *Comenius: A Critical Reassessment of his Life and Work* (Cambridge, 1995)

Neidiger, Hans: 'Die Entstehung der evangelisch-reformierten Gemeinde in Nürnberg als rechtsgeschichtliches Problem', *Mitteilungen des Vereins für Geschichte der Stadt Nürnberg* 43 (1952), 1-153

Newman, William: 'Thomas Vaughan as an Interpreter of Agrippa von Nettesheim', *Ambix* 29 part 3 (November 1982), 125-40

- 'Newton's *Clavis* as Starkey's *Key*', *Isis* 78 (1987), 564-74

- 'Prophecy and Alchemy: The Origin of Eiranæus Philalethes', *Ambix* 37 (1990), 97-115.

- *Gehennical Fire: The Lives of George Starkey, An Alchemist of Harvard in the Scientific Revolution* (Harvard, 1994)

Norbrook, David: '"The Masque of Truth": Court Entertainments and International Protestant Politics in the Early Stuart Period', *The Seventeenth Century Journal* 1 (1986), 81-110

O'Brien, J.J.: 'Commonwealth Schemes for the Advancement of Learning', *British Journal of Education Studies* 16 (1968), 30-42

Ong, Walter J.: *Ramus, Method and the Decay of Dialogue: From the Art of Discourse to the Art of Reason* (Cambridge, Mass., 1958).

Otte, Wolf-Dieter: 'Ein Einwand gegen Johann Valentin Andreæs Verfasserschaft der Confessio Fraternitatis R.C.', *Wolfenbüttler Beiträge* 3 (1978), 97-113

Pagel, Walter: *Paracelsus: An Introduction to Philosophical Medicine in the Era of the Renaissance* (Basel and New York, 1958)

- 'The Spectre of Van Helmont and the Idea of Continuity in the History of Chemistry', *Changing Perspectives in the History of Science*, ed. Mikulás Teich and Robert Young (London, 1973), 100-9

- *Joan Baptista Van Helmont: Reformer of Science and Medicine* (Cambridge, London, New York, New Rochelle, Melbourne and Sidney, 1982)

[Pages, Georges]: *The Thirty Years War, 1618-1648*, trans. David Maland and John Hooper (London, 1970).

Parker, Geoffrey: *Europe in Crisis* 1598-1648 (London, 1980)

- *The Thirty Years War* (London, Boston, Melbourne and Henley, 1984)

Parker, T.H.L.: *John Calvin* (London, 1975)

Peuckert, Will-Erich: *Die Rosenkreuzer: Zur Geschichte einer Reformation* (Jena, 1928)

Pietsch, Erich: 'Johann Rudolph Glauber: Der Mensch, sein Werk und seine Zeit', *Deutsches Museum Abhandlungen und Berichte* 24, Heft 1 (1956), 1-64

Pilz, Kurt: 'Die Entstehung der evangelisch-reformierten Gemeinde in Nürnberg', *Mitteilungen des Vereins für Geschichte der Stadt Nürnberg* 43 (1952), 1-153

Ploss, Emil Ernst, Heinz Rosen-Runge and Heinrich Schipperges: *Alchimia: Ideologie und Technologie* (Munich, 1970)

[Polisensky, J.V.]: *The Thirty Years* War, trans. Robert Evans (Berkely and Los Angeles, 1971)

Popkin, Richard H.: *The Third Force in Seventeenth Century Thought* (Leiden, 1992)

Porter, Roy and Mikulás Teich (eds.): *The Scientific Revolution in National Context* (Cambridge, 1992)

Prestwich, Menna (ed.): *International Calvinism 1541-1715* (Oxford, 1985)

Pumfrey, Stephen, Paolo L. Rossi and Maurice Slawinsky (eds.): *Science, Culture and Popular Belief in the Renaissance* (Manchester, 1991)

Purver, Margery: *The Royal Society: Concept and Creation* (London, 1967)

Pust, R.: 'Über Valentin Andreæs Anteil an der Sozietätsbewegung des 17. Jahrhunderts', *MCG* 14 (1905), 240-8

Rattansi, P.M.: 'Paracelsus and the Puritan Revolution', *Ambix* 11 (1963), 24-32

268

BIBLIOGRAPHY

- 'The Helmontian-Galenist Controversy in Restoration England', *Ambix* 12 (1964), 1-23
- 'Some Evaluations of Reason in Sixteenth and Seventeenth Century Natural Philosophy', *Changing Perspectives in the History of Science*, ed. Mikulás Teich and Robert Young (London, 1973), 148-66

Raylor, Timothy: 'New Light on Milton and Hartlib', *Milton Quarterly* 27 (1993), 19-31.

Read, John: *Prelude to Chemistry: An Outline of Alchemy, Its Literature and Relationships* (London, 1936)

Repgen, Konrad: 'Seit wann gibt es den Begriff "Dreißgjährigen Krieg"?', *Weltpolitik, Europagedanke, Regionalismus: Festschrift für Heinz Gollwitzer 1982*, ed. Heinz Dolliger (Aschendorff and Münster, 1982)
- 'Noch einmal zum Begriff "Dreißigjährigen Krieg"', *Zeitschrift für historische Forschung* 9 (1982), 347-52

Righini Bonelli, M.L. and William R. Shea (eds.): *Reason, Experiment and Mysticism in the Scientific Revolution* (London and Basingstoke, 1975)

Rocke, A.J.: 'Agricola, Paracelsus and "Chymia"', *Ambix* 32 (1985), 37-45.

Rood, Wilhelmus: *Comenius and the Low Countries: Some Aspects of the Life and Work of a Czech Exile in the Seventeenth Century* (Amsterdam, 1970)

Rosenkranz, A.: *Das evangelische Rheinland: ein rheinisches Gemeinde- und Pfarrerbuch* (Düsseldorf, 1956-8)

[Rossi, Paolo]: *Francis Bacon: From Magic to Science*, trans. Sacha Rabinovitch (Chicago, 1968)
- *Clavis universalis* (Bologna, 1983)

Salmon, Vivian: *The Study of Language in Seventeenth-Century England (Amsterdam Studies in the Theory and History of Linguistics Series 3: Studies in the History of Linguistics*: vol. 17) (Amsterdam, 1979)

Schama, Simon: *The Embarrassment of Riches: An Interpretation of Dutch Culture in the Golden Age* (Berkeley, Los Angeles and London, 1988)

Schilling, Heinz (ed.): *Die Reformierte Konfessionalisierung in Deutschland - Das Problem der 'Zweiten Reformation' (Wissenschaftliches Symposion des Vereins für Reformationsgeschichte* Bd. 195) (Gütersloh, 1986)

Schneider, Heinrich: *Joachim Morsius und sein Kreis: Zur Geistesgeschichte des Siebzehnten Jahrhunderts* (Lübeck, 1929)

Schneider, Walter: *Adam Boreel: Sein Leben und seine Schriften* (Giessen, 1911)

Scholem, Gershom: *Kabbalah* (Jerusalem, 1974)

Shapiro, Barbara J.: *Probability and Certainty in Seventeenth-Century England: A Study of the Relationships between Natural Science, Religion, History, Law and Literature* (Princeton, 1983)

Sheppard, H.J.: 'Chinese and Western Alchemy: the Link through Definition', *Ambix* 32 (1985), 32-7

Skalweit, Stephan: *Reich und Reformation* (Berlin, 1967)

Soliday, Gerald Lymon: *A Community in Conflict: Frankfurt Society in the Seventeenth and Early Eighteenth Centuries* (Hanover, New Hampshire, 1974)

Sprunger, Keith L.: *Dutch Puritanism: A History of English and Scottish Churches in the Netherlands in the Sixteenth and Seventeenth Centuries (Studies in the History of Christian Thought* vol. 31) (Leiden, 1982)

Starck, Caspar Heinrich: *Lübeckische Kirchen-Geschichte* (Hamburg, 1724)

Teich, Mikulás and Robert Young (eds.): *Changing Perspectives in the History of Science: Essays in Honour of Joseph Needham* (London,1973)

Thomas, Keith: *Religion and the Decline of Magic: Studies in Popular Beliefs in Sixteenth and Seventeenth Century England* (London, 1971, 4th. ed. 1980)

Thompson, Edward H.: 'Oeconomy, Government and Economy in a Seventeenth Century Utopia' (delivered at Durham University Centre for Seventeenth Century Studies Biennial Conference 1993, draft text kindly supplied by the author)

BIBLIOGRAPHY

Tillyard, E.M.W.: *The Elizabethan World Picture* (London, 1943)

Toischer, W.: 'Die Didaktik des Elias Bodinus', *Mitteilungen der Gesellschaft für deutsche Erziehungs- und Schulgeschichte* 9 (1899), 209-29

Toon, Peter (ed.): *Puritans, the Millennium and the Future of Israel: Puritan Eschatology 1600-1660* (Cambridge and London, 1970)

Trevor-Roper, Hugh: *Archbishop Laud, 1573-1645* (London, 1940)

- *Religion, the Reformation and Social Change* (London, 1967)
- *Catholics, Anglicans and Puritans: Seventeenth Century Essays* (London, 1987)

Turnbull, George: *Samuel Hartlib: A Sketch of his Life and his Relations to J. A. Comenius* (London, 1920)

- *Hartlib, Dury and Comenius: Gleanings from Hartlib's Papers* (Liverpool, 1947)
- 'Samuel Hartlib's Connection with Sir Francis Kynaston's "Museum Minervæ"', *Notes and Queries* 197 (1952), 33-7
- 'Samuel Hartlib's Influence on the Early History of the Royal Society', *Notes and Records of the Royal Society* 10 (1953), 101-30
- 'John Hall's Letters to Samuel Hartlib', *Review of English Studies* New Series 4 (1953), 221-33.
- 'Peter Stahl, the First Public Teacher of Chemistry at Oxford', *Annals of Science* 9 (1953), 265-70
- 'Johann Valentin Andreæs Societas Christiana', *Zeitschrift für deutsche Philologie* 73 (1954), 407-41
- 'Robert Child', *Colonial Society of Massachusetts Transactions* 38 (1959), 21-53
- 'George Stirk, Philosopher by Fire', *Publications of the Colonial Society of Massachusetts* 38 (1959), 219-51

Vaughan, Robert: *The Protectorate of Oliver Cromwell* (London, 1839)

Wall, E.G.E. Van Der: *De Mystieke Chiliast Petrus Serrarius (1600-1669) en zijn Wereld* (Leiden, 1987)

Watson, Foster: *Vives on Education* (Cambridge, 1913)

Webster, Charles: 'English Medical Reformers of the Puritan Revolution: A Background to the "Society of Chymical Physitians"', *Ambix* 14 (1967), 16-41

- 'The Origins of the Royal Society' (essay review of Purver, *The Royal Society: Concept and Creation*, q.v.), *History of Science* 6 (1967), 106-28
- *The Great Instauration: Science, Medicine and Reform 1626-1660* (London, 1975)
- *Utopian Planning and the Puritan Revolution: Gabriel Plattes, Samuel Hartlib and Macaria* (Oxford, 1979)
- *From Paracelsus to Newton: Magic and the Making of Modern Science* (London, 1982)

Wedgwood, C.V.: *The Thirty Years War* (London, 1938)

Westin, G.: *Negotiations about Church Unity 1628-1634* (Upsala, 1932)

Whaley, Joachim: *Religious Toleration and Social Change in Hamburg 1529-1819* (Cambridge Eng., London, New York, New Rochelle, Melbourne and Sydney, 1985)

J.C. Whitebrook: 'Dr John Stoughton the Elder', *Transactions of the Congregational Historical Society* 6 (1913-15), 89-107 and 177-84.

Wilkinson, Ronald Stearne: 'George Starkey, Physician and Alchemist', *Ambix* 11 (1963), 121-52

- 'The Problem of the Identity of Eirenæus Philalethes', *Ambix* 12 (1964), 24-43
- 'The Hartlib Papers and Seventeenth-Century Chemistry', *Ambix* 15 (1968), 54-69 and 17 (1970), 85-110

Willey, Basil: *The Seventeenth Century Background: Studies in the Thought of the Age in Relation to Poetry and Religion* (London, 1934)

Wittop Koning, Dirk: 'J.R. Glauber in Amsterdam', *Jaarboek van het Genootschap Amstelodamum* 43 (1949), 1-6

Wolters, Ernst Georg: 'Paul Felgenhauers Leben und Wirken', *Jahrbuch der Gesellschaft für Niedersächsische Kirchengeschichte* 54 (1956), 63-84, and 55 (1957), 54-94

Yates, Frances A.: *Giordano Bruno and the Hermetic Tradition* (London, 1964)

BIBLIOGRAPHY

- *The Art of Memory* (London, 1966)
- *The Rosicrucian Enlightenment* (London, 1972)
- *Astræa: The Imperial Theme in the Sixteenth Century* (London, 1975)

Index

INDEX

INDEX

INDEX

Münster, Johann Friedrich,
16

Neefen, Peter, 16
Nürnberg, 3, 13-14, 15
Nuysement, Jacques, 234,
236, 237

Office of Address (Council
of Learning), xi, 59,
201, 218, 219, 249
Oughtred, William, 39,
116
Oxenstierna, Axel, 135

Paracelsus, Theophrastus,
156, 157, 166, 184,
186, 236
Pell, John, 22, 37, 50, 59,
113-17, 119, 124-5,
165, 248, 249, 250
Idea of Mathematics,
114-17
Pepys, Samuel, 57
Pergens family, 10
Pergens, Jacob, 10, 221
Petty, William, 198, 200,
202, 218, 221-2
Pfaff, Nikolaus, 16
Phinor, Jacob, 12
Plattes, Gabriel, 24, 110,
158, 160-61
Pöhmer, Johann Abraham,
102, 105
Poleman, Joachim, 62, 76,
78, 81, 159, 162-3,
171, 203, 204, 205,
206, 238
Poniatovská, Christina,
132
Popp, Johann, 167
Potter, Francis, 87
Potter, William, 126
Pruvost, Pierre le, 237
Prynne, William, 90
Pym, John, 128, 129

Rakóczi, Gÿorgÿ, Prince of
Transylvania, 84, 123
Ramus, Petrus, 5
Rand, William, 51
Rasch, Erasmus, 202, 205,
206, 238

Raselius, Christoph
Andreas, 17
Ratke, Wolfgang, 103
Rave, Christian, 37, 41,
44, 49, 64
Reeve, Richard, 51
Ridgely, Thomas, 199
Ripley, George, 158
Rittangel, Johann Stephan,
44-6, 48, 249
Rosicrucianism, 7, 17, 18-
19, 21, 156-7
Rulice (Rulitius), Johann,
59, 84, 121-2, 123,
134, 248
Rushworth, John, 153

Sadler, John, 59, 78, 198,
219, 248
Schlezer, Johann Friedrich,
169
Schöfler, 205
Schönborn, Johann
Philipp, Elector and
Archbishop of Mainz,
193
Schütgens, minister in
Cologne, 9
Sefer Yezirah, 45, 46
Sendivogius, Michael, 228,
234, 236, 237
Serrarius, Petrus, 11, 41-2,
82, 83, 87, 197, 219
Sevi, Sabatai, 42
Shapira, Nathan, 41-2
Sictor, Jan, 122
Sommer, Georg, 20, 122
Sorbière, Samuel de, 196-
7, 201
Sotherby, 50, 199
Stahl, Peter, 51, 62, 81
Stapula, 169
Starkey (Stirk), George,
49, 75, 79-80, 154,
156, 157, 158, 164,
174, 206, 228-29,
230, 231, 238, 250
Stoffgen, Christian, 9
Stoughton, John, 87
Strafford, Earl of, 79, 129,
133
Streso, Caspar, 122, 123

INDEX

Printed and bound by CPI Group (UK) Ltd, Croydon, CR0 4YY

22/10/2024

01777623-0016